Prevention and Societal Impact of Drug and Alcohol Abuse

Prevention and Societal Impact of Drug and Alcohol Abuse

Edited by

Robert T. Ammerman
*MCP-Hahnemann University
and Allegheny General Hospital*

Peggy J. Ott
Ralph E. Tarter
University of Pittsburgh School of Medicine

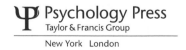

Psychology Press
Taylor & Francis Group

New York   London

First Published by
Lawrence Erlbaum Associates, Inc., Publishers
10 Industrial Avenue
Mahwah, NJ 07430

Transferred to Digital Printing 2009 by Psychology Press
270 Madison Ave, New York NY 10016
27 Church Road, Hove, East Sussex, BN3 2FA

Cover design by Kathryn Houghtaling Lacey

Library of Congress Cataloging-in-Publication Data

Prevention and societal impact of drug and alcohol abuse / edited by Robert T.
Ammerman, Peggy J. Ott, Ralph E. Tarter.
                  p. cm.
Includes bibliographical references and indexes.
ISBN 0-8058-3157-6 (cloth : alk. paper) — ISBN 0-8058-3158-4 (pbk. : alk. paper).
1. Drug abuse—Prevention. 2. Drug abuse—Social aspects. 3. Alcoholism—Prevention. 4.
Alcoholism—Social aspects. 5. Drug abuse—Treatment. 6. Alcoholism—Treatment. I.
Ammerman, Robert. T. II. Ott, Peggy, J. III. Tarter, Ralph E.
HV5801.P69   1999
362.29'17—dc21   98-42313
                                          CIP

Publisher's Note
The publisher has gone to great lengths to ensure the quality of this reprint
but points out that some imperfections in the original may be apparent.

Contents

Part IV: Intervention: Primary and Secondary Prevention

Preface

Substance use and abuse is in the forefront of societal problems. It is a pervasive problem, affecting directly or indirectly the overwhelming majority of persons. The deleterious impact of alcohol and drugs is devastating. Financially, significant resources are devoted to drug control, stopping crime related to drug trafficking, substance abuse treatment, and rehabilitation. The human cost is equally startling. Substance use and abuse undermines individuals, families, and communities. It is generally acknowledged that the most cost effective means of curtailing alcohol and drug abuse is prevention. Providing interventions to at-risk individuals before they develop serious problems with substance use is the most important component of the "war on drugs." Fortunately, the past decade has seen a dramatic increase in the quantity and quality of scientific research on those areas crucial to the advancement of prevention science. Progress has been made in explicating the impact and consequences of substance use and abuse, understanding the causes of alcohol and drug abuse, identifying precursors to use, understanding the developmental progress of alcohol and drug use disorders, and designing prevention programs that successfully avert substance use and abuse.

The original idea for *Prevention and Societal Impact of Drug and Alcohol Abuse* emerged from our desire to compile the tremendous amount of information on this topic that has accumulated in recent years. We are convinced that the field has matured to a point where such a book is warranted and needed. Future progress in prevention science will emanate from the theoretical advances and empirical achievements of recent years. Documenting these accomplishments and setting the stage for future efforts comprise the focus of *Prevention and Societal Impact of Drug and Alcohol Abuse.*

The book is divided into four sections. Section 1 contains introductory chapters addressing current issues in prevention science and characteristics of abusable substances. Section II, Historical Overview and Health Effects, includes chapters on the historical contexts of substance abuse, and the deleterious health consequences of alcohol and other drugs. Section III focuses on the impact of drug and alcohol abuse on society. Included are chapters on alcohol and drug abuse and driving, infectious illness, disability, managed care, the criminal justice system and adolescents and adults, sale and distribution, the media, and community responses. Finally, Section IV consists of chapters on prevention in specific settings and with certain populations. The following topics are covered in this section: schools, the workplace, the community, the military, prisons, and medical service systems.

We thank the contributors for sharing their expertise and insights with us in compiling the book. We also acknowledge the valuable help provided to us by Pat Park, Erika Newcomer, and Cindy DeLuca. Finally, we thank Larry Erlbaum, Judith Amsel, and Sara Scudder at LEA for their support and patience in bringing this effort to fruition. This book emanates from the Center for Education and Drug Abuse Research (CEDAR), a center funded by the National Institute on Drug Abuse, and a consortium of Western Psychiatric Institute and Clinic (University of Pittsburgh School of Medicine) and St. Francis Medical Center. We thank our colleagues for their support of this endeavor.

Finally, we are saddened by the death of one of the contributors, Dr. David N. Nurco. He was an important figure in the substance abuse field, and he will be greatly missed by his colleagues. We extend our condolences to his family, friends, and colleagues.

—Robert T. Ammerman
—Peggy J. Ott
—Ralph E. Tarter

INTRODUCTION

1

Critical Issues in Prevention of Substance Abuse

Robert T. Ammerman
MCP-Hahnemann University and Allegheny General Hospital

Peggy J. Ott
Ralph E. Tarter
University of Pittsburgh School of Medicine

Timothy C. Blackson
The Pennsylvania State University

Substance abuse is one of the most challenging problems facing society in the late 1990s. The prevalence of substance use and abuse is staggering. Alcohol consumption is commonplace, with approximately 140 million Americans using alcohol in 1995 (Office of Applied Studies, 1995). An additional 13 million persons used illicit drugs in at least 1 month during 1994 (U.S. Department of Health and Human Services, 1995). The consequences of alcohol and drug abuse are equally disconcerting, as evidenced by the link between substance abuse and acute and chronic health problems, car-related injuries and deaths, poor work performance and attendance, psychosocial maladjustment, and involvement in criminal activity. Considerable financial expenditures also result from substance use and abuse, involving the health care system, law enforcement, the criminal justice system, and lost economic efficiency. Substance use typically emerges in adolescence. For a significant proportion of individuals, problems with drugs and alcohol will continue through adulthood. As with many social ills, treatment of affected individuals is expensive and has a limited rate of success. Accordingly, it is almost universally acknowledged that the most effective approach to decreasing substance abuse is prevention. Curtailing the full clinical expression of substance use disorders preserves resources currently allocated to treatment and other forms of intervention (e.g., law enforcement) and mitigates the harmful impact of substance abuse on individuals, families, communities, and society.

Coie et al. (1993) coined the term *prevention science* to describe the systematic and empirically driven approach to studying the averting of psychological and behavioral disorders, including substance abuse. They noted the multidisciplinary nature of this "new" discipline, joining together the combined expertise of psychology, psychiatry, public health, sociology, criminology, education, and human development. In the past decade, prevention science has coalesced into a vibrant and informative domain of study. Reflections of this include the founding of professional organizations devoted to prevention science (such as the Society for Prevention Research), special editions of journals devoted to prevention, and the plethora of recent journal articles focusing on prevention of mental health problems in general, and substance abuse in particular. Clearly, this is a field that has emerged from its nascent stage to a new level of scientific maturity and sophistication.

The purpose of this chapter is to succinctly review the major issues in the prevention science of substance abuse. We begin by briefly recounting the impact of substance use and abuse, because this documents the negative consequences of the phenomenon and provides an important starting point from which prevention efforts can be explored. After an overview of current issues in the conceptualization of prevention science, we examine important elements of efficacious prevention programs. Finally, we end with a summary and proposed template to guide the future directions that research and practice might take. It should be noted that, although substance abuse prevention efforts have been implemented across the life span, much of the work in the field has focused on children and adolescents, and this population is the primary focus of this chapter. The reasons for this are compelling. First, exposure to and initiation of substance use typically occurs in adolescence. Second, a sizable proportion of substance use problems (including the development of abuse and dependence) begin in adolescence and extend into adulthood. Third, the goal of prevention is to intervene with individuals *before* they begin using and develop problems with alcohol and drugs, thus necessitating an emphasis on children and youth. And fourth, childhood and adolescence are times of dynamic change and development in psychological and physical domains. It is desirable to influence these more malleable developmental processes before they become entrenched and more resistant to intervention.

IMPACT OF SUBSTANCE ABUSE

The damaging consequences of alcohol and drug abuse impact individuals, families, and the systems in which they live. They can be expressed in financial terms: it has been estimated that federal, state, and local drug control policies substance abuse cost the United States approximately $20 billion per year (Office of National Drug Control Policy, 1996). It can also be expressed in the incalculable suffering and lost potential of those afflicted with substance use disorders. Prevention is clearly the most cost-effective means of mitigating the negative effects of substance abuse.

Substance abuse undermines physical health. For example, chronic alcohol abuse is associated with diseases of the liver, central nervous system, and heart (see Goodwin & Gabrielli, 1997). Often, as in the case of the brain disorder Korsakoff's syndrome, the damage resulting from alcohol abuse is irreversible. Additional health problems stemming from the use of other substances are well documented (see Lowinson, Ruiz, Millman, & Langrod, 1997). Well-known examples are lung cancer caused by smoking, and pervasive central nervous system damage resulting from the inhaling of solvents. In addition, many substances are toxic in excessive doses, resulting in numerous acute and chronic effects on physical health, potentially leading to permanent disability or death. Finally, substance abuse increases the risk for acquiring other health-related problems, such as HIV, sexually transmitted diseases, or trauma secondary to accidents while under the influence of psychoactive substances.

Mental health disorders often occur with substance abuse. Comorbidity is relatively common, with up to one third of individuals with psychiatric disorders reporting a lifetime history of substance abuse disorders as well (Helzer & Pryzbeck, 1998). In some instances, psychiatric disorder precedes or even contributes to the development of substance abuse, whereas in others, emotional and behavioral disturbances arise within the context of alcohol and drug use problems. A large body of research has delineated the disproportionate representation of psychological dysfunction in substance abusers (see Tarter, Ammerman, & Ott, 1998). Included are problems in personality, mood, self-esteem, coping, behavior, and social functioning. Once again, some of these psychological difficulties may be evident prior to the onset of substance abuse, although psychological functioning often worsens over time in individuals with substance use disorders.

Abuse of specific substances may also contribute to relatively unique psychological presentations, such as the amotivational state that has been linked to chronic marijuana use (see Grinspoon & Bakalar, 1997). Other psychological effects of substance abuse are directly linked to the biological impact of psychoactive substances (such as anxiety and irritability stemming from withdrawal) and the behaviors that result from dependence on drugs and alcohol (such as craving and preoccupation with obtaining desired substances).

The family, too, is significantly impacted by substance abuse. Behavioral patterns that often accompany addiction (e.g., preoccupation with obtaining drugs or alcohol, engaging in criminal activities to financially support addiction, lying, involvement in dangerous and risky activities, educational and vocational underachievement) can put tremendous strain on the emotional and financial resources of affected families. Moreover, because substance abuse (particularly when it occurs during adolescence) is more likely to emerge in families that are already distressed or dysfunctional, stress arising from a family member's addiction may further tax already compromised coping capabilities. Drug and alcohol use in parents can contribute to child abuse and neglect (Peterson, Gable, & Saldana, 1996), couples violence (Hotaling & Sugarman, 1986), and poor communication and lack of support and cohesion within the family.

The cost of substance abuse to the community is also of concern. There is a strong association between substance abuse and crime (Bureau of Justice Statistics, 1993), especially involving illicit substances that are highly addictive (such as crack cocaine and heroin). As the disorder progresses, persons dependent on such drugs often turn to crime to obtain sufficient quantities of drugs to maintain their addictions. Up to 75% of the prison population regularly uses alcohol or drugs, or has been incarcerated for substance-related offenses (see Kleber, Califano, & Demers, 1997). Moreover, addiction also increases the risk of being a victim of crime. Drug activity (such as selling) further undermines the community by exposing children to drugs, providing easy accessibility to illicit substances, and facilitating gang and other organized crime infiltration. Finally, substance abuse deprives the community of human resources that might otherwise be used to strengthen and enhance neighborhood vitality.

The deleterious effects of substance abuse are also seen at the societal level. Substance abusers are likely to perform inefficiently at work, and have higher rates of absenteeism (see Kleber et al., 1997). It is estimated that lost work hours and poor performance costs employers $35 billion per year (Rice, 1995). Additional employer costs are incurred through employee assistance programs for addicted workers, and premiums paid to insurance providers to cover substance abuse treatment. At both the local, state, and federal levels, a tremendous amount of human and financial resources is devoted to lowering the supply and accessibility of drugs. These efforts have only limited success (see Kleber et al., 1997), further underscoring the value of prevention in decreasing the incidence and prevalence of substance abuse.

CONCEPTUAL FOUNDATIONS OF PREVENTION SCIENCE IN ALCOHOL AND DRUG USE

The conceptual roots of prevention science reach back to the early stages of theoretical and empirical emergence of child development, developmental psychopathology, psychiatry, community psychology, and public health (see Institute of Medicine, 1994). However, the clear articulation of principles to guide prevention science is relatively recent. Kelly (1966) outlined four principles of ecological psychology that form the bedrock on which prevention science has been propagated: interdependence, cycling of resources, adaptation, and succession. *Interdependence* refers to the synergistic, bidirectional influences of systems comprising the individual's environment. Changes in one system necessarily affect and alter other systems. *Cycling of resources* reflects the fact that changes in the availability of resources in one system have a subsequent impact on resources needed and used in others. *Adaptation* is the reaction of individuals to changes in influential factors and resources within and between ecological systems. Altering the features of one or more systems will elicit responses in individuals that constitute adaptations to these changes. Finally, *succession* describes the fact that ecological systems are dynamic and in a state of flux. Changes in systems, therefore, are likely to be temporary. Taken together, Kelly's principles underscore the fact that individuals live in environments that are complicated, mutually dependent, and susceptible to change. In order to be effective, prevention programs must be constructed to reflect these characteristics of ecological systems.

The ecological model, originally proposed by Bronfenbrenner (1977) and expanded and refined by others (e.g., Belsky, 1993), draws on Kelly's (1966) formulation of ecological systems. This conceptualization proposes four levels of influence on the individual's psychological development and functioning. These systems, each nested one within the other in a hierarchical fashion, consist of the microsystem, mesosystem, exosystem, and macrosystem. The *ontogenetic* represents characteristics of the individual, including temperament, personality, and physical features. The *microsystem* describes settings where individuals spend the majority of time, such as family, school, and peer groups. The *exosystem* consists of the neighborhood and community where individuals reside. Finally, the *macrosystem* comprises the social and cultural forces that emanate from and, in turn, reciprocally influence the other systems. Included at this level are cultural values, shared beliefs, and economic events that have pervasive influence (e.g., economic depression). Bronfenbrenner highlighted the importance of ecological validity in social and behavioral research. Specifically, he argued that empirical investigations of individuals must take into account (and, ideally, directly measure and simultaneously examine) the systems in which they lived and developed, or else risk ignoring the complexity of development and psychosocial adjustment. Moreover, according to the implicit assumptions of the ecological model, magnitude of change and durability of intervention effects are directly linked to the degree to which prevention efforts target multiple systems and levels of ecological influence.

Iterations of the ecological model emphasize the transactional interplay of risk and protective factors in the etiology of social, emotional, and behavioral disturbance (e.g., Cicchetti & Rizley, 1981; Sameroff & Chandler, 1975). These formulations distinguish between risk factors, which increase the likelihood that psychopathology will develop, and protective factors, which serve as buffers that decrease the probability of psychosocial maladjustment. Consistent with the ecological approach, risk and protective factors can emerge from the multiple systems affecting the individual. In addition, risk and protective factors can be stable and unchangeable (e.g., family history of a disorder), or temporary (e.g., loss of a job). Risk factors interact and combine in dynamic and mutually interdependent ways. Protective factors can serve as buffers, offsetting the negative influences of risk factors and their combinations. The relevance and salience of given risk and protective factors varies across development. As children and adolescents pass through different and sequential stages of cognitive, emotional, behavioral, and social development, those factors that are most important in promoting or protecting against the emergence of maladaptation may differ in both quantity and quality. As a result, the timing of the occurrence of influencing variables is critical to determining developmental course and outcome.

Tarter and Vanyukov (1994) proposed a liability model for alcohol abuse that is a logical extension of the ecological model and its derivatives. Specifically, they argue that some individuals are born with a genetic vulnerability to developing alcohol use disorders, and that the degree of vulnerability is variable within the population. This genetic liability is expressed in a variety of behaviors and traits (e.g., difficult temperament, emotional and behavioral dysregulation, compromised attentional capacities) that increase the likelihood of subsequently exhibiting alcohol problems in adolescence. The developmental trajectory toward alcohol abuse and dependence is propelled by the influence of environmental factors (e.g., low parental monitoring, affiliation with deviant peers) that interfere with normal adjustment and adaptation (Blackson, Tarter, Loeber, Ammerman, & Windle, 1996). Likewise, other variables strengthen the individual's functioning, and reverse this negative trajectory, thereby offsetting the vulnerability to alcohol use disorders reflected in the genetic liability. As with the ecological and transactional models, the number, order, time of occurrence, and strength of risk and protective factors is important in determining developmental outcome. The liability model of alcohol use problems has considerable heuristic appeal because it (1) incorporates genetic vulnerability, a well-documented contributor to the etiology of alcohol abuse and dependence (see Vanyukov, Neale, Moss, & Tarter, 1996); (2) invokes the importance of development in understanding the emergence of alcohol use problems; and (3) incorporates the multisystem and transactional conceptualization of the ecological approach. Although Tarter and Vanyukov originally presented the liability model from the perspective of alcohol use problems, it is equally applicable to other substances of abuse. Indeed, it provides a useful framework for conceptualizing other psychiatric disorders and psychopathologies, as well.

RISK FACTORS AND ETIOLOGIC CONTRIBUTORS TO ALCOHOL AND DRUG ABUSE

As noted above, those factors that contribute to negative developmental outcomes in general, and substance abuse in particular, exert their influence in complicated and multidetermined ways. No single factor or subset of factors has been identified that uniquely and consistently predicts the development of substance abuse. Rather, it is the timing, intensity, duration, interaction, and combination of contributory factors that leads to the clinical manifestations of alcohol and drug abuse. However, a number of variables have been identified as important in the etiology of, or serve as risk factors for, substance abuse. These are presented in Table 1.1, and categorized

TABLE 1.1
Risk Factors and Etiologic Contributors to Alcohol and Drug Abuse

Individual	Genetic liability to alcohol and/or drug abuse
	Early onset of puberty
	Cognitive impairment
	Affective and behavioral dysregulation
	Temperament and personality traits (e.g., sensation seeking)
	Psychopathology and psychiatric disorder (e.g., conduct disorder)
	Coping and problem-solving skills deficits
	Interpersonal skills deficits
Family, School, and Peers	Parental alcohol and/or drug abuse
	Exposure to alcohol and/or drug use
	Acceptance and valuing alcohol and/or drug use
	Poor communication and low cohesion
	Inconsistent and harsh discipline
	Inadequate monitoring
	Physical abuse and neglect
	Affiliation with alcohol and drug using peers
	Affiliation with delinquent peers
Neighborhood and Community	Crime
	Poverty
	Inadequate housing
	Inadequate community resources
	Drug activities
	Accessibility of substances
Society and Culture	Acceptance of alcohol and drug use
	Incorporation of alcohol and drug use in cultural rituals and practices
	Media images and advertisements encouraging substance use

using the four-level schema of the ecological model. Although this is not an exhaustive list of potentially causative variables, those factors that have been consistently linked to substance abuse, and are thought to be important determinants of alcohol and drug use problems, are represented. (Comprehensive reviews of the etiology of alcohol and drug abuse are found in Hawkins, Catalano, & Miller, 1992; Hawkins, Kosterman, Maguin, Catalano, & Arthur, 1997; Institute of Medicine, 1996; Tarter & Vanyukov, 1994). Ideally, prevention efforts should be structured to alter and reverse those etiologic mechanisms that move individuals along a developmental trajectory toward substance use and abuse. To this end, factors listed in Table 1.1 should be addressed and targeted for change in prevention programs.

It is noteworthy that Coie et al. (1993) outlined a similar constellation (as that presented in Table 1.1) of risk and causative factors for mental health problems in children and youth in general, highlighting the fact that substance abuse often presents concurrently (and shares etiologic pathways) with other problem behaviors and psychopathologies (see Jessor & Jessor, 1977). Therefore, prevention programs that focus on altering causative mechanisms for substance abuse are also likely to simultaneously impact other social, emotional, and behavioral problems.

COMPONENTS OF SUCCESSFUL PREVENTION PROGRAMS

The concept of prevention originally emerged from a public health model (Commission on Chronic Illness, 1957). Within this framework, prevention was divided into three categories: primary, secondary, and tertiary. Primary prevention describes interventions designed to decrease the number of new cases (i.e., incidence) of a disease or disorder. Secondary prevention focuses on lowering the rate (i.e., prevalence) of identified cases of a disease or disorder in the population. Finally, tertiary prevention seeks to decrease the amount of disability in identified cases.

As our understanding of the complicated etiology of disease and illness increased, this approach to characterizing prevention has given way to one that is based on the link between known causes and intervention. Gordon (1987) proposed a classification system that reflects the relation between risk for acquiring a disorder and the type of prevention initiative that is optimal. Universal prevention is desirable and relevant for almost everyone in a given population. Examples from public health include using seat belts, prenatal care, and obtaining immunizations (see Institute of Medicine, 1994). Selective prevention targets individuals thought to be at greater risk for developing the disorder relative to the general population. Illustrative are cancer screenings for breast cancer in women, condom usage in groups at greater risk for acquiring HIV, and parent training for teenage mothers and fathers. Finally, indicated prevention seeks to reach individuals who have characteristics or conditions that make them highly likely to develop the condition or disease. Examples are reducing heart attacks by targeting persons with hypertension, weight reduction in persons with diabetes, and preventing alcohol use problems in conduct disordered youth. There are several implications of Gordon's classification system. First, in contrast to earlier conceptualizations, the focus is on the population to be served rather than the disease or condition to be prevented. Second, there is an implicit cost-benefit examination in determining the need for universal, selective, and indicated strategies. That is, the cost of implementing the program is weighed against the risk for developing the disorder (and the subsequent cost and impact of the disorder) in a given population. And third, this approach is based on a knowledge of probabilities of acquiring the disorder in a given population. As a result, an understanding of etiologic mechanisms is essential to the efficient and effective design and implementation of prevention programs.

The goals of substance abuse prevention are relatively straightforward. They include: (1) delay onset of first use of illicit substances, (2) limit the number and types of substances used, (3) circumvent the transition from substance use to abuse and dependence, and (4) diminish the negative consequences of those individuals who engage in substance use and/or eventually exhibit clinically significant manifestations of substance use disorders (i.e., harm reduction). Fully achieving these goals, however, has been elusive. Although the aforementioned conceptual models provide guidelines for the design, implementation, and evaluation of prevention programs, a gap remains between our theoretical appreciation of the etiologic complexity of substance use and abuse and the practical application of prevention interventions. This stems, in large part, from the incomplete understanding of the causes of substance use problems, and our inability at this point in time to precisely predict specific developmental trajectories for individuals and populations. As a result, we are far from the ideal of being able to identify those individuals at greatest risk, assess their unique needs, and design and implement an optimal intervention based on an assessment. Rather, we are at a stage where we can identify populations at greater or lesser risk, conduct assessments that measure functioning in important areas (but not necessarily in all domains) relevant to the individual, and carry out programs that address broad areas of need (but not necessarily the specific and unique needs of the individual). This state of affairs is not unique to the substance abuse field. In fact, it accurately characterizes current limitations in carrying out psychological interventions for both children (Kazdin & Weisz, 1998) and adults (DeRubeis & Crits-Christoph, 1998).

Despite these limitations, a number of important advances have occurred in prevention science in the past decade. In addition to more accurately elucidating the mechanisms by which substance use and abuse emerge, and identifying subgroups at greater risk for developing substance abuse problems, several specific prevention programs have been empirically proven to decrease substance use and the subsequent development of substance use disorders (e.g., Botvin, Baker, Dusenbury, Botvin, & Diaz, 1995; Donaldson, Graham, & Hansen, 1994; Hawkins et al., 1992; Pentz et al., 1989). Broadly speaking, prevention initiatives focus on (1) altering the psychological characteristics of the individual that predispose or protect persons from developing problematic drug and alcohol use, (2) changing the environmental contexts that augment or mitigate risk, and (3) modifying the interaction between these variables (cf. Tarter & Vanyukov, 1994). Botvin and Botvin (1997) further categorize prevention as falling into five strategies: (1) information dissemination approaches, (2) affective education approaches, (3) alternatives approaches, (4) social resistance skills approaches, and (5) broader competency training programs. Each of these strategies has been represented in universal, selected, and indicated programs (see Botvin & Botvin, 1997; Hawkins et al., 1997; Institute of Medicine, 1996). Although it has only been recently that prevention programs have been subjected to systematic empirical evaluation (e.g., Botvin et al., 1995), a clearer understanding of essential characteristics of successful prevention efforts has appeared.

NIDA Recommendations

The National Institute on Drug and Alcohol Abuse (NIDA) recently published a summary of recommendations for key elements of successful prevention programs for children and adolescents (1997). These recommendations, or "principles," are derived from the scientific literature on prevention, and are presented in Table 1.2. They are entirely consistent with the conceptualizations of prevention science that define the theoretical cutting-edge of the field (e.g., Coie et al., 1993; Hawkins et al., 1997). In particular, they emphasize (1) a developmental approach; (2) intervention at the individual, peer, family, and community levels; (3) diminishing the impact of risk factors and enhancing the positive influences of protective factors; and (4) the importance of adapting prevention programs to the unique needs of groups of individuals who are at greater risk. Although these principles are specifically directed toward programs involving children and adolescents, the majority of them are also applicable for prevention of alcohol and drug use in adults. These principles will each be reviewed in turn.

The enhancement of protective factors and diminishment of risk factors should serve as a foundation on which prevention programs are designed and implemented. To this end, the social ecology (Bronfenbrenner, 1977) and liability (e.g., Tarter & Vanyukov, 1994) perspectives provide the work-

TABLE 1.2
Preventive Principles for Children and Adolescents

- Prevention programs should be designed to enhance "protective factors" and move toward reversing or reducing known "risk factors."
- Prevention programs should target all forms of drug abuse, including the use of tobacco, alcohol, marijuana, and inhalants.
- Prevention programs should include skills to resist drugs when offered, strengthen personal commitments against drug use, and increase social competency (e.g., in communications, peer relationships, self-efficacy, and assertiveness), in conjunction with reinforcement of attitudes against drug use.
- Prevention programs for adolescents should include interactive methods, such as peer discussion groups, rather than didactic teaching techniques alone.
- Prevention programs should include a parents' or caregivers' component that reinforces what the children are learning—such as facts about drugs and their harmful effects—and that opens opportunities for family discussions about use of legal and illegal substances and family policies about their use.
- Prevention programs should be long-term, over the school career with repeat interventions to reinforce the original prevention goals. For example, school-based efforts directed at elementary and middle school students should include booster sessions to help with critical transitions from middle to high school.
- Family-focused prevention efforts have a greater impact than strategies that focus on parents only or children only.
- Community programs that include media campaigns and policy changes, such as new regulations that restrict access to alcohol, tobacco, or other drugs, are more effective when they are accompanied by school and family interventions.
- Community programs need to strengthen norms against drugs use in all drug abuse prevention settings, including the family, the school, and the community.
- Schools offer opportunities to reach all populations and also serve as important settings for specific subpopulations at risk for drug abuse, such as children with behavior problems or learning disabilities and those who are potential dropouts.
- Prevention programming should be adapted to address the specific nature of the drug abuse problems in the local community.
- The higher the level of risk of the target population, the more intensive the prevention effort must be and the earlier it must begin.
- Prevention programs should be age-specific, developmentally appropriate, and culturally sensitive.

From National Institute on Drug Abuse. (1997). *Preventing drug use among children and adolescents: A research-based guide*. NIH Publication No. 97-4212.

ing framework for program development. Designers of prevention programs should be aware that risk and protective factors vary in a population in terms of both type and quantity, and also differentially impact individuals depending on developmental level, chronological age, and social contexts. Moreover, some factors can be directly modified in an intervention (e.g., teaching adolescents social skills to resist peer pressure), while others will be relatively inaccessible and are only influenced indirectly (e.g., genetic liability to substance abuse). Prevention programs, therefore, must be constructed to address risk and protective factors that are most salient for participants given their age, development, and the environmental settings in which they live.

Because the etiologic mechanisms of alcohol and drug abuse often overlap, it is critical that prevention programs target multiple forms of substance use. For example, several risk factors are important to both alcohol and cannabis abuse, such as exposure to substance-using peers (Brook, Whiteman, & Finch, 1992), being the offspring of substance-abusing fathers (see Hawkins et al., 1992a), and exhibiting behavioral and emotional dysregulation (Martin et al., 1994). Moreover, it has been demonstrated that adolescents typically use cigarettes and alcohol prior to engaging in use of illicit substances (Kandel, Kessler, & Margulies, 1978). By targeting adolescent of these initial, "gateway" substances, it is likely that subsequent use and abuse of other drugs can be curtailed.

Most of the empirically demonstrated efficacious prevention programs utilize behavior change technologies and emphasize the training of selected skills to enhance psychological and interpersonal competence. This is consistent with recent research demonstrating the effectiveness of psychological interventions for children and adolescents in general, and those that use learning principles in particular (see Kazdin & Weisz, 1998). Illustrative skills that are core features of empirically tested prevention programs involve the following domains: resistance to peer influences, interpersonal competence, and coping and problem-solving. Skills-building and attitude change are the two primary objectives of most prevention interventions, and the scientific literature supports the utility and success of behavioral and cognitive-behavioral approaches in achieving these goals (see Ammerman, Hersen, & Last, 1999).

Similarly, preventive interventions with children and adolescents should include interactive elements rather than relying solely on didactic training methods. The empirical literature supporting this principle is extensive and compelling. Numerous outcome studies of psychological interventions demonstrate the increased effectiveness of active rather than passive therapeutic and skills-training strategies. Examples include role playing and other interactive therapeutic modalities. These methods allow practice and rehearsal of newly learned skills. Also, use of active prevention approaches permits observation of participant performance in the intervention setting, thereby providing opportunities for trainers to deliver feedback.

Incorporation of parents and other caregivers into prevention interventions is an important ingredient of success. Indeed, because family characteristics may contribute to the risk for substance use and abuse (through low parental monitoring, inadequate supervision of children's activities, and coercive interactional processes), failure to address family issues in prevention programs will ensure limited success. Moreover, at risk families may undermine efforts of prevention programs by providing information and reinforcing beliefs and attitudes contrary to that put forth in prevention programs. By forming partnerships with families, and directly involving them in prevention programs, the likelihood of successful prevention is greatly enhanced.

Prevention is an ongoing effort, and intermittent "booster" sessions are required after completion of formal programs in order to maintain gains achieved during that period. Additional sessions administered intermittently post-treatment have become an integral part of psychological interventions. Such an approach is essential for two reasons. First, without regular and consistent practice, learned skills dissipate over time. To the extent that skills important to substance abuse prevention (e.g., refusal skills) are unlikely to be naturally reinforced in the adolescent's environment (e.g., peers may respond to refusals with increased pressure), it is critical that they be practiced in a formal and structured program. And second, many of the factors that augment risk and vulnerability to substance use will continue to exert their influence throughout development. For example, adolescents will be exposed to substance-using peers throughout their school experience, and long after time-limited prevention programs have ended. Skills that are maintained because of periodic booster sessions add to the overall protective resources available to children and adolescents as they grow older, thereby offsetting those forces and liabilities that potentiate alcohol and drug abuse.

NIDA (1997) notes that family-focused interventions, rather than programs targeting parents and children separately, are more likely to be successful. Coordinated prevention efforts that target systems in which children and adolescents live are preferable to those that focus on individuals in piecemeal fashion. It is noteworthy that several prevention efforts that have been systematically evaluated and found to be efficacious include a family intervention. Concentrating on the family as a system promotes uniform acquisition of skills across family members that protect children and adolescents from the development of substance abuse, and provides a long-term, stable, and durable buffer for youth as they grow and mature.

Universal prevention efforts utilizing public service messages or other media approaches are more likely to be effective if they are combined with individual and family-focused interventions. Although universal prevention initiatives have the advantage of reaching large numbers of individuals, they fall short in meeting the unique needs of children and adolescents who are especially vulnerable to substance use problems. Public service approaches, in isolation, are unlikely to successfully disrupt those mechanisms that contribute to substance use and abuse in high-risk youth. Accordingly, combining public service initiatives with more intensive efforts targeting such populations is the most desirable prevention strategy.

An especially important goal of prevention programs is establishing normative standards and attitudes in individuals, families, and communities that discourage substance use and abuse. Attitudes about drug and alcohol abuse are important precursors to subsequent use and abuse. Incorrect information about the nature of substance abuse and the potentially negative consequences of use, beliefs that promote or encourage the use of illicit substances, and normative standards and values that are accepting of alcohol and drug use, all increase the likelihood that children and adolescents will become involved with drugs and alcohol. Moreover, attitudes and beliefs about alcohol and drug use are readily susceptible to change, and there is considerable evidence that association with substance abusing peers can alter adolescents' views in the direction of embracing and valuing alcohol and drug use (Oetting & Beauvais, 1990). If drugs and alcohol are also widely used and visible in families and communities, adolescent beliefs and attitudes about illicit substances will be more accepting. The proximal influence of these factors undermine and sabotage (often successfully) the information provided by public service messages that warn about the dangers of substance use and abuse.

Schools are among the most important settings where prevention programs are carried out. There are several reasons for this. First, children and adolescents spend much of their time at school. As schools have taken on an increased role in providing activities for children after the traditional end of the school day (e.g., afterschool programs), the time that many children and youth spend in schools has also risen. Logistically and practically, this the easiest base from which prevention programs are delivered. Second, learning is the primary focus of schools, and there is a clear partnership between the learning of academic material and acquiring skills essential for health and well-being, such as those taught in substance abuse prevention programs. And third, a significant proportion of contact with peers occurs at schools. Because of the importance of peer influences in exposure to and development of attitudes and beliefs about alcohol and drugs, it is logical to implement prevention programs in settings where children and adolescents interact.

The community contexts where drug and alcohol use occur should dictate the design of prevention programs. Generic, "one size fits all" prevention programs will fail if contextual factors interfere with or undermine the effectiveness of the intervention. It is especially important that substance abuse programs address the unique needs of the community and its residents. Such an approach will promote the forming of partnerships with community leaders, ensure the acceptance and adoption of the program by residents, and enhance the relevance and applicability of the program to participants. Program design should be guided by cultural norms and practices. In the absence of cultural and contextual awareness and sensitivity, failure of prevention efforts is all but assured.

And finally, intensity of the prevention effort should parallel the level of risk exhibited by the targeted population. This is a relatively new concept in the substance abuse field, and grows out of the increased understanding of the relationship between risk factors and the subsequent development of substance abuse problems (Tarter & Vanyukov, 1994). In addition, it is now recognized that those children and adolescents who are most susceptible to substance abuse disorders are unlikely to fully benefit from the types of universal prevention programs that have, until relatively recently, characterized most prevention efforts. Accordingly, those individuals at greatest risk for substance use problems will require more varied, comprehensive, and intensive programs than those at low or average risk.

SUMMARY AND FUTURE DIRECTIONS

Prevention of substance abuse has made great progress in the past decade. Conceptual formulations have been developed that elucidate the complex interplay of risk and protective factors. There has been an increasing appreciation of substance abuse as emerging from development processes, thereby lending support to the importance of early intervention and prevention during childhood and adolescence. Specific prevention programs have been subjected to empirical evaluation with increasingly more sophisticated methodological rigor. As a result, several prevention programs have emerged as promising, and a clearer delineation of essential components to prevention has been obtained (National Institute on Drug Abuse, 1997).

Although the recent advances in prevention science are encouraging, much work remains to be done. There are three issues that should be the focus of attention and research in the coming years. First, there is a need for a stronger linkage between etiology and prevention. Historically, these two areas in substance abuse have progressed independently. Prevention programs have been greatly influenced by practical and logistical limitations (hence the emphasis on universal prevention efforts), and etiological research has been conducted with minimal consideration of the real world impediments faced by practitioners. There has been considerable progress in the past 5 years in bringing these two subdisciplines together, although much work remains to be done.

A second, and related issue, is the need for indicated prevention efforts that focus on individuals at particularly high risk for alcohol and drug abuse. Currently, children and adolescents at greatest risk for substance abuse are likely to receive only circumscribed benefits from universal and selected prevention efforts. There are multiple pathways by which risk leads to subsequent substance abuse, and specialized (and even individualized) prevention programs are needed to target these especially vulnerable populations. Although such programs are labor intensive and expensive, they have considerable potential to be cost effective in the long run.

And finally, a third goal for the future is the design of prevention programs that are dynamic and flexible, changing over time to meet the unique needs of individuals at different stages of development across the lifespan. This approach takes into account the fluctuating presence and influence of risk and protective factors throughout development, and maximizes the likelihood that prevention will be relevant to and effective for program participants. As we continue to amass data documenting essential components of prevention programs, a flexible and integrated strategy for prevention becomes more of a possibility for the future.

ACKNOWLEDGMENT

Preparation of this chapter was supported in part by a Center Grant from the National Institute on Drug Abuse (P50-DA05605).

REFERENCES

Ammerman, R. T., Hersen, M., & Last, C. L. (1999). A prescriptive approach to treatment of children and adolescents. In R. T. Ammerman, M. Hersen, & C. L. Last (Eds.), *Handbook of prescriptive treatments for children and adolescents, 2nd ed* (pp. 1–9). Boston: Allyn & Bacon.

Belsky, J. (1993). Etiology of child maltreatment: A developmental-ecological analysis. *Psychological Bulletin, 114*, 413–434.

Blackson, T. C., Tarter, R. E., Loeber, R., Ammerman, R. T., & Windle, M. (1996). The influence of paternal substance abuse and difficult temperament in fathers and sons on sons' disengagement from family to deviant peers. *Journal of Youth and Adolescence, 25*, 389–410.

Botvin, G. J., Baker, E., Dusenbury, L., Botvin, E. M., & Diaz, T. (1995). Long-term followup results of a randomized drug abuse prevention trial in a white middle-class population. *Journal of the American Medical Association, 273*, 1106–1112.

Botvin, G. J., & Botvin, E. M. (1997). School-based programs. In J. H. Lowinson, P. Ruiz, R. B. Millman, & J. G. Langrod (Eds.), *Substance abuse: A comprehensive textbook* (pp. 764–774). Baltimore: Williams & Wilkins.

Bronfenbrenner, U. (1977). Toward an experimental ecology of human development. *American Psychologist, 32*, 513–531.

Brook, J. S., Whiteman, M. M., & Finch, S. (1992). Childhood aggression, adolescent delinquency and drug use: A longitudinal study. *Journal of Genetic Psychology, 153*, 369–383.

Bureau of Justice Statistics. (1993). *Survey of state prison inmates, 1991*. Washington, DC: U.S. Department of Justice.

Cicchetti, D., & Rizley, R. (1981). Developmental perspectives on the etiology, intergenerational transmission, and sequelae of child maltreatment. *New Directions for Child Development, 11*, 31–35.

Coie, J. D., Watt, N. F., West, S. G., Hawkins, J. D., Asarnow, J. R., Markman, H. J., Ramey, S. L., Shure, M. B., & Long, B. (1993). The science of prevention: A conceptual framework and some directions for a national research program. *American Psychologist, 48*, 1013–1022.

Commission on Chronic Illness. (1957). *Chronic illness in the United States*. Vol. 1. Published for the Commonwealth Fund. Cambridge: Harvard University Press.

DeRubeis, R. J., & Crits-Christoph, P. (1998). Empirically supported individual and group psychological treatments for adult mental disorders. *Journal of Consulting and Clinical Psychology, 66,* 37–52.

Donaldson, S. I., Graham, J. W., & Hansen, W. B. (1994). Testing the generalizability of intervening mechanism theories: Understanding the effects of adolescent drug use prevention interventions. *Journal of Behavioral Medicine, 17,* 195–216.

Goodwin, D. W., & Gabrielli, W. F., Jr. (1997). Alcohol: Clinical aspects. In J. H. Lowinson, P. Ruiz, R. B. Millman, & J. G. Langrod (Eds.), *Substance abuse: A comprehensive textbook* (pp. 142–148). Baltimore: Williams & Wilkins.

Gordon, R. (1987). An operational classification of disease prevention. In J. A. Steinberg & M. M. Silverman (Eds.), *Preventing mental disorders* (pp. 20–26). Rockville, MD: Department of Health and Human Services.

Grinspoon, L., & Bakalar, J. B. (1997). Marijuana. In J. H. Lowinson, P. Ruiz, R. B. Millman, & J. G. Langrod (Eds.), *Substance abuse: A comprehensive textbook* (pp. 199–206). Baltimore: Williams & Wilkins.

Hawkins, J. D., Catalano, R. F., & Miller, J. Y. (1992). Risk and protective factors of alcohol and other drug problems in adolescence and early adulthood: Implications for substance abuse prevention. *Psychological Bulletin, 112,* 64–105.

Hawkins, J. D., Catalano, R. F., Morrison, D. M., O'Donnell, J., Abbott, R. D., & Day, L. E. (1992). The Seattle Social Development Project: Effects of the first four years on protective factors and problem behaviors. In J. McCord & R. Tremblay (Eds.), *The prevention of anti-social behavior in children* (pp. 139–161). New York: Guilford.

Hawkins, J. D., Kosterman, R., Maguin, E., Catalano, R. F., & Arthur, M. W. (1997). Substance use and abuse. In R. T. Ammerman & M. Hersen (Eds.), *Handbook of prevention and treatment with children and adolescents* (pp. 203–237). New York: Wiley.

Helzer, J. E., & Pryzbeck, T. R. (1988). The co-occurrence of alcoholism with other psychiatric disorders in the general population and its impact in treatment. *Journal of Studies in Alcohol, 49,* 219–224.

Hotaling, G., & Sugarman, D. (1986). An analysis of risk markers in husband to wife violence: The current state of knowledge. *Violence and Victims, 1,* 101–124.

Institute of Medicine. (1994). *Reducing risks for mental disorders: Frontiers for preventive intervention research.* Washington, DC: National Academy Press.

Institute of Medicine. (1996). *Pathways of addiction: Opportunities in drug abuse research.* Washington, DC: National Academy Press.

Jessor, R., & Jessor, S. L. (1977). *Problem behavior and psychosocial development: A longitudinal study of youth.* New York: Academic Press.

Kandel, D. B., Kessler, R. C., & Margulies, R. Z. (1978). Antecedents of adolescent initiation into stages of drug use: A developmental analysis. *Journal of Youth and Adolescence, 7,* 13–40.

Kazdin, A. E., & Weisz, J. R. (1998). Identifying and developing empirically supported child and adolescent treatments. *Journal of Consulting and Clinical Psychology, 66,* 19–36.

Kelly, J. G. (1966). Ecological constraints on mental health services. *American Psychologist, 21,* 535–539.

Kleber, H. D., Califano, J. A., & Demers, J. C. (1997). Clinical and societal implications of drug legalization. In J. H. Lowinson, P. Ruiz, R. B. Millman, & J. G. Langrod (Eds.), *Substance abuse: A comprehensive textbook* (pp. 855–864). Baltimore: Williams & Wilkins.

Lowinson, J. H., Ruiz, P., Millman, R. B., & Langrod, J. G. (Eds.). (1997). *Substance abuse: A comprehensive textbook.* Baltimore: Williams & Wilkins.

Martin, C., Earleywine, M., Blackson, T., Vanyukov, M., Moss, H., & Tarter, R. (1994). Aggressivity, inattention, hyperactivity, and impulsivity in boys at high and low risk for substance abuse. *Journal of Abnormal Child Psychology, 22,* 177–201.

National Institute on Drug Abuse. (1997). *Preventing drug use among children and adolescents: A research-based guide.* NIH Publication No. 97-4212.

Oetting, E. R., & Beauvais, F. (1990). Adolescent drug use: Findings of national and local surveys. *Journal of Consulting and Clinical Psychology, 58,* 385–394.

Office of Applied Studies. (1995). *National household survey on drug abuse: Population estimates 1994.* Rockville, MD: Substance Abuse and Mental Health Services Administration.

Office of National Drug Control Policy. (1996). *The national drug control strategy: 1996, budget summary.* Washington, DC: U.S. Government Printing Office.

Pentz, M. A., Dwyer, J. H., MacKinnon, D. P., Flay, B. R., Hansen, W. B., Wang, E. Y., & Johnson, C. A. (1989). A multi-community trial for primary prevention of adolescent drug abuse: Effects on drug use prevalence. *Journal of the American Medical Association, 261,* 3259–3266.

Peterson, L., Gable, S., & Saldana, L. (1996). Treatment of maternal addiction to prevent child abuse and neglect. *Addictive Behaviors, 21,* 789–801.

Rice, D. (1995). *The economic costs of alcohol and drug abuse and mental illness: 1995.* Washington, DC: U.S. Department of Health and Human Services.

Sameroff, A. J., & Chandler, M. J. (1975). Reproductive risk and the continuum of caretaking casualty. In F. D. Horowitz, M. Hetherington, S. Scarr-Salapatek, & G. Siegel (Eds.), *Review of child development research* (vol. 4, pp. 187–244). Chicago: University of Chicago Press.

Tarter, R. E., Ammerman, R. T., & Ott, P. J. (1998). *Handbook of substance abuse: Neurobehavioral pharmacology.* New York: Plenum.

Tarter, R. E., & Vanyukov, M. (1994). Alcoholism: A developmental disorder. *Journal of Consulting and Clinical Psychology, 62,* 1096–1107.

U.S. Department of Health and Human Services. (1995). *Preliminary estimates from the 1994 National Household Survey on Drug Abuse.* Washington, DC: Author.

Vanyukov, M. M., Neale, M. C., Moss, H. B., & Tarter, R. E. (1996). Mating assortment and the liability to substance abuse. *Drug and Alcohol Dependence, 42,* 1–10.

2

What Constitutes a Drug of Abuse?

Peter R. Giancola
Ralph E. Tarter
University of Pittsburgh School of Medicine

Substance abuse is a devastating disorder that has insidiously contaminated and destroyed the lives of millions of Americans. Findings from large epidemiological studies reveal that between 16.7% to 26.6% of Americans qualify for a lifetime diagnosis of a substance use disorder (Kessler et al., 1994; Regier et al., 1990). Substance abuse carries with it a legion of undesirable consequences. In 1990, the total economic costs associated with alcohol abuse were estimated at $98.6 billion, a 40% increase from just 5 years prior (Rice, 1993). Given that this value is restricted to alcohol abuse, the costs for all substance use disorders is certainly much higher. Drug use decreases work productivity and the probability of being employed (Mullahy & Sindelar, 1992), while increasing work-related injuries and absenteeism (Podolsky & Richards, 1985). Finally, substance abuse also engenders a myriad of socially destructive effects such as firearm assaults, sexual assaults, homicides, and motor vehicle fatalities (Murdoch, Pihl, & Ross, 1990), to say nothing of its harmful medical and health-related concomitants (Sands, Knapp, & Ciraulo, 1993).

Given the pervasive damaging consequences of substance abuse to both the individual and society, efforts aimed at designing intervention strategies to treat and prevent this social menace are receiving increasing attention and support. Nevertheless, before any disorder can be adequately treated, a full understanding of its underlying etiological mechanisms must be secured (Tarter, 1992). Complicating matters further, when a disorder involves the "abuse" of a drug (i.e., addiction), the etiology of that disorder cannot be fully discerned without an appreciation of why the drug is addictive. This is simply because a major portion of understanding the nature of drug addiction involves a determination of how the addictive properties of drugs interact, biologically and psychologically, within the individual to produce the disorder. The first step in attempting to comprehend why a drug is addictive is the formulation of a clear definition describing the necessary criteria that constitute a *drug of abuse* (i.e., a drug with addiction potential). Although we state that a *drug of abuse* is one with *addiction potential*, we do not intend to use the latter term as a definition for the first; this would obviously represent circular logic. The inclusion of the term *addiction potential* is not intended to define, but merely to clarify the intended meaning of the term "drug of abuse."

DEFINITIONS

Before proceeding any further in attempting to answer our question, the terms *substance* and *drug* must be defined. For the purposes of this chapter, *substances* or *drugs* will be defined as any physical compounds, whether in a solid, liquid, or gaseous state, that can be taken into the body via at least one route of administration (e.g., oral, nasal, intramuscular, intravenous). As such, candy, chicken soup, cigarette smoke, benzodiazepines, opioids, antidepressants, and even antibiotics would fit these parameters. However, not all of these compounds are *drugs of abuse*. Nonetheless, when we typically think of a person as being addicted to drugs, we are usually referring to drugs of abuse. Therefore, we beg the question, what is it that distinguishes all drugs/substances from drugs of abuse?

Unfortunately, the introduction of the term *abuse* creates even further definitional quandaries. Generally speaking, and in its loosest sense, the term *substance abuse* is usually meant to imply a destructive and maladaptive pattern of drug use and the possibility of drug addiction. However, according to standard medical and psychiatric nosological systems, particular terms have been designated to specifically describe differing patterns of pathological drug use and drug addiction. The fourth edition of the *Diagnostic and Statistical Manual of Mental Disorders* (DSM-IV; American Psychiatric Association, 1994) has put forth two general diagnoses for substance use disorders: *substance abuse* and *substance dependence*. Both are defined as "maladaptive patterns of substance use leading to clinically significant impairment or distress." The diagnosis of substance abuse is made if the individual qualifies for one, or more, of four symptom criteria within a 12-month period, whereas that of substance dependence is made if the individual qualifies for three or more of seven symptom criteria within a 12-month period. Clinically, substance abuse is considered to be a milder form of substance dependence, the latter being characterized by tolerance

TABLE 2.1
DSM-IV Diagnostic Criteria for Substance Use Disorders

Substance Dependence	Substance Abuse
Tolerance	Recurrent substance use resulting in failing to fulfill major role obligations at work, school, or home
Withdrawal	Recurrent substance use in situations in which it is physically hazardous
Substance taken in larger amounts or over longer period of time than intended	Recurrent substance-related legal problems
Persistent desire or unsuccessful attempts to reduce or control intake of the substance	Continued substance use despite having persistent or recurrent social or interpersonal problems caused or exacerbated by the substance
Great deal of time spent trying to obtain the substance	
Reduction or elimination of important social, occupational, or recreational activities	
Continued use of substance despite knowledge of having a physical or psychological problem that is likely caused or exacerbated by the substance	

and withdrawal symptoms. DSM-IV symptoms for both substance abuse and dependence are presented in Table 2.1.

CRITERIA FOR A "DRUG OF ABUSE"

Now that we have clarified the meanings of the terms *substance*, *drug*, and *abuse*, at least for the purposes of this chapter, we attempt to describe the essential properties that a substance must possess in order to qualify as *a drug of abuse*. In our opinion, in order to fall under this rubric a drug must contain the following three properties: (1) its initial usages must produce rewarding effects, and (2) its discontinuation must yield aversive withdrawal effects, and (3) it must lead to a strong craving for the drug.

Rewarding Effects

It is well known that after a drug addiction has begun its course, many addicts continue to administer the drug in order to avoid the aversive withdrawal symptoms that accompany discontinuation of use. However, what are the factors that cause the individual to use the substance before discontinuation would produce withdrawal symptoms? One logical answer would seem to be that the drug has pleasurable or rewarding effects. Whereas curiosity or peer pressure may instigate the initial use of a drug, subsequent usages are likely due to the initial pleasurable experiences induced by the drug. Sedatives, including benzodiazepines, barbiturates, and alcohol, are known for their calming and tension-reducing effects. Stimulants such as amphetamines, cocaine, and nicotine are known for their arousing and mood-elevating properties, and hallucinogens such as LSD, psilocybin, and marijuana, are known for their positive alterations of consciousness and affect.

Although each of these drug classes produces different effects, they all appear to have one outcome in common. At least initially, they all tend to alter mood, cognitive functioning, and physiological arousal in a manner that is interpreted as positive and pleasurable. For example, many of these drugs tend to produce behaviorally disinhibiting effects. The socially anxious individual, frustrated with his or her inability to have normal social interactions, may decide to take a sedative drug with the hopes that it will relieve his or her interpersonal fears. If he or she experiences the drug's intended effects, the resultant gratification of a reduction in cognitive, emotional, and anxious physiological arousal, and concurrent facilitation of social interactions will increase the probability of further use. Another example is the individual who, out of curiosity, tries cocaine and experiences a highly pleasurable and arousing after effect with concomitant feelings of well being, security, invulnerability. Unless bound by the typical concerns that preclude others from trying cocaine (which would have inhibited him or her from taking the drug in the first place), the highly succorous effect he or she will have found in the company of this substance will most certainly predict continued use.

Before concluding this section, we broach the issue of individual differences in predisposition to drug abuse. In presenting our first criteria, we may have given the impression that all individuals who experience the rewarding properties of drugs are destined to a life of drug addiction. This is obviously not the case. There exist many individuals who have experienced pleasurable and rewarding effects during an initial drug use episode and have not taken the drug again. There also exist those who experience pleasurable effects, but only use the drug sparingly without developing a clinical addiction. However, it should be mentioned that these cases almost exclusively involve the use of drugs whose rewarding effects are relatively mild in magnitude. That is, the pleasurable effects of crack cocaine are much stronger than those of marijuana; therefore, crack cocaine has a much higher addiction potential than marijuana. Nevertheless, the answer to why certain individuals follow destructive paths toward drug addiction after an initial attempt whereas others do not is unknown at this time. However, the solutions lie in the study of individual differences: the study of what factors distinguish a person who tries a drug once, finds it pleasurable, but does not use it again, from another who experiences the same amount of pleasure but then proceeds toward a diagnosis of substance dependence.

Withdrawal Effects

Once a drug of abuse has been consumed on a sufficient number of occasions, the individual will experience a number of biological and psychological alterations. Biological alterations can occur in the form of changes in the production of various neurochemicals, changes in neurotransmitter receptor binding sites, and changes in autonomic physiological arousal. Psychological alterations can include changes in expectancies about the effects of drugs, as well as changes in cognition, mood, and motivation.

These, and many other modifications, will affect the individual in such a manner that now requires the continual administration of the drug to maintain a state of biological and psychological equilibrium. That is, in the absence of the drug, these alterations will produce what are typically known as *withdrawal symptoms*, which are highly aversive in nature. Withdrawal symptoms include watery eyes, runny nose, weakness, tremors, anxiety, nausea, agitation, headaches, abdominal cramps, insomnia, tachycardia, disorientation, hallucinations, delusions, and convulsive seizures (O'Brien & Chafetz, 1982). The *opponent process theory of motivation* proposed by Solomon and Corbit (1974) provides an excellent theoretical framework for explaining how the manifestation of withdrawal symptoms develops from the rewarding properties of drugs.

The theory states that the biological and psychological effects of a drug follow a developmental trajectory that is characterized by four general phases. This first involves the manifestation and peaking of the drug's initially pleasurable effects. The second involves the attainment of a time-limited systemic stabilization of the drug, which also produces pleasurable effects. The third phase involves the metabolism of the substance whereby blood levels begin to decline until the drug is expelled from the system. It is at this time that an aversive effect, opposite in direction to that experienced during the first and second phases, begins to take place. Withdrawal symptoms typically occur during this phase. The severity of the symptomatology is determined by the degree of addiction to the substance. Finally, the fourth phase involves the return of the system to a drug-free equilibrium.

Proximal to the nadir of the curve's trajectory (i.e., the withdrawal phase), the individual's choice to initiate further use of the drug will determine whether or not an addictive process will manifest itself. It is at this time that the most negative and aversive effects of the drug are experienced. The individual must now make a choice. Whether to abstain from the substance until the negative withdrawal effects subside, or to avoid these negative effects all together by readministering the drug and therefore recapitulating the cycle. Unfortunately, the problem with choosing the latter option is that the peak pleasure experience of the drug will not be as potent as the previous administration (i.e., tolerance), and the negative experience of the opposing force will be much stronger (i.e., withdrawal symptoms). Therefore, according to the theory, unless the cycle is broken, constant readministrations of the drug will only serve to attenuate the positive and intensify the negative effects of the curve until the individual is compelled by overpowering physical and psychological forces to continue using the drug in order to avoid what are essentially strengthening withdrawal effects.

Craving

Craving can be defined as a compelling and overwhelming edacity for a particular substance. Strictly speaking, according to the parameters of the opponent process theory, craving might be interpreted as a feature of the third phase of the curve (i.e., withdrawal effects). However, we have chosen to treat it as a separate entity for two conceptual reasons. First, whereas withdrawal effects represent the negative consequences of discontinuing the use of a drug after an addictive process has begun, we believe that craving is neither a positive nor a negative consequence. It is merely an unconditioned motivational response to a particular set of biological and psychological circumstances that signal the individual that he or she requires a particular substance in order to relieve the aversive withdrawal state. Second, from a phylogenetic perspective, craving can be viewed as an evolutionary adaptation designed to alleviate various aversive conditions. It is adaptive in the sense that humans are genetically preprogrammed to crave substances that help them sustain life (i.e., food and water). To extend this argument to substance abuse, if the maintenance of life is viewed as a positive or rewarding condition, then challenges to its survival (i.e., thirst and hunger) may produce similar, but not identical states, to drug withdrawal. As such, drug abuse may simply represent an unfortunate marriage of a biological adaptation and an assortment of environmental agents (drugs of abuse).

If chosen to be interpreted in this manner, craving should not be viewed as a component of withdrawal effects. Whereas withdrawal effects are the organism's negative reaction to the discontinuation of a drug it now depends on, craving is a hardwired biological adaptation possibly designed for life sustaining purposes. Therefore, the artificial activation of the craving response by a drug with addictive potential would then be inconsistent with the original life sustaining purpose of the craving adaptation.

NECESSARY AND SUFFICIENT?

The presentation of these criteria begs the question of whether they are necessary and sufficient in their ability to define the parameters of a drug of abuse. We will first consider the criteria that drugs of abuse must have rewarding effects. If the neophyte drug user does not experience rewarding or pleasurable effects during her initial encounters with a particular substance, the chances of a sustained relation between the two are highly doubtful. For example, how many people have developed a clinical dependency on carrot juice? Mostly likely none. Why? Probably because the reinforcing or pleasurable effects of carrot juice are minimal, if there are any at all. Whereas experiencing the rewarding effects of a drug is not a sufficient criteria to define a drug of abuse, it is certainly necessary. Second, as they are closely related, withdrawal effects and craving will be examined together. Given human biological and psychological reactions to prolonged drug administrations, withdrawal effects are a natural consequence of a sudden discontinuation of the drug and craving is the motivational state that provides the incentive to avoid the aversive withdrawal effects. Therefore, in the absence of withdrawal symptoms, the individual would not experience craving and therefore, would not engage in a vicious cycle of drug administration. As with reward, withdrawal effects and craving are not sufficient criteria for defining a drug of abuse, but they too are indeed necessary. Nevertheless, as can been derived from these arguments, when all three of the criteria are combined, it would appear that they do provide a combination of variables that are necessary and sufficient for determining whether a substance qualifies as a drug of abuse.

CONCLUSIONS

In conclusion, it can be argued that rewarding effects, withdrawal effects, and craving are three necessary and sufficient criteria to distinguish drugs of abuse from nonaddictive substances. We believe that this distinction is important because it can serve as an heuristic guide for the multidisciplinary study of the etiology of drug addiction. For example, chemists may wish to study the chemical properties of drugs that produce rewarding effects. Neurobiologists may then attempt to understand how these chemical properties behave in the brain and how they interact with endogenous neurochemicals. Biopsychologists would then try to discern how these brain occurrences affect the individual's mood, cognitions, and behaviors. Finally, those skilled in theories of learning would contribute to the solution by describing the contextual factors that delimit where, when, and in whom the properties of these drugs are likely to be most prominent. These same individuals would then investigate the concomitant effects of withdrawal and craving. Complicating matters even further, if one subscribes to a transactional model of drug addiction, the whole group of investigators would then be prompted to work together in pursuit of how occurrences in each of their respective areas affect the addiction process at other levels. As we stated at the beginning of this chapter, in order to successfully prevent and treat drug addition, one must have a full appreciation of the etiology of the disorder. However, the attainment of such a goal involves a comprehensive and interdisciplinary research approach that is guided by a clear definition of the disorder and the chemical catalysts of that disorder.

REFERENCES

American Psychiatric Association. (1994). *Diagnostic and statistical manual of mental disorders. 4th ed.* Washington, DC: Author.

Kessler, R. C., McGonagle, K. A., Zhao, S., Nelson, C. B., Hughes, M., Eshleman, S., Wittchen, H. U., & Kendler, K. S. (1994). Lifetime and 12-month prevalence of DSM-III-R psychiatric disorders in the United States: Results from the national comorbidity survey. *Archives of General Psychiatry, 51*, 8–19.

Mullahy, J., & Sindelar, J. (1992). Effects of alcohol on labor market success: Income, earnings, labor supply, and occupation. *Alcohol Health and Research World, 16*, 134–139.

Murdoch, D., Pihl, R., & Ross, D. (1990). Alcohol and crimes of violence: Present issues. *International Journal of the Addictions, 25*, 1065–1081.

O'Brien, R., & Chafetz, M. (1982). *The encyclopedia of alcoholism.* New York: Facts on File.

Podolsky, D. M., & Richards, D. (1985). Investigating the role of substance abuse in occupational injuries. *Alcohol Health and Research World, Summer*, 42–45.

Regier, D. A., Farmer, M. E., Rae, D. S., Locke, B. Z., Keith, S. J., Judd, L. L., & Goodwin, F. K. (1990). Comorbidity of mental disorders with alcohol and other drug abuse: Results from the epidemiologic catchment area (ECA) study. *Journal of the American Medical Association, 264*, 2511–2518.

Rice, D. P. (1993). The economic cost of alcohol abuse and alcohol dependence: 1990. *Alcohol Health and Research World, 17*, 10–11.

Sands, B. F., Knapp, C. M., & Ciraulo, D. A. (1993). Medical consequences of alcohol-drug interactions. *Alcohol Health and Research World, 17*, 316–320.

Solomon, R. L., & Corbit, J. D. (1974). An opponent-process theory of motivation: Temporal dynamics of affect. *Psychological Review, 81*, 119–145.

Tarter, R. E. (1992). Prevention of drug abuse: Theory and application. *The American Journal on Addictions, 1*, 2–20.

II

HISTORICAL OVERVIEW
AND HEALTH EFFECTS

3

Historical Overview of Alcohol Abuse

David J. Hanson
State University of New York

Any alcohol consumption that is perceived as being a problem constitutes alcohol abuse. Therefore, the extent of alcohol abuse is difficult to gauge historically, because its identification depends not only on societal norms regarding alcohol but also on who does the labeling.

Societal views of alcohol and its consumption have changed dramatically over time. During Prohibition, most consumption of alcohol was defined as abuse by many people, just as today members of certain religious groups define any level of consumption as abuse. On the other hand, many college students and members of the military view heavy episodic drinking as acceptable or even expected. Therefore, the abuse of alcohol cannot be properly understood as constituting some specific quantity or frequency of consumption. To understand abuse, one must not examine simply the behavior of the drinker, but also the historical time, the social context of the drinking, and the demographic characteristics of the drinker. What many people today would consider acceptable drinking behavior at a New Year's Eve party, they would not consider to be acceptable at a business reception. Many would consider consuming a glass of wine with dinner acceptable by a 21-year-old, but would reject the exact same behavior by a 20-year-old. Moreover, most would modify their judgment if the drinker were pregnant or a recovering alcoholic.

This chapter details changing definitions of alcohol abuse in America over time, describes major developments regarding alcohol abuse since the Great Depression, and concludes by presenting contrasting approaches to conceptualizing and preventing the abuse of alcohol.

THE EARLY YEARS

As the Puritans loaded provisions onto the Mayflower before casting off for the New World, they brought on board more beer than water (Royce, 1981, p. 38). This reflected their traditional drinking beliefs, attitudes, and behaviors. They saw alcohol as a natural and normal part of life.

Upon their arrival in the New World, the colonists quickly began brewing beer and ale. They also learned to make a wide variety of wines from fruits, vegetables, and even oak leaves. Following the introduction of apples, cider became a popular beverage (Mendelson & Mello, 1985, pp. 9–10). A brewery was one of Harvard College's first construction projects, so that a steady supply of beer could be served in the student dining halls (Furnas, 1965, p. 20), and Connecticut required each town to ensure that a place could be made available for the purchase of beer and ale (Krout, 1925, p. 7).

Moderation Was the Norm

Alcohol was viewed positively although its abuse was condemned. In 1673, Increase Mather praised alcohol, saying that "Drink is in itself a creature of God, and to be received with thankfulness" (Mendelson & Mello, 1985, p. 10). Consistent with that belief, toddlers drank beer, wine, and cider with their parents and regular use was seen as healthful for everyone (Asbury, 1968, pp. 3–4; Popham, 1978, pp. 267–277; Sinclair, 1962, pp. 36–37). Rorabaugh in 1979 pointed out that:

> Alcohol was pervasive in American society; it crossed regional, sexual, racial and class lines. Americans drank at home and abroad, alone and together, at work and at play, in fun and in earnest. They drank from the crack of dawn to the crack of dawn. At nights taverns were filled with boisterous, mirth-making tipplers. Americans drank before meals, with meals, and after meals. They drank while working in the fields and while travelling acrose half a continent. They drank in their youth, and, if they lived long enough, in their old age. They drank at formal events, such as weddings, ministerial ordinations, and wakes, and on no occasion—by the fireside of an evening, on a hot afternoon, when the mood called. From sophisticated Andover to frontier Illinois, from Ohio to Georgia, in lumber camps and on satin settees, in log taverns and at fashionable New York hotels, the American greeting was, "Come, Sir, take a dram first." Seldom was it refused. (pp. 20–21)

In colonial America, informal social controls helped maintain conformity to the expectation that the abuse of alcohol was unacceptable. There was a clear consensus that although alcohol was a gift from God its abuse was "from the Devil." "Drunkenness was condemned and punished, but only as an abuse of a God-given gift. Drink itself was not looked on as culpable, any

TABLE 3.1
Apparent Mean Consumption of Absolute Alcohol in
U.S. Gallons per Capita of the Drinking-Age Population

Year	Mean Consumption	Year	Mean Consumption
1710	5.1	1890	2.1
1770	6.6	1895	2.1
1785	6.1	1900	2.1
1790	5.8	1905	2.3
1795	6.2	1910	2.6
1800	6.6	1915	2.4
1805	6.8	1920	0.9
1810	7.1	1925	0.9
1815	6.8	1930	0.9
1820	6.8	1935	1.5
1825	7.0	1940	1.6
1830	7.1	1945	2.0
1835	5.0	1950	2.0
1840	3.1	1955	1.9
1845	1.8	1960	2.0
1850	1.8	1965	2.2
1855	2.0	1970	2.5
1860	2.1	1975	2.7
1865	2.0	1980	2.8
1870	1.9	1985	2.6
1875	1.8	1990	2.5
1880	1.9	1992	2.4
1885	2.0		

Adapted from Williams, Clem, and Dufour, 1994; Rorabaugh, 1979.

more than food deserved blame for the sin of gluttony. Excess was a personal indiscretion" (Aaron & Musto, 1981, p. 132).

Informal social controls operated both in the home and in the larger community. Tavern owners, for example, were expected not only to dispense food, drink, and hospitality, but also to monitor behavior and keep their customers in check (Aaron & Musto, 1981, pp. 132–133). Although drunkenness was observed, moderation was clearly the norm.

When informal controls failed, there were always legal ones. Alcohol abuse was treated with rapid and sometimes severe punishment. Habitual drinkers "were whipped or forced to wear a mark of shame. Once so labeled, they could be refused the right to purchase liquor. During the 17th century, all of the colonies specified a fine or prescribed the stocks for the first drunkenness offense. Repeat offenders often received sentences to hard labor or corporal punishment" (Krout, 1925, pp. 27–28; Mendelson & Mello, 1985, p. 11). Although infractions did occur, the general sobriety of the colonists suggests the effectiveness of their system of informal and formal controls in a population in which the average consumption per person was about three and a half gallons of absolute alcohol per year (Rorabaugh, 1991, p. 17). This was dramatically higher than the present rate of consumption.

Change and Revolution Created Problems

When the colonies grew from a rural society into one with more towns and cities, drinking patterns began to change, with rum becoming increasingly popular. As the American Revolution approached, economic change and urbanization were accompanied by increasing poverty, unemployment, and crime. These emerging social problems were often blamed on drunkenness. Alcohol, which had been the "good creature of God" was becoming "Demon rum."

Following the Revolutionary War, the new nation experienced cataclysmic social, political, and economic changes that affected every segment of the new society. Social control over alcohol abuse declined, antidrunkenness ordinances were relaxed, and alcohol problems increased dramatically. Drinking, which had been controlled by the tightly knit family and social fabric in the colonial period, increasingly became an individualistic activity associated with masculine aggression and antisocial behavior by the early 19th century (Peele, 1987). It became segregated by gender and age, which encouraged excessive consumption, and concern was frequently expressed over immoderate drinking. As life in the colonies "became less cohesive and structured, the social sanctions that had kept drunkenness to a minimum began to lose their power" (Schlaadt, 1992, p. 9).

When British blockade disrupted the production of rum, a substitute was found in whiskey. In 1810, it was estimated that 14,171 distilleries produced more than 25 million gallons of whiskey (Krout, 1925, p. 99). By the 1820s, whiskey sold for 25¢ a gallon, making it cheaper than beer, wine, coffee, tea, or milk (Rorabaugh, 1991, p. 17). Annual consumption may have been as high as 10 gallons per person (Asbury, 1968, p. 12; Clark, 1976, p. 20). This level of consumption was several times higher than the current rate: "the period from the 1790s to the early 1830s was probably the heaviest drinking era in the nation's history" (Lender & Martin, 1982, p. 46). "Instead of a morning coffee break, Americans stopped work at 11:00 a.m. to drink. A lot of work went undone but in this slow paced, preindustrial age this was not always a problem. A drunken stage coach driver posed little threat, since the horses knew the route and made their own way home" (Rorabaugh, 1991, p. 17). But not all was well. The famous observer of American life, Tocqueville, suggested that the sudden disappearance of traditional boundaries left people bereft and disoriented (Aaron & Musto, 1981, p. 136), with negative consequences for social control.

By the early 1800s, the frontier was advancing across the Mississippi River. Many on the frontier were uprooted individuals, vagabonds, or those whose jobs kept them migrant and isolated for long periods of time. They included fur trappers, cowboys, miners, and federal troops. Such individuals lived isolated hard lives, without constraining social obligations and controls (Lender & Martin, 1982, p. 48). As described by Lender and Martin (1982):

> frontier drinking could be highly unrestrained and often was associated with gambling, fighting, and whoring. Drinking bouts tended to come after long dry spells; that is, after days or weeks—and in some cases months—in the mountains, on the trail, or in mining digs, where opportunities for drinking or other amusements were virtually nil. So at a mountain man's semiannual "rendezvous," a cowtown, or any other potential site of entertainment (which could have been only a settler's wagon with a whiskey barrel), the impulse was to cut loose and make a trapper, miner, soldier, and cowboy blow their entire pay on a weekend debauch in towns with evocative names like Tombstone, Gomorrah, and Delirium Tremens. It was, in short, often a rude and individualistic group that pushed the frontier forward, often with personal and drinking behavior to match. (p. 48)

With the settling of the West (which brought the moderating influence of the family, the church, and other social institutions), alcohol abuse became less acceptable. As social conditions improved, there was a greater capacity for a reasonable family life and alcohol was used less as a relief from intolerable conditions. At the same time, the level of emotionalism attached to drinking, particularly the concept of machismo—male superiority shown in the capacity to hold liquor—began to drop (Zinberg & Fraser, 1985, p. 467). Although alcohol was an integral part of the farmer's daily life, disruptive drinking was a threat. Frequent intoxication diverted too much time and effort from maintaining a homestead and was a luxury the average struggling farmer could not afford (Lender & Martin, 1982, p. 51).

Economic development brought other changes back East, such as, "middle- and upper-class Americans cut back their drinking drastically because it was no longer considered appropriate for an industrious life. As alcohol was eliminated from the ordinary daily routines of the middle class, when people did drink, they were more likely to go on binges where they drank all out" (Peele, 1989, p. 36).

The Beginnings of Temperance

An eminent physician of the period, Dr. Benjamin Rush, argued that the excessive rise of distilled spirits was injurious to physical and psychological health and urged abstinence from ardent spirits and moderation in the consumption of fermented beverages (Katcher, 1993). "He envisioned a healthy American people bursting with beer, light wines, and happiness" (Asbury, 1968, p. 28).

By the early 1800s, an organized temperance movement was underway. Its members advocated temperance or moderation rather than abstinence. The American Temperance Society was formed in 1826 and benefitted from a renewed interest in religion and morality. Within 10 years it claimed more than 8,000 local groups and over 1,500,000 members (Furnas, 1965, p.55). By 1839, 15 temperance journals were being published (Cherrington, 1920, pp. 98–123). Simultaneously, many Protestant churches were beginning to promote temperance.

From Temperance to Total Abstinence

Between 1830 and 1840, most temperance organizations began to argue that the only way to prevent drunkenness was to eliminate the consumption of alcohol. The Temperance Society became the Abstinence Society. The Independent Order of Good Templars, the Sons of Temperance, the Templars of Honor and Temperance, the Anti-Saloon League, the National Prohibition Party and other groups were formed and grew rapidly (Blocker, 1985, pp. 67–72). With the passage of time "the temperance societies became more and more extreme in the measures they championed" (McConnell, 1963, p. 569). Although it began by advocating the temperate or moderate use of alcohol, the movement now insisted that no one should be permitted to drink any alcohol in any quantity, and it did so with religious fervor and increasing stridency (Royce, 1981, p. 40; Sheehan, 1984). Even when compared to the sophisticated use of mass media today, the temperance movement still rivals the best in terms of scope, commitment, and response (Wallack, 1981).

After the Civil War, the Women's Christian Temperance Union (WCTU) was founded. Of course, the organization did not promote moderation or temperance but rather prohibition. It saw the value of education in promoting its views and its agenda and ultimately came to control the content of alcohol education in the public schools of every state and federal territory.

Temperance materials made no distinction between drinking and alcohol abuse, and they were portrayed as one and the same. A typical poster presented the virtue and blessings of the abstainer on one side and the sin and misery of the drinker (synonymous with the drunk) on the other. A temperance pamphlet, summing up allegedly accepted findings, stated that "the offspring of parents both of whom drink are invariably either insane, tuberculous or alcoholic" and cited cases of "small children with an hereditary yen for alcohol so strong that the mere sight of a bottle shaped like a whiskey flask brought them whining for a nip" (Furnas, 1965, p. 194). Some temperance writers even implied that merely inhaling alcohol vapors might lead to defective offspring through their descendants for at least three generations (Ploetz, 1915, p. 29).

The WCTU's Department of Scientific Temperance Instruction promoted as scientifically proved the facts that:

- The majority of beer drinkers die from dropsy.
- When it (alcohol) passes down the throat it burns off the skin leaving it bare.
- It causes the heart to beat many unnecessary times and after the first dose the heart is in danger of giving out so that it needs something to keep it up and, therefore, the person to whom the heart belongs has to take drink after drink to keep his heart going.
- It turns the blood to water.
- [Referring to invalids], a man who never drinks liquor will get well, where a drinking man would surely die. (Kobler, 1973, p. 143)

The approved textbooks appear to have been written with the purpose of frightening children into avoiding all contact with alcohol. One can only speculate as to how many children unnecessarily suffered anxiety and emotional trauma as they watched their parents enjoy a glass of wine (poison) or a beer (poison) with their dinner. But the WCTU was unalterably opposed to moderation. Kobler (1973) pointed out that:

Nowhere in all this gallimaufry of misguidance . . . aimed at children, or in any of the prohibition literature and talk addressed to adults, did there linger the ghost of a suggestion that perhaps one might drink moderately without damage to oneself or to others. The very word "moderation" inflamed the WCTU and the Prohibition Party. It was "the shoddy life-belt, which promotes safety, but only tempts into danger, and fails in the hour of need . . . the fruitful fountain from which the flood of intemperance is fed. . . . Most men become drunkards by trying to drink moderately and failing." Even conceding that a rare few could conceivably imbibe in moderation at no risk to themselves, they should nevertheless refrain lest they set a bad example for the weaker majority of the human race. (p. 140)

Thus, approved textbooks asserted that "to drink fermented liquors moderately has led to the hopeless ruin of untold thousands" and "that it is the nature of alcohol to make drunkards" (Billings, 1903, pp. 30–31).

By defining any consumption of alcohol as alcohol abuse, the temperance movement and those it influenced saw abuse as serious and widespread. Unfortunately, social research of that period is essentially useless in clarifying the situation. At best, it tended to provide crude evidence of the perceptions held by various observers or respondents. Several such studies were conducted in Massachusetts. For example, one investigator sent a mail survey to all asylums in the state in 1875 requesting a count of the patients whose "insanity was caused by intemperance" and concluded that "on the average, intemperance is the cause of insanity" in 7% of the cases (Babor & Rosenkrantz, 1991, p. 270). Interviews with 1,600 mental patients in Massachusetts during the same time period concluded that a lower proportion of insanity was "due to the use of intoxicating liquors" among the native-born (33.6% of men and 9.1% of women) than the naturalized and alien patients (44.3% of men and 15.2% of women) (Babor & Rosenkrantz, 1991, p. 271). Another report at the time concluded that public intoxication accounted for 68% of the 18,232 criminal convictions made during a 12-month period (Babor & Rosenkrantz, 1991, p. 271). Personal interviews of all paupers admitted to Massachusetts welfare institutions in 1894–1895 led to the conclusion that 19.7% of adult men and 6.6% of adult women were excessive drinkers, defined as "all who are completely under the influence of the drinking habit—who are, in fact, common drunkards" (Babor & Rosenkrantz, 1991, p. 271). A nationwide survey of charity organizations in 1909 concluded that 45.2% of the male paupers' poverty was caused by their intemperance or that of a parent or spouse and 43.2% of the females' poverty was similarly caused (Babor & Rosenkrantz, 1991, pp. 272–273).

These studies all uncritically accepted the 19th-century assumption (and the temperance assumption) that alcohol abuse is the cause, rather than the result, of social, psychological or other problems. For decades, alcohol had been blamed for almost all human misery or misfortune and Prohibition had been touted as the almost magical solution to the nation's poverty, crime, violence, and other ills (Aaron & Musto, 1981, p. 157). On the eve of National Prohibition in 1920, the famous evangelist Billy Sunday preached on the benefits of the "noble experiment . . . the rein of tears is over. . . . the slums will soon be only a memory. We will turn our prisons into factories and our jails into storehouses and corncribs" (Asbury, 1968, pp. 144–145). Because alcohol was to be banned, and because it was seen as the cause of most, if not all, crime, some communities actually sold their jails (Anti-Saloon League of America, 1920, p. 28).

Unfortunately, the "great experiment" of Prohibition (1920–1933) proved to be a failure. The actual consequences ranged from unfortunate to deadly. Not only did it fail to prevent the consumption of alcohol, but it led to the extensive production of unregulated and untaxed alcohol, the development of organized crime empires, increased violence, massive political corruption, and widespread contempt for law (Asbury, 1968, ch. 9–14; Englemann, 1979; Everest, 1978; Grant & Ritson, 1983, p. 21; Kobler, 1973, ch. 10–13; Nelli, 1985; Sinclair, 1962, ch. 9–15).

Bootleg alcohol was often a cause of disability and even death. Many stills used lead coils or lead soldering, which gave off acetate of lead, a dangerous poison. Some bootleggers used recipes that included iodine, creosote, or even embalming fluid (Asbury, 1968, pp. 272–273 and 283). Another serious problem (Mendelson & Mello, 1985) was that highly toxic wood alcohols found their way into much of the available bootleg liquor. When denatured industrial alcohol was not sufficiently diluted, or was consumed in large quantities, the result was paralysis, blindness and death. In 1927, almost twelve thousands deaths were attributed to alcohol poisonings, many of these among the urban poor who could not afford imported liquors. In 1930, U.S. public health officials estimated that fifteen thousand persons were afflicted with "jake foot," a debilitating paralysis of the hands and feet brought on by drinking denatured alcohol flavored with ginger root. (p. 87)

In addition to being ineffective, Prohibition was counterproductive in that it encouraged the heavy and rapid consumption of high-proof distilled spirits in secretive, nonsocially regulated and controlled ways; that is, "people did not take the trouble to go to a speakeasy, present the password, and pay high prices for very poor quality alcohol simply to have a beer. When people went to speakeasies, they went to get drunk" (Zinberg & Fraser, 1985, p. 468). Those authors conclude that removing "alcohol from the norms of everyday society increased drinking problems. Without well-known prescriptions for use and commonly held sanctions against abuse, Prohibition drinkers were left almost as defenseless as were the South American Indians in the face of Spanish rum and brandy" (p. 470). They suggested that Prohibition "may have curtailed that growth of the responsible drinking practices that had emerged during the 25 or so years preceding Prohibition" (p. 470).

Near the end of Prohibition, an observer wrote that "since 1920 the changed attitudes of woman toward liquor has been one of the most influential factors in the encouragement of lawless drinking. Drinking in 1910 was a man's game. . . ." He explained that "[d]rinking today is a man-and-woman's game. . . . In all former times the man got drunk and came home to his disgusted and long-suffering wife. Today they sometimes get drunk together and try to slip into the house as quietly as possible, so as not to wake the children" (Asbury, 1968, p. 159).

As the problem caused by Prohibition continued to grow, popular opinion turned strongly against it and the end of the "noble experiment" was decisive. By a three-to-one popular vote, the American people rejected Prohibition; only two states opposed repeal (Childs, 1947, pp. 260–261; Merz, 1969). Happy throngs sang "Happy Days Are Here Again!" and President Roosevelt would soon look back to what he called "the damnable affliction of Prohibition" (Blocker, 1976, p. 242). But not all were happy. The Anti-Saloon League declared "War . . . NO PEACE PACT—NO ARMISTICE," and warned that temperance forces would soon be ready to launch the offensive against the liquor traffic (Lender & Martin, 1982, p. 135).

These threats were not idle, and the temperance movement clearly continued to wield much influence. Eighteen states continued Prohibition at the state level and almost two-thirds of all states adopted some form of local option that enabled residents in political subdivisions to vote for or against local Prohibition. Therefore, despite the repeal of prohibition at the national level, 38% of the nation's population lived in areas with state or local prohibition (Mendelson & Mello, 1985, p. 94). Not surprisingly, alcohol consumption failed to rebound dramatically. A substantial minority of the population maintained its strongly antialcohol sentiments and many tried to use World War II as an excuse to reimpose Prohibition to whatever degree possible (Childs, 1947; Rubin, 1979). Although its goal was largely defeated, the temperance movement continued to promote its cause and to influence public policy. Writing shortly after World War II, Childs (1947, p. 229) observed that, according to national opinion surveys, "about one-third of the people in the United States favor national prohibition."

MAJOR DEVELOPMENTS AND ISSUES

Alcoholics Anonymous, developed in 1935, spread slowly at first but in less than 50 years, 500,000 Americans had joined and spinoff groups had formed. Al-Anon is for the families of alcoholics and Ala-Teen is for teenage children of alcoholics (Kurtz, 1979).

The creation of the Yale University Center of Alcohol Studies in the late 1930s was a major development in the study of alcohol problems. The Center (now at Rutgers University) launched the *Journal of Studies on Alcohol* in 1940 and popularized the disease theory of alcoholism. It also facilitated the organization of the National Council on Alcoholism in 1944 (Blocker, 1989). In 1943, the first corporate effort to assist rather than discharge employees experiencing drinking problems was established. Today, there are many thousands of employee assistance programs. In 1944, the U.S. Public Health Service identified alcoholism as the fourth largest public health problem in the country (Masi, 1984).

By the mid-1950s, both the American Medical Association and the American Hospital Association passed resolutions accepting the disease concept of alcoholism. In the mid-1960s, several court cases (*Driver v. Hinnaut, Easter v. District of Columbia*, and *Powell v. Texas*) provided legal support for the disease theory (Grad, Goldberg, & Shapiro, 1971, pp. 10–13). However, courts upheld the legality of arrests for public intoxication or for operating vehicles or machinery while intoxicated. In spite of the possibly self-serving resolutions of medical groups, the disease theory of alcoholism remains controversial and many scholars dispute its legitimacy and utility (Fingarette, 1988; Peele, 1989; Schaler, 1995). It should be noted that, depending on time and place, deviant drinking has been considered by society to be sinful, criminal, or sick, and deviant drinkers have consequently been shunned, punished, or treated (Conrad & Schneider, 1980).

But much more important controversies exist. There is not even agreement as to the extent of drinking problems. The existence of the National

Institute of Alcoholism and Alcohol Abuse (NIAAA), the federal Center for Substance Abuse Prevention (CSAP), and state alcohol abuse agencies have been beneficial in many ways. They have "engendered bureaucratic incentive for convincing the people and members of Congress (who appropriate funds) of the perils and dangers of contemporary alcohol problems" (Mendelson & Mello, 1985, pp. 98–99). The welfare, if not the survival, of the alcohol agencies depends largely on promoting the widespread belief that alcohol problems are enormous, that they are growing, and that they are a serious burden on the economy.

During the 1980s, advocacy groups such as the Center for Science in the Public Interest, the National Coalition for the Prevention of Impaired Driving and National Council on Alcoholism and Drug Dependency pressed for legislation to limit and reduce the consumption of beverage alcohol (Engs, 1991). By 1987, political pressure led to a federally mandated (under threat of withholding highway funds) expansion of alcohol Prohibition in all states to all citizens under the age of 21. This was followed by a federal tax increase on alcohol beverages in 1991, and to state laws reducing the acceptable blood alcohol content for driving. Reduction-of-consumption policies have led to a dramatic decrease in beer, wine, and spirits consumption since 1980 (Hanson, 1995b). But lower is never low enough. As a reduction-of-consumption advocate wrote, "the slogan for the new temperance is, regarding alcohol, 'less is better' " (Beauchamp, 1987, p. 62). Nor is there any reason to expect alcohol abuse to decline when consumption declines or to increase when consumption increases. Alcohol abuse is more closely related to attitudes, beliefs, and norms than to consumption levels (Hanson, 1995a).

Importantly, there is controversy over the best way to reduce alcohol problems. The reduction-of-consumption approach tends to assume that:

1) The substance of alcohol is in and of itself the complete and total cause of all drinking problems.

2) The availability of alcohol determines the extent to which it will be consumed.

3) The quantity of alcohol consumed (rather than the manner in which it is consumed, the purpose for which it is consumed, the social context in which it is consumed, etc.) determines the extent of drinking problems.

4) Educational efforts should be directed toward stressing the problems that alcohol consumption can cause and encourage abstinence.

The more traditional reduction-of-consumption approach called for the complete and total prohibition of the manufacture, distribution, sale, possession, or consumption of any and all beverage alcohol. Given the clear failure of Prohibition, supporters of the reduction-of-consumption model now more typically call for a variety of measures designed to discourage consumption. These include such practices as:

- imposing higher taxes on alcohol beverages
- limiting or reducing the number of sales outlets
- restricting even more the permissible locations for sales outlets
- limiting the alcohol content of beverages
- prohibiting or restricting the promotion of alcohol (through sponsorship of athletic events, sponsoring events on college campuses, giving free samples, etc.)
- requiring the use of warnings with all advertisements and commercials
- requiring the use of stronger warning labels on all beverage containers
- requiring the display of stronger warning signs in establishments that sell or serve alcohol beverages
- limiting the days or hours during which alcohol can be sold
- increasing server liability for subsequent problems associated with the misuse of alcohol
- limiting the sale of alcohol to people of specific ages
- decreasing the legal blood alcohol content level for driving vehicles or operating equipment
- eliminating the tax deductibility of alcohol as a business expense

The reduction-of-consumption approach assumes that the problem is alcohol rather than the abuse of alcohol. Therefore, it attempts to discourage or prevent people from consuming alcohol rather than trying to prevent them from using alcohol irresponsibly.

A study of per capita alcohol consumption found that consumption rose 11.8% between 1967 and 1984. However, few drinking problems increased over the same time (Hilton & Clark, 1991). And, conversely, now that consumption has been decreasing, there is little evidence that most drinking problems have declined.

The sociocultural approach to alcohol tends to assume that

1) It is the misuse of alcohol, not alcohol itself, that is the source of drinking problems.
2) It is important to distinguish between alcohol use and abuse.
3) The misuse of alcohol can be reduced by educating individuals to make one of two decisions: one decision is to abstain, the other decision is to drink responsibly.

4) Because many individuals will choose to drink alcohol, it is important that societal norms regarding what is acceptable and unacceptable behavior for those who choose to drink be clear and unambiguous.

5) People who are going to drink as adults should gradually learn how to drink. Preferably, this should occur first in the home from the parents and then be reinforced through formal education in schools.

The sociocultural approach is based on the experience of Italians, Jews, Greeks, and many other groups around the world that use alcohol extensively with few problems. Research tends to support the sociocultural approach (Hanson, 1995a). However, until such time as scientific consensus is reached, public policy is likely to continue alternating between the two approaches.

REFERENCES

Aaron, P., & Musto, D. (1981). Temperance and Prohibition in America: A historical overview. In M. H. Moore & D. R. Gerstein (Eds.), *Alcohol and public policy: Beyond the shadow of prohibition* (pp. 127–181). Washington, DC: National Academy Press.

Anti-Saloon League of America. (1920). *Anti-Saloon League of America yearbook* (p. 20). Westerville, OH: American Issue Press. Cited by H. A. Mulford (1965), *Alcohol and alcoholism in Iowa* (p. 9). Iowa City: University of Iowa Press.

Asbury, H. (1968). *The great illusion: An informal history of prohibition.* New York: Greenwood.

Babor, T. F., & Rosenkrantz, B. G. (1991). Public health, public morals, and public order: Social science and liquor control in Massachusetts, 1880–1916. In S. Barrows & R. Room (Eds.), *Drinking: Behavior and belief in modern history* (pp. 265–286). Berkeley: University of California Press.

Beauchamp, D. E. (1987). Alcohol-abuse prevention through beverage and environmental regulation: Where we have been and where we are going. In H. D. Holder (Ed.), *Advances in substance abuse: Behavioral and biological research* (pp. 53–63). Supplement 1. Greenwich, CT: JAI.

Billings, J. S. (1903). *Physiological aspects of the liquor problem.* Boston: Houghton Mifflin.

Blocker, J. S. (1976). *Retreat from reform.* Westport, CT: Greenwood.

Blocker, J. S. (1985). *"Give to the winds thy fear": The Women's Temperance Crusade, 1873–1874.* Westport, CT: Greenwood.

Blocker, J. S. (1989). *American temperance movements: Cycles of reform.* Boston: Twayne.

Cherrington, E. H. (1920). *The evolution of prohibition in the United States of America.* Westerville, OH: American Issue Press.

Childs, R. W. (1947). *Making repeal work.* Philadelphia: Pennsylvania Alcohol Beverage Study.

Clark, N. H. (1976). *Deliver us from evil: An interpretation of American prohibition.* New York: Norton.

Conrad, P., & Schneider, J. (1980). *Deviance and medicalization.* St. Louis, MO: Mosby.

Engelmann, L. (1979). *Intemperance: The lost war against liquor.* New York: The Free Press.

Engs, R. C. (1991). Resurgence of a new "clean living" movement in the United States. *Journal of School Health, 61*, 155–159.

Everest, A. S. (1978). *Rum across the border: The prohibition era in northern New York.* Syracuse, NY: Syracuse University Press.

Fingarette, H. (1988). *Heavy drinking*. Berkeley: University of California Press.

Furnas, J. C. (1965). *The life and times of the late Demon Rum*. New York: Putnam.

Grad, F. P., Goldberg, A. L., & Shapiro, B. A. (1971). *Alcoholism and the law*. Dobbs Ferry, NY: Oceana.

Grant, M., & Ritson, B. (1983). *Alcohol: The prevention debate*. New York: St. Martin's Press.

Hanson, D. J. (1995a). *Preventing alcohol abuse: Alcohol, culture, and control*. Westport, CT: Praeger.

Hanson, D. J. (1995b). The United States of America. In D. B. Health (Ed.), *International handbook on alcohol and culture* (pp. 301–315). Westport, CT: Greenwood.

Hilton, M. E., & Clark, W. B. (1991). Changes in American drinking patterns and problems, 1967–1984. *Journal of Studies on Alcohol, 48*, 515–522.

Katcher, B. S. (1993). Benjamin Rush's educational campaign against hard drinking. *American Journal of Public Health, 83*, 273–281.

Kobler, J. (1973). *Ardent spirits: The rise and fall of prohibition*. New York: Putnam.

Krout, J. A. (1925). *The origins of prohibition*. New York: Knopf.

Kurtz, E. (1979). *Not-God: A history of Alcoholics Anonymous*. Center City, MN: Hazelden Educational Services.

Lender, M. E., & Martin, J. K. (1982). *Drinking in America: A history*. New York: The Free Press.

MacAndrew, C., & Edgerton, R. (1969). *Drunken comportment: A social explanation*. Chicago: Aldine.

Masi, D. A. (1984). *Designing employee assistance programs*. New York: American Management Association.

McConnell, D. W. (1963). Temperance movements. In E. R. A. Seligman & A. Johnson (Eds.), *Encyclopedia of the social sciences* (vol. 14, pp. 567–570). New York: Macmillan.

Mendelson, J. H., & Mello, N. K. (1985). *Alcohol: Use and abuse in America*. Boston: Little, Brown.

Merz, C. (1969). *The dry decade*. Seattle: University of Washington Press. (Contains a new introduction by the author. Original work published 1930)

Nelli, H. S. (1985). American syndicate crime: A legacy of prohibition. In D. E. Kyvig (Ed.), *Law, alcohol, and order: Perspectives on national prohibition* (pp. 123–138). Westwood, CT: Greenwood Press.

Peele, S. (1987). The limitations of control-of-supply models for explaining and preventing alcoholism and drug addiction. *Journal of Studies on Alcohol, 48*, 61–70.

Peele, S. (1989). *The diseasing of America: Addiction treatment out of control*. Lexington, MA: Lexington.

Ploetz, A. J. (1915). *The influence of alcohol upon the race*. Westerville, OH: American Issue Press.

Popham, R. E. (1978). The social history of the tavern. In Y. Israel, F. B. Glazer, H. Kalant, R. E. Popham, H. Schmidt, & R. G. Smart (Eds.), *Research advances in alcohol and drug problems* (vol. 4, pp. 255–302). New York: Plenum.

Rorabaugh, W. J. (1979). *The alcoholic republic: An American tradition*. New York: Oxford University Press.

Rorabaugh, W. J. (1991). Alcohol and alcoholism. In M. K. Cayton, E. J. Gorn, & P. W. Williams (Eds.), *Encyclopedia of American social history* (vol. 3, pp. 2135–2142). New York: Scribner's.

Royce, J. E. (1981). *Alcohol problems and alcoholism: A comprehensive survey*. New York: The Free Press.

Rubin, J. L. (1979). American liquor control, 1941–1945. In J. S. Blocher, Jr. (Ed.), *Alcohol, reform and society: The liquor issue in social context* (pp. 235–258). Westport, CT: Greenwood.

Schaler, J. (1995, November). *Thinking about drinking: The power of self-fulfilling prophecies*. Paper presented at the conference on Alternative Approaches to Addiction and Destructive Habits, Edmonton, Alberta.

Schlaadt, R. G. (1992). *Alcohol use and abuse*. Guilford, CT: Dushkin.

Sheehan, N. M. (1984). National pressure groups and provincial curriculum policy: Temperance in Nova Scotia schools, 1800–1930. *Canadian Journal of Education, 9*, 73–88.

Sinclair, A. (1962). *Prohibition: The era of excess*. Boston: Little, Brown.

Wallack, L. M. (1981). Man media campaigns: The odds against finding behavior change. *Health Education Quarterly, 8*, 209–260.

Williams, G. D., Clem, D. A., & Dufour, M. C. (1994). *Apparent per capita consumption: National, state, and regional trends, 1977–1992*. Surveillance Report #31. Washington, DC: National Institute on Alcohol Abuse and Alcoholism.

Zinberg, N. E., & Fraser, K. M. (1985). The role of the social setting in the prevention and treatment of alcoholism. In J. H. Mendelson & N. K. Mello (Eds.), *The diagnosis and treatment of alcoholism* (2nd ed., pp. 457–483). New York: McGraw-Hill.

4

Historical Overview of Other Abusable Drugs

J. Bryan Page
University of Miami

Humankind has identified hundreds of preparations that, when absorbed by the body, alter its functions in ways that make the user feel transformed. The word preparation seems appropriate to denote the range of things that otherwise carry the names *drug, substance, chemical, narcotic, stimulant, sedative, hallucinogen,* and *anxiolytic,* among others, because they require varying degrees of preparation before the user ingests them. The process of getting a drug (the most broadly understandable of the commonly used terms) ready for consumption may involve actions as simple as finding a plant or mushroom and eating it, or as elaborate as chemical extraction of specific alkaloids from plant-derived liquids, modification of the alkaloid, dilution in water, and hypodermic injection into the vein. The idea that drugs require preparation should prove especially useful in examining the history of drugs other than alcohol, because it causes us to imagine how our ancestors developed present-day forms of drugs.

This chapter explains the distinctions among four widely disseminated drugs, in terms of psychotropic properties, chemical development, and social, economic, and political processes that accompanied discovery and diffusion. It also lists the major drugs other than alcohol in the world pharmacopeia and explain how they came to world prominence.

INVENTING A DRUG

Anthropologists learn early in their required archaeology courses that accident is the true mother of invention, and this view of invention certainly applies to most of the preparations described here. The varieties of accidents responsible for discovering the mind-altering properties of plants, the primary sources of drugs, fall into two categories: a) direct exposure to effects of plants through accidental or experimental ingestion, and b) observation of the plants' effects on animals that consume them. Tobacco and betel are associated with legends that describe the former process, and coffee and amanita muscaria are associated with origin legends that describe the latter (Knipe, 1995; Ray, 1983).

This, however, only identifies the plant source of the drug. Next comes a process of modification that renders the drug consumable by humans. The red, sap-filled berries of the coffee shrub may have caused goats to frisk on the hillside, but they are removed by several preparative steps from the dark, hot fluid consumed on Turkish streetcorners. The first of these removes the red outer husk and drains off the viscous fluid around the beans. The beans are dried, graded, and then roasted. Finally, after grinding the beans to a powdery consistency and allowing hot water to flow through the grounds, the brown liquid that results is ready for human ingestion.

Similar processes, usually requiring centuries of development after accidental discovery, apply to most of the drugs currently in use. Once developed, these drugs either diffused to other populations or did not. The factors that affected the diffusion or nondiffusion of specific drugs receives attention in the succeeding pages.

THE PROCESS OF DIFFUSION

Drug use takes place within complexes of human behavior that vary greatly in how they apply identified drugs to the human body. In some cultural traditions, people restrict taking of drugs to highly circumscribed ritual contexts for purposes of divination and curing, such as *ayahuasca* or *datura* (Harner, 1974), while in others drug-taking facilitates social interaction, as in the cases of *coca* or *qat* (Burchard, 1978; Weir, 1985). With the possible exception of the volatile hydrocarbon inhalants, whose users sometimes discover their properties spontaneously, learning how to use drugs requires instruction in some sort of patterned behavior, usually conducted by an experienced older person. Becker's (1953) studies of marijuana users in Chicago exemplify this process of learning. Use of cannabis seems an especially good example because users report wide varieties of drug effects. What the new user learns about a drug like marijuana helps predict the effects that user will report as a consequence of smoking (Becker, 1953; Page & Carter, 1980).

The same principle obtains for most other drugs, although their effects may be more clearly defined than those of marijuana. For example, the opiates' effects correspond to direct interaction between the drug and the nervous system's own chemical receptors. Still, the novice drug user's expectations, shaped by his or her instructor, will have influence on the kinds of effects reported for whatever drug he or she takes. Beyond expectation of effects, users also need to learn the basic skills, such as rolling marijuana "joints," holding the smoke in their lungs, cooking opium, or finding veins for injection of "speedball" that enable them to obtain the effects they have learned to expect. This learning process begins with whatever motivates a user to try a drug in the first place, and then moves into the social environment in which the new user must receive some kind of instruction, whether directly or indirectly. This instruction is the most basic principle of how patterns of drug use spread: diffusion occurs when a population that uses a drug comes into contact with a population that does not, and members of the latter group begin to use that drug. Drugs do not diffuse in the absence of clear behavioral examples of how people consume them. Whether under the tutelage of an older peer who gives detailed instructions on what effects to expect and how to apply the dose, or through the example of a user observed through a door slightly ajar, the novice must have an example to emulate.

THE ARRAY OF DRUGS

Four varieties of drugs receive most of the emphasis in this discussion, because the preparations derived from them have established populations of users all over the world: tobacco, coca leaf and its derivatives, the opiates, and cannabis. Furthermore, they account for the vast majority of health problems related to drugs other than alcohol. Table 4.1 gives brief descriptions of each variety of drug and its preparations, origins, and variety of effects. Two originated in the Western Hemisphere and two in the Eastern Hemisphere.

Tobacco

Native American populations had great familiarity with tobacco (several species of the genus *Nicotiana*, including *tabacum*, *bigelovii*, and *attenuata*, among others) at the time of Columbus' arrival, setting in motion the most rapid and thorough process of drug diffusion in human history. In four centuries, its use became custom for people in hundreds of different cultural traditions on all continents. Unfortunately, there are no written records of tobacco's discovery and diffusion in North and South America, but it certainly was thorough, based on what is known (Driver & Massey, 1957). European explorers encountered tobacco use among the Arawak and Caribe islanders, Timucuan in Florida, Aztec in Mexico, Plains Indians in the central

TABLE 4.1

Preparation Name, Process, Route of Ingestion, Invention Site & Cultural Tradition, Date of Invention, Effects

Preparation Name	Process	Route of Ingestion	Invention Site & Cultural Tradition	Date of Invention	Effects
Tobacco and Its Preparation					
Cigar	leaves dried, cured, chopped, wrapped with whole leaf into cylindrical shape	smoke in mouth, nose	Americas, Amerind[a]	3000 B.P.[b]	mild sedative, but depends on intensity of ingestion; can cause convulsions if inhaled
Chewing strips and plugs	leaves dried, cured, cut into strips, flavor added, pressed into bars or plugs	chewed	Americas, Amerind	3000 B.P.	mild sedative
Cut for smoking (pipes)	leaves dried, cured, chopped, flavored	smoke in mouth, nose	Americas, Amerind	3000 B.P.	mild sedative
Cigarette	leaves dried, cured, chopped, rolled into small cylinder with paper wrapper	smoke in lungs	Europe, Northwestern	1700s	mild sedative
Snuff	leaves dried, cured, ground into powder	insufflated in nose, or held in mouth	America, Amerind	3000 B.P.	mild sedative
Coca Leaf and Its Preparations					
Coca	leaves gathered, sorted, dried	chewed bolus of leaves, quicklime added	South America; Andean	3800 B.P.	numb mouth, resistance to cold, hunger
Mate coca (coca tea)	leaves gathered, sorted, dried, steeped in hot water	drunk	South America; Andean	3800 B.P.	resistance to effects of altitude

Cocaine (base, toco, bazuco)	leaves gathered, sorted, dried, mashed with petroleum, precipitated with sulfuric acid, precipitate dried, cut, sold to users	smoked in pipes or tobacco cigarettes	South America; Urban Andean	late 1900s (ca. 1970)	stimulant to central nervous system, brief ecstatic "rush" when first inhaled
Cocaine (hydrochloride)	base washed with acetone, ether, hydrochloric acid, resulting water soluble powder sold to users	insufflation in nose, hypodermic injection	Europe; German & Italian	1800s	numbness at point of ingestion, stimulant to central nervous system, ecstatic "rush" when injected
Crack (rock, base bazuco)	hydrochloride cooked with baking soda and water, sold in chunks to users	smoked in pipes or tobacco cigarettes	Southern California	late 1900s (ca. 1983)	stimulant to central nervous system, brief ecstatic "rush" when smoked

Opium and Its Preparation

Opium	plant's seed pod scored, sap seeps through scoring, collected, dried, cooked before smoking	smoke in mouth, nose, lungs	Middle East; Sumerian	6500 B.P.	sedation, pleasure
Morphine	raw opium cooked to dissolve in water, skimmed of impurities, calcium hydroxide added, liquid filtered, cooled, ammonium chloride added, precipitate washed with hydrochloric acid (HCl) or sulfuric acid, resulting powder used medicinally or refined into heroin	oral, topical, hypodermic injection	Germany	1804	sedation, pleasure, relief of pain
Heroin	morphine base treated with acetic anhydride under low heat, precipitate dried, HCl added	nasal insufflation, hypodermic injection	Germany	1900s	sedation, pleasure, relief of pain

(Continued)

TABLE 4.1
(Continued)

Preparation Name	Process	Route of Ingestion	Invention Site & Cultural Tradition	Date of Invention	Effects
Pharmaceutical Opiates	morphine base further treated to produce oxycodone, hydromorphone (Percodan, Dilaudid)	oral, hypodermic injection	United States	1900s	sedation, pleasure, relief of pain
Codeine	separate active alkaloid, removed in early stage of refining morphine	oral	United States	1900s	sedation, pleasure, relief of pain
Cannabis and Its Preparations					
Bhang	leaves gathered, sorted, dried, ground into powder, mixed with water, honey, or other sweeteners	drunk	Asian Subcontinent; Hindu	5000 B.P.	mild sedative, varied cognitive effects
Ganja, Marijuana, Kif	leaves gathered, sorted, dried, tops and flowers selected, crumbled, placed in pipes or rolled into cigarettes or cigars, often mixed with tobacco	smoke in mouth, nose, lungs	Asian Subcontinent; Hindu	5000 B.P.	mild to strong sedative, varied cognitive effects
Hashish, Charas	resin expressed by plants collected, dried	smoked in pipes or inserted in tobacco cigarettes	Asian Subcontinent; Hindu	5000 B.P.	mild to strong sedative, varied cognitive effects

[a] Amerind refers to Native American cultures before arrival of Europeans.
[b] B.P. denotes Before Present.

continent, and among the Tupi and other inhabitants in the Brazilian jungles (Billings, 1875). The 16th century simply marked the next big step in tobacco's spread, the opening of four new continents and Oceania.

The spread of tobacco to all corners of the world represents the most remarkable and inexorable example of a drug's diffusion, yet the chronicles of that spread give few clues as to why it occurred with such rapidity and universality. The European explorers who bridged the passage of tobacco to Europe and set themselves up as promoters in the rest of the world did not seem particularly fascinated by its use among the people they encountered in the New World. Their accounts hardly sang the praises of tobacco. Columbus noticed natives whiffing what appeared to be smoldering firebrands, and later described a man in a canoe who had with him "... some dry leaves which must be a thing very much appreciated among them, because they had already brought me some as a present at San Salvador ..." (Brooks, 1952). Bartolomé de Las Casas described smoking as he saw it in 1535 (Brooks, 1952):

> ... their smokes, which are some dry herbs put in a certain leaf, also dry, in the manner of a musket made of paper ... and having lighted one part of it, by the other they suck, absorb, or receive that smoke inside with the breath, by which they become numbed and almost drunk, and so it is said that they do not feel fatigue. These muskets, as we will call them, they call tobacco (*tabacos*). ... (pp. 14–15)

Perhaps the drug's mundane, unprepossessing appearance and usage constituted an advantage for rapid diffusion. Its effects did not engender drunkenness or outrageous comportment, yet they complemented the effects of alcohol well. Tobacco's routes of ingestion, puffed or inhaled smoke or chewing, only encounter brief coughing and sneezing reactions before the mild narcotic effects become easily attainable by the novice. Once the new user succeeded in obtaining agreeable effects of tobacco, however, he (men were always first to have access to this new drug) usually wanted more. This may have contributed most strongly to the spread of tobacco, especially if the commerce-minded Europeans recognized the property of addiction with any clarity at all. A product that one must burn to consume and to which the customer essentially commits for life had especially strong appeal to those seeking to profit from their adventures in the New World. Nevertheless, recognition of these virtues does not appear clearly articulated in the chronicles of tobacco's early promotion in the Old World. Songs composed in the 16th century in England foreshadowed the commercial jingles of the 20th century:

> Love maketh lean the fat mann's tumor
> So doth tobacco.
> Love still dries up the wanton humour

So doth tobacco.
Love makes men sail from shore to shore
So doth tobacco.
'Tis fond love often makes men poor
So doth tobacco.
(From "Tobacco Is Like Love," in Greenberg, 1962)

By the end of the 17th century, planters in the North American and Cuban colonies had established tobacco as a reliable moneymaker. By the end of the 18th century, substantial segments of population among the sensibly resistant Chinese had taken up tobacco smoking. In the succeeding two centuries, people as disparate as Micronesians and Zulus also began consuming tobacco. This process combined persistent trade overtures, military bullying, and a product that seems to draw people into regular consumption.

As with most drugs, the appeal of tobacco alone could not have driven the drug's relentless march across all of the lands inhabited by human beings. In 1792, when the mandarins balked at the English attempts to establish tobacco trade in China, the British navy helped to assure that Chinese consumers could satisfy their desires for tobacco (Knipe, 1995).

The predominant forms of ingestion practiced during the first two and a half millennia of humankind's interaction with tobacco did not change appreciably from the smoking of chopped leaves, chewing of compressed leaves, and the intranasal insufflation of snuff, a powdered form. The Europeans found this a genteel way to consume tobacco without smoke or offensive spittle juice. Snuff became especially popular among gentry and nobility and caused the development of cottage industries for production of elegant boxes for carrying and storing it, as well as handkerchiefs for catching sneezes caused by the powder.

Later the Spanish invented small papers for rolling small quantities of smoking tobacco into small *papelates*, which had become popular in 18th-century Spain, and the French apparently began mass-producing little cigars or "cigarettes" wrapped in paper (Goodman, 1993). These involved such small quantities of tobacco that they could be inhaled without the nausea and discomfort associated with inhalation of cigar and pipe tobacco. The seemingly simple innovation of wrapping less tobacco in light paper resulted eventually in a worldwide business of immense impact on world economics and public health, especially when the tobacco producers offered them to the consumers ready-made, without the trouble of wrapping them. Cigarettes offered a lightweight, convenient vehicle for consumption of tobacco that produced less overpowering smoke than did pipes or cigars. In fact, they seemed so comparatively innocuous that women, who typically had avoided all forms but snuff, began to smoke in the late 19th and early 20th centuries.

By the middle of the 20th century, large populations in Europe, Asia, South and North America, Africa, and Australia had taken up cigarette smoking, and the production, marketing, and exportation of cigarettes had grown into a multibillion-dollar international business. By 1950, cigarettes accounted for more than half of tobacco consumption worldwide (Goodman, 1993). Large-scale media of communications, including print, radio, television, and motion pictures played major roles in presenting cigarette smoking in the most glamorous, desirable light possible. In fact, they supplanted the less subtle means of assuring markets for tobacco employed in previous centuries, and proved considerably more effective. Generations of adolescents practiced in front of mirrors in attempts to look like the models and movie stars whose images they wanted to emulate through inhaling smoke through a small cylinder of tightly rolled, chopped leaves. The result of this amounted to an almost universal acceptance of cigarettes, with 35% of the United States' adult population and hundreds of millions throughout the world chronically smoking them.

Tobacco use began to attract medical attention in the 1940s and 1950s in the United States, because its consumers seemed to have high rates of cancer, heart disease, and respiratory problems (Goodman, 1993, p. 125). By 1964, the U.S. Surgeon General deemed the evidence convincing enough to begin initiatives to prevent tobacco use and to set in motion the process of establishing warnings of tobacco related health risks to all consumers. This led to some mass media campaigns against smoking, the placement of a warning on cigarette packets, and the eventual ban of cigarette advertisement on television in 1973.

The latter development, oddly, grew out of the tobacco industry's own initiative. Television campaigns against cigarettes in the middle and late 1960s had begun to have measurable effects by 1970, with reductions in new smokers and increases in numbers of people who quit smoking. The tobacco industry offered to refrain from advertising on television, if television would stop airing antismoking ads. Print media and billboards became the primary vehicles for cigarette ads, with few competing messages against smoking, and the market for cigarettes had a resurgence for the next two decades.

Worldwide, the tobacco industry continues to develop new markets by targeting youth and women. Its success at this could be seen in front of any high school in the mid-nineties, despite setbacks in the form of regulations forbidding people to smoke in government buildings, commercial airplanes, and other public places, and growing numbers of lawsuits over mortality due to effects of cigarette smoking.

Coca Products

Archaeological evidence indicates that Native Americans in the Andean region of South America knew about coca, the leaves of the plant *Erythroxylon coca* and held it in high regard as early as 3800 B.P. (Dobkin de Rios, 1984). For the next 3650 years, two preparations dominated the use of coca leaves:

tea made from steeping the leaves in boiling water, and leaves chewed and balled into the cheek, with quicklime added. These uses had both ritual and practical significance to people living in the Andean highlands. They represented a gift from the deities, but they also helped people to resist the thin air and cold of their mountainous home.

The Spanish conquistadors who arrived in the region in the 16th century dismissed coca chewing as the repulsive habit of ignorant Indians, although they tolerated its use among laborers who claimed that the coca helped them to work longer hours under difficult conditions (Carter & Mamani, 1986). Studies in the 20th century (Bolton, 1976; Burchard, 1975, 1976, 1978) attempted to explain this perception of coca's effects in terms of the leaf's water-soluble alkaloids that are theorized to aid in the digestion and metabolization of complex carbohydrates.

One alkaloid that does not dissolve in water, however, attracted attention of the European chemists who attempted to unlock the secret of the coca leaf's powers during the 19th century. At least two chemists, Neuman in Germany and Mariani in Italy, apparently developed the technique of extracting cocaine from coca leaf and adding a hydrochloride radical in order to make cocaine hydrochloride, a water-soluble delivery system for cocaine (Ray, 1983). The amount of cocaine in the few leaves chewed by indigenous coca chewers delivered very little cocaine to the nervous system. Chemical extraction, on the other hand, used large quantities of leaf to produce a highly potent alkaloid that soon became a major component of patent medicines and elixirs, including Mariani's Famous Coca Wine, and (until 1909) Coca-Cola.

The properties of cocaine attracted attention of physicians (for its topical anaesthetic effects), psychiatrists (for its ability to lift the spirits of depressed patients), and even authors of mysteries (A. Conan Doyle wrote it into Sherlock Holmes's personal habits as a stimulator of hyperactive analytic acumen) during the 19th century. By the early 20th century, however, the brief euphoria over cocaine's ability to stimulate gave way to news of people's inability to stop using it, as well as onset of depression when they cannot get any more. Some reports of violent crime in connection with cannabis use further jaundiced the public image of cocaine. In the activity prior to the framing of the Harrison Act and its passage in 1914, cocaine's reputation as a cause of problems became bad enough to lead to its inclusion as a controlled substance in that legislation (Musto, 1987). For the next 60 years, cocaine use in the United States had devotees only among those willing to participate in behaviors driven underground by the laws against the importation, sale and use of that drug (i.e. the street-based users of illegal drugs).

The social ferment of the middle and late 1960s included questioning of laws against use of drugs outlawed by the Harrison Act and subsequent legislation. Cocaine became one of the drugs that came under the scrutiny of the experimental users of that era. New users, largely from the American and European middle classes, began to experiment with cocaine in the early 1970s, and by the middle of that decade, centers for treatment of drug abuse began to recognize that people presenting for treatment had problems with heavy, regular use of cocaine hydrochloride. Documentaries, television melodramas, and news reports began to feature stories of the downfall of substantial businessmen and professionals caused by obsessive use of cocaine.

Heavy use of cocaine can rapidly lead to a total collapse of the user's social and economic resources, in as few as 4 to 6 months. Perhaps the short duration of its effects, combined with the user's depressed view of the world after the effects wear off engender this rapid progression and depletion among users of cocaine. Whatever the reason for the proliferation of stories about personal collapse associated with cocaine use, the popularity of cocaine among advantaged segments of the U.S. population stopped growing by 1980, and by 1984, use of cocaine had stabilized.

In South America, however, a pattern of cocaine smoking had been developing since the early 1970s (Jerí, 1978). Some of the raw material used for manufacturing cocaine hydrochloride had been diverted to street use in South American cities. The preparation used in this way consisted of pure coca base in a sulfur dioxide precipitate that had to be smoked to be ingested. Its consumers reportedly became so obsessed with procuring more of the drug that they exhausted all of their resources on the drug called *bazuco* in Bogota and *toco* in La Paz. This smoked form of cocaine fortunately was not exported to the United States. Unfortunately, in 1984, a different form of smokeable cocaine began to appear in the United States, a preparation made by combining baking soda and cocaine hydrochloride with a little water and cooking it until it formed a pebble-like clump.

This preparation of cocaine made the drug accessible to a different segment of the population than had been possible before. The minimum units of sale in the hydrochloride market tended to be $20 or $30, but the minimum unit of this new product, called base, rock, or crack, sold for $5, and in some cases $3. New users among the poor and the very young took up this new drug with startling rapidity. The next 6 years brought truly unprecedented developments in patterns of street drug use, fueled by the properties of crack cocaine that the effects of coca paste in Latin America foreshadowed (Chitwood, Rivers, & Inciardi, 1995; Inciardi, 1993). Among these were an intensification of the sex trade, increase in violent crime, and pervasive involvement of youth in trafficking.

As seems to happen with cocaine in other historical contexts, crack's popularity crested and subsided among most youthful and adult users by the early 1990s. Its use ceased to grow, and in fact shrank, so that by 1995, the epidemic of crack use had subsided. The impoverished sectors of inner cities continued to have traffic and consumption of crack cocaine on an endemic basis, but use of that preparation only occurred infrequently in other segments of the United States' population.

Opiates

Prehistoric humans in Europe and Asia apparently discovered that the opium poppy (*Papaver somniferum*) offered edible leaves and seeds long before the plant's psychotropic properties became known (Merlin, 1984). Inferences of human familiarity with the drug effects of opium come from Sumerian tablets of cuneiform writing that associate the poppy with "joy," or "rejoicing," as early as 6500 B.P. (Lindesmith, 1968; Merlin, 1984).

For the next 6300 years, the collected sap from scorings on the seed pod of the poppy was the only preparation used to produce the sedative or euphoric effects of opium. During that time, the full range of uses for the poppy became known throughout the Middle East and Europe, as well as parts of Asia (Lindesmith, 1968; Merlin, 1984).

In 1804, a European chemist, Friedrich Wilhelm Adam Serturner, after considerable tinkering with raw opium, isolated its principal active ingredient, morphine. This became the strong analgesic of choice soon after its entry into the Western pharmacopeia. In water-soluble form, this drug could be drunk, dusted directly on open wounds, or injected with a hypodermic syringe. As with cocaine, it became a popular ingredient for patent medicines, and it attracted large numbers of consumers in Europe and the United States during the 19th century. In the United States, morphine and its derivatives dominated the pharmaceutical analgesics throughout the 19th and early 20th centuries, but in those times, the use of opiates tended to attract women of privileged classes, while some men in the criminal underworld smoked opium (Lindesmith, 1968).

Nearly a century after the isolation of morphine (1898), chemists for the Bayer laboratories isolated a more refined and potent version of morphine, called diacetyl morphine, or more commonly, heroin. Ironically, its developers thought that the new version of morphine would obviate the problems associated with the old, especially addiction (Ray, 1983). As often happens in humankind's pharmacological tinkering, they were wrong.

Heroin gave users an easily transportable, highly potent preparation for obtaining the euphoric effects of opium. Still, during the first years after its identification, heroin primarily had pharmaceutical applications. By 1900, officials in the United States had come to perceive use of opiates as a problem, and initiatives to enact federal legislation and international treaties to control production, trafficking, and consumption of opiates began to take form. The passage of the Harrison Act in 1914, primarily on the strength of the United States' commitment to control opiate consumption, ushered in an era of increased control over opiates (Musto, 1987; Platt, 1986).

At the time of the first laws attempting to control them, opiates' primary routes of ingestion were oral and hypodermic. At that time, most users of opiates could be classified as self-medicators, either to calm nerves or to alleviate chronic pain. O'Donnell (1969) identified a population of opiate injectors living in Kentucky who as late as 1965 had depended on personal physicians for the bulk of their morphine supplies. Between 1920 and 1950, morphine and heroin users were forced, through increased enforcement of laws intended to control opiate use, to change their ways of obtaining and injecting their drugs of choice (O'Donnell & Jones 1968). Instead of depending on "scrip doctors" for prescriptions of morphine, increased vigilance over dispensing of opiates led these users to resort to the illicit street market. Instead of injecting into a muscle the relatively large amounts of drugs that their doctors had prescribed, the users experimented with injecting into the vein in order to achieve an effect comparable to that of an intramuscular injection of pharmaceutical quality morphine. Heroin bought on the street tended to have high proportions of adulterants, and this made the intravenous route necessary. O'Donnell and Jones (1968) traced these developments through interviews with long-time opiate users at the Lexington Addiction Treatment facility, and found that, as the enforcement of drug control laws continued, injection of opiates shifted from intramuscular to intravenous. Furthermore, the new users tended to emphasize the "rush" of euphoria experienced after an intravenous shot, rather than the analgesic effects of the drug.

During all of these developments, the population of injecting opiate users remained small and restricted to poor urban neighborhoods in large cities. As with cocaine, the social upheaval of the 1960s resulted in a massive questioning of the proscriptions against opiates, and consequently, the United States and Western Europe experienced what came to be called a drug epidemic. Between 1967 and 1971, thousands of people between the ages of 16 and 25 began to experiment with opiates, including heroin (Hunt & Chambers, 1976). This produced a cohort of users that proceeded to overload all of the infrastructure for control and treatment that existed at that time. In response to that epidemic, the United States instituted unprecedented federal funding of treatment for addiction, including the strategy of maintenance through use of a synthetic opiate analog called methadone. Heroin users who wished to stop using street opiates could enroll in methadone programs that would either titrate the dose gradually down to nothing or administer a steady dose indefinitely. During the next 30 years, methadone would become established as an option in the repertoire of treatments for drug abuse problems.

The segment of the drug epidemic cohort that survived into the 1980s became part of the AIDS pandemic, especially in the United States. Its decimation by AIDS because of contamination of needles and syringes (Page,

Smith, & Kane, 1990) may have provided a motive for intravenous users of cocaine and opiates to seek other ways to ingest their drugs of choice. One method involves smoking heroin in a style that users call *chasing the dragon*, in which a small ball of heroin is heated with flame as it rolls down a chute made of metal foil. As of the mid-1990s, this practice had not yet become widespread in the United States.

Cannabis

Like the opium poppy, cannabis' two major species, *sativa* and *indica*, probably entered ancient peoples' menus and wardrobes long before it became a drug. After originating in central Asia, it appears to have spread to China by 4900 B.P. as a foodstuff (oily seeds) and source of fiber. Chronicles of psychotropic use appeared considerably later, and these uses of the plant probably began at least a thousand years later in India, the land with the most elaborate, multileveled patterns of preparing the plant as a drug (Chopra & Chopra, 1957). Its diffusion toward Western Europe possibly began with the Hellenic extensions to western India 2300 years ago, although somewhat earlier, Herodotus briefly described what might have been cannabis use among the Scythians. Mohammed's injunction against the use of alcohol seemed to provide some stimulus for the spread of cannabis use in the Arab world from the 9th to the 13th centuries. Despite the extensive contact between Europeans and Arabs (and, in the 17th century, English and Indians) during and after that period, however, there is little evidence of cannabis use among Europeans until the 19th century. Even when Europeans finally came to use cannabis, the drug had few devotees outside of artists and literati.

Why, with extensive opportunities for diffusion to Western Europe and the New World, would cannabis fail to attract the attention of Europeans? First, in contrast to tobacco, its smoke is acrid and harsh. In fact, most users of cannabis combine it in one way or another with tobacco. Second, its effects are highly variable, and can be frightening, especially in early exposures to the drug. Costa Rican heavy users often reported a phenomenon that they called "white death" in which the user feels cold, sweaty, nauseous, and near death. It often happens to novices (Page & Carter, 1980). Third, the preparations of cannabis consumed by current users do not differ from those invented primarily in India at least 3500 years ago, strong evidence that European chemists found little desirable in a drug that they must have known about for at least 700 years.

Most of the chemical knowledge about the pharmacologically active alkaloids in cannabis stems from research that began in the 1940s. This interest grew out of a politically motivated campaign by a single bureaucrat, Harry Anslinger. In 1937, he pushed through legislation that scheduled marijuana as a dangerous drug and carried out a publicity campaign to galvanize voters' opinions in favor of his antimarijuana position. According to this campaign, which included among its products the film *Reefer Madness*, marijuana was threatening the cream of America's innocent youth and causing crime, insanity, and suicide among youthful users.

The arrival of cannabis in the New World had some influence on this view, not because of the drug's effects, but because of who brought it. Although the Spanish were planting *cañamo* for maritime cordage as early as the 16th century, no evidence of psychotropic use of marijuana appears in any histories until the 19th century (Carter, Page, Doughty, & Coggins, 1980). The influx of a sizeable population of drug users and their subsequent exposure to the host population held the key to the diffusion of cannabis. In the 1840s, East Indian indentured servants provided the human vehicle for spread of cannabis use in the Caribbean area. The use of the term *ganja* as a synonym for marijuana provides linguistic evidence of this process.

Jamaicans and Trinidadians who descended from Africans apparently learned uses of ganja and subsequently emigrated to places around the Caribbean that needed skilled and semiskilled labor, such as the Panama Canal, the railroad projects in Costa Rica, and the sugar refineries of Cuba (Carter et al., 1980; Page, 1982). One of the effects of this process was that wherever cannabis showed up in the Caribbean area, it came with newcomers who contrasted racially and culturally with the host population. This made them the objects of social disapproval, and their customs likewise were suspect. Effectively, in all points of arrival for cannabis smoking, its carriers were objects of prejudice and discrimination. Once cannabis arrived in the United States, it came with Mexican and Caribbean stevedores, field hands, and sugar technicians. As long as it remained among them, the smoking of marijuana or ganja would attract little attention from the host population. Once cannabis developed a following among white youth, however, it excited xenophobic responses that a politician like Anslinger, somewhat desperate about his flagging career, found too tempting to pass up.

Perhaps the most ruinous aspect of this sequence of events came during the drug epidemic of the 1960s. Anslinger's films became major hits among the drug experimenting youth of the time, and its egregious exaggerations and hyperboles led these youth to question other aspects of drug information that may have been valid. The experimentation of that generation with heroin and cocaine can partly be attributed to the disinformation campaign about cannabis carried out in the 1930s.

In the United States and Europe, marijuana became so widespread and entrenched that it will probably never disappear. As of the mid-1990s, approximately 40 million North Americans had tried marijuana at some time in their lives and regular users numbered in the millions.

CONCLUSIONS

Properties of the drugs themselves, tinkering by Western biochemists, trade initiatives backed up with military force, political maneuvers, and social prejudice against newcomers all played parts in the development and diffusion of the drugs reviewed in this chapter. Knowledge of these processes and their implications for current patterns of use should play a part in how we deal with these drugs in the future.

Of these four, tobacco has the most inexorable history of spread and eventual impact on public health. Cocaine fads seem to have a cyclical course that depends on how quickly word gets around that the drug has negative effects. We might expect future cocaine fads to have shorter duration because of the increasing speed of communication. Opiates have strong impact on the population of regular users, although whether or not that impact is attributable to the drugs themselves may be subject to debate. Furthermore, the population of regular users remains small, with minor fluctuations due to changes in supply. Cannabis use requires extensive contact between user and novice, and given the large population of established users worldwide, the pedagogical process of learning to use marijuana has large numbers of potential teachers. We would do well to pay close attention to scientific findings on the effects of this drug and apply them assiduously to policy concerning its control. We especially need to differentiate between xenophobia-driven demagoguery and scientific study when making these kinds of determinations about any of the drugs described in this chapter.

REFERENCES

Becker, H. (1953). Becoming a marijuana user. *American Journal of Sociology, 59*, 235–242.

Billings, E. R. (1875). *Tobacco: Its history, varieties, culture, manufacture, and commerce*. Hartford, CT: American Publishing Company.

Bolton, R. (1976). Andean coca chewing: A metabolic perspective. *American Anthropologist, 78*, 630–633.

Brooks, J. E. (1952). *The mighty leaf: Tobacco through the centuries*. Boston: Little, Brown.

Burchard, R. E. (1975). Coca chewing: A new perspective. In V. Rubin (Ed.), *Cannabis and culture* (pp. 463–484). The Hague: Mouton.

Burchard, R. E. (1976). *Myths of the sacred leaf: Ecological perspective on coca and peasant biocultural adaptation in Peru*. University of Michigan, Michigan.

Burchard, R. E. (1978). Una nueva perspectiva sobre la masticación de la coca. *América Indígena, 38*, 123–130.

Carter, W. E., & Mamani P. M. (1986). *Coca en Bolivia*. La Paz, Bolivia: Liberal Editorial "Juventud."

Carter, W. E., Page, J. B., Doughty, P. L., & Coggins, W. J. (1980). Marijuana in Costa Rica. In W. E. Carter (Ed.), *Cannabis in Costa Rica* (pp. 12–40). Philadelphia: ISHI Press.

Chitwood, D. D., Rivers, J. E., & Inciardi, J. A. (Eds.). (1995). *The American pipe dream.* New York: Harcourt Brace College Publishers.

Chopra, I. C., & Chopra, R. N. (1957, January–March). The use of cannabis drugs in India. *Bulletin on Narcotics,* 4–29.

Dobkin de Rios, M. (1984). *Hallucinogens: Cross-cultural perspectives.* Albuquerque: University of New Mexico Press.

Driver, H. E., & Massey, W. C. (1957). Comparative studies of North American Indians. *Transactions of the American Philosophical Society, 47,* 165–456.

Goodman, J. (1993). *Tobacco in history: The cultures of dependence.* New York: Routledge.

Greenberg, N. (1962). *An Elizabethan songbook.* New York: Ford Foundation.

Harner, M. J. (1974). *Hallucinogens and shamanism.* New York: Oxford University Press.

Hunt, L. G., & Chambers, C. (1976). *Heroin epidemics.* New York: Spectrum.

Inciardi, J. A. (Ed.). (1993). *The crack pipe as pimp.* New York: Harcourt Brace College Publishers.

Jerí, R. F. (1978). The syndrome of coca paste. *Journal of Psychedelic Drugs, 10,* 361–370.

Knipe, E. (1995). *Culture, society, and drugs.* Prospect Heights, IL: Waveland.

Lindesmith, A. R. (1968). A sociological theory of addiction. *American Journal of Sociology, 43,* 593–613.

Merlin, M. D. (1984). *On the trail of the ancient opium poppy.* London: Associated University Presses.

Musto, D. F. (1987). *The American disease: Origins of narcotic control.* New York: Oxford University Press.

O'Donnell, J. A. (1969). *Narcotic addicts in Kentucky.* U.S. Public Health Service Publication No. 1881. Chevy Chase, MD: National Institute of Mental Health.

O'Donnell, J. A., & Jones, J. P. (1968). Diffusion of intravenous techniques among narcotic addicts in the U.S. *Journal of Health and Social Behavior, 9,* 120–130.

Page, J. B. (1982). A brief history of mind-altering drug use in pre-revolutionary Cuba. *Cuban Studies/Estudios Cubanos, 12,* 56–71.

Page, J. B., & Carter, W. E. (1980). Smoking environment and effects. In W. E. Carter (Ed.), *Cannabis in Costa Rica* (pp. 116–144). Philadelphia: ISHI Press.

Page, J. B., Smith, P. C., & Kane, N. (1990). Venous envy: The importance of having usable veins. *Journal of Drug Issues, 20,* 291–308.

Platt, J. J. (1986). *Heroin addiction: Theory, research, and treatment.* Malabar, FL: Robert E. Krieger.

Ray, O. (1983). *Drugs, society, and human behavior.* St. Louis, MO: Mosby.

Weir, S. (1985). *Qat in Yemen: Consumption and social change.* London: British Museums Publications.

5

Health Effects of Alcohol

Mark A. Korsten
Mount Sinai School of Medicine
and Bronx V.A. Medical Center

J. S. Wilson
Prince of Wales Hospital

Few parts of the body are immune to the deleterious effects of alcoholism. In general, chronic alcohol consumption alters health by one of the following mechanisms: 1) effects of alcohol oxidation on intermediary metabolism, 2) effects mediated by toxic breakdown products such as acetaldehyde, 3) effects due to coexistent malnutrition, and 4) effects that are a secondary consequences of alcohol-induced organ injury per se. This review begins with a discussion of the liver and pancreas, as these organs are most likely to be injured by alcohol exposure and functional alterations in the digestive system have profound ramifications on other parts of the body.

HEPATIC EFFECTS OF ALCOHOL

This is probably the most common and potentially the most serious medical complication associated with excess consumption of alcohol. Alcohol abuse remains the major cause of cirrhosis in Western society.

Pathogenesis

Liver damage is clearly related to the degree and duration of ethanol consumption (Lelbach, 1976), although other environmental and genetic factors may modulate the development of serious liver disease. The liver is the major organ for metabolism of ethanol and it is this metabolism, with subsequent altered cellular homeostasis, that is thought to be central to the pathogenesis of alcoholic liver disease (Lieber, 1995). Metabolism of ethanol results in the production of a toxic metabolite, acetaldehyde, that can bind irreversibly to cellular proteins and enzymes. In addition, complexes of acetaldehyde with various cellular proteins (acetaldehyde adducts) may form the basis of a cellular immune response directed toward the hepatocyte (Hoerner et al., 1988). Metabolism of ethanol also results in the production of hydrogen, with subsequent interference with carbohydrate metabolism and mitochondrial function contributing to accumulation of fat within the liver (alcoholic fatty liver), and possibly also alcoholic hyperlipidemia (Lieber, 1995).

Alcohol dehydrogenase (ADH) is the major enzyme mediating alcohol metabolism. However, after prolonged use of ethanol, or at high blood ethanol levels, a second system becomes increasingly important. This is the cytochrome P-450 2E1 (CYP2E1) system. This system is located in the endoplasmic reticulum of the hepatocyte. It is inducible (i.e., its activity increases after chronic ethanol exposure; this is in contradistinction to the ADH system which is not inducible), and is more active at higher blood ethanol concentrations. Activity of the CYP2E1 pathway may have a number of adverse consequences for the liver cell via production of acetaldehyde and generation of reactive oxygen species (such as hydroxyl radical), which are capable of disrupting biological membranes (Lieber, 1995).

It has long been recognized that only a minority of heavy drinkers (15–20%) develop alcoholic liver disease. The reasons for this individual susceptibility are largely unknown but may include coexistent infection with hepatitis B or C, ingestion of other hepatotoxins such as acetaminophen, individual variations in immune responsiveness, and genetic polymorphism of the enzymes of ethanol metabolism including ADH, aldehyde dehydrogenase, and CYP2E1.

Although the majority of patients with alcoholic liver disease are males over 40 (a reflection of the increased incidence of ethanol abuse among men), females appear to be more susceptible (Wilkinson, Santamaria, & Rankin, 1969). This may relate to decreased body water space in females or to decreased gastric metabolism of ethanol (DiPadova, Frezza, & Lieber, 1988), both resulting in higher blood ethanol concentrations after a given dose of ethanol.

The Spectrum of Alcoholic Liver Disease

Histopathologically, three major categories of alcoholic liver disease have been identified. These are alcoholic fatty liver, alcoholic hepatitis, and alcoholic cirrhosis. They are overlapping conditions with two, or perhaps all three, often being identified in an individual patient. Each condition can be clinically silent and evident only on liver biopsy, or it can result in a symptomatic patient with clinical signs of liver disease.

Alcoholic fatty liver is an early, reversible condition, characterized by the accumulation of macrovesicular fat within liver cells. There may be an element of associated pericentral and sinusoidal fibrosis, and those individuals who manifest this change are thought to be at increased risk of progressing to alcoholic cirrhosis.

Alcoholic hepatitis is a more severe condition characterized by liver cell necrosis, neutrophilic infiltration, and the accumulation of Mallory's hyalin within hepatocytes. Mallory's hyalin is an amorphous eosinophilic material thought to be derived from the cytoskeleton; its presence helps to confirm alcohol as an etiologic factor, although it can also be seen (albeit rarely) in other liver conditions.

Alcoholic cirrhosis is characterized by disruption of liver architecture with extensive fibrosis, formation of nodules of hepatocytes with derangement of the normal relationship between portal tracts and central veins, and evidence of liver regeneration. In cirrhosis, the size of the nodules can vary but alcoholic cirrhosis tends to be micronodular in type.

Classically, alcoholic hepatitis has been regarded as an essential prerequisite for the development of alcoholic cirrhosis. Recently, this concept has been challenged with evidence from animal studies that alcoholic fatty liver can progress directly to cirrhosis without going through a hepatitic phase.

Depressed hepatic function in alcoholic liver disease can result in a number of defects including decreased production of albumin with consequent depression of serum albumin levels, decreased production of clotting factors with subsequent coagulopathy, and decreased biliary excretion of bilirubin with subsequent jaundice. Derangement of liver architecture in cirrhosis obstructs the flow of portal venous blood through the liver with a consequent increase of pressure in the portal venous system—portal hypertension. Portal hypertension has a number of sequelae including dilatation of portal-systemic venous collaterals (resulting in esophageal and gastric varices), splenomegaly, gastric mucosal congestion (portal gastropathy), ascites, and hepatic encephalopathy.

The cause of ascites is multifactorial. Portal hypertension leads to increased hydrostatic pressure in peritoneal capillaries. There is usually increased sodium and water retention by the kidney due to alterations in systemic blood flow resulting in secondary hyperaldosteronism. Finally, hypoalbuminemia may contribute to the development of ascites by decreasing plasma oncotic pressure and favoring the transudation of fluid into the peritoneum.

The pathophysiology of hepatic encephalopathy is incompletely understood. In simple terms, it results from inadequate detoxification by the liver (because of impaired liver function and the presence of portal-systemic collaterals allowing blood from the gut to bypass the liver) of nitrogenous substances produced in the gut with subsequent impairment of cerebral function.

Clinical Features

The patient with alcoholic steatosis is generally asymptomatic. Physical examination reveals hepatomegaly, which is usually nontender. Serum biochemistry can reveal elevated levels of gamma-glutamyl transpeptidase (GGT). The hepatic synthesis of this enzyme is induced by chronic alcohol consumption. If this increased production is associated with hepatocyte membrane injury, then elevated levels may be observed in the serum. Serum transaminases may also be mildly elevated. An aspartate transaminase (AST) / alanine transaminase (ALT) greater than 1 suggests an alcoholic etiology. Other blood tests may be used to corroborate excess consumption of alcohol. These include measurement of the mean corpuscular volume of red cells with a macrocytosis suggesting the presence of excess alcohol ingestion. Currently, carbohydrate deficient transferrin (CDT) levels in the serum are thought to be the most accurate way of detecting excess consumption of alcohol (Rosman & Lieber, 1992).

Alcoholic hepatitis may also be an asymptomatic condition but, more often, the patient is clinically ill with anorexia, jaundice, fever, and right upper quadrant pain. Alcoholic cirrhosis may also be present. The patient may manifest signs of hepatic encephalopathy, coagulopathy and portal hypertension.

Blood tests are generally more deranged than with simple fatty liver. The serum bilirubin is often elevated. Transaminases may be elevated but the elevation is only moderate and not to the degree seen in acute viral hepatitis. Levels of transaminases of approximately 300 IU/L are commonly seen. Again, an AST/ALT ratio greater than 1 would suggest an alcoholic etiology. The GGT level may also be elevated and a GGT elevation out of proportion to serum alkaline phosphatase levels suggests an alcoholic etiology. A depressed serum albumin level suggests the coexistence of alcoholic cirrhosis. Hematologically, a neutrophilic leucocytosis is typical with the elevation of the white cell count being proportional to the severity of the underlying liver disease. A macrocytosis due to alcohol consumption may be present, and thrombocytopenia may be observed because of hypersplenism and a reversible direct suppressant effect of ethanol on platelet production by the bone marrow. The prothrombin time may be prolonged because of impaired production of clotting factors by the liver.

Alcoholic cirrhosis is an irreversible condition. Like alcoholic fatty liver and alcoholic hepatitis, it can be clinically silent. Clinical features include fatigue, jaundice, hepatomegaly (although in advanced, end-stage disease, the liver may be of normal size or small), splenomegaly, ascites, and encephalopathy. Peripheral stigmata of chronic liver disease, including Dupuytren's contracture, palmar erythema, and spider nevi, may be present.

The patient with advanced alcoholic cirrhosis often presents with gastrointestinal bleeding. This is as a result of portal hypertension and can arise from either esophageal or gastric varices or as a result of portal gastropathy.

Treatment

Complete abstinence from alcohol is the cornerstone of treatment. Without this, other therapeutic endeavors are often futile. Abstinence has been shown to prolong survival in patients with alcoholic cirrhosis (Powell & Klatskin, 1968).

Because malnutrition is a frequent accompaniment of alcoholic liver disease, attention has focused on nutritional supplementation. Several studies have suggested that enteral and parenteral nutrient supplementation in patients with severe alcoholic liver disease may result in improvement in nitrogen balance and biochemical variables of liver injury, and perhaps also mortality (Cabre et al., 1990; Mezey, Caballeria, & Mitchell, 1991). Such an approach should be reserved for those people with advanced disease.

There have been many trials of corticosteroids in patients with alcoholic hepatitis. The results of these trials have varied, with only a minority showing a beneficial effect. In a meta-analysis that included 11 randomized trials of hospitalized patients (Imperiale & McCullogh, 1990), corticosteroids appeared to improve the outcome of alcoholic hepatitis with a reduction in mortality. The greatest effect was seen in those individuals with hepatic encephalopathy without gastrointestinal bleeding.

The complications of alcoholic liver disease present major challenges for the clinician. Bleeding varices (most commonly esophageal) are treated by resuscitation of the patient by blood transfusion and replacement of clotting factors, infusion of octreotide (a somatostatin analog that has been shown to decrease portal pressure) and by endoscopically guided injection sclerotherapy or banding of varices. Continued variceal bleeding may require the use of tamponade with a Sengstaken-Blakemore or Minnesota tube. Once acute variceal bleeding has been controlled, the varices can be obliterated on an elective basis by endoscopic sclerotherapy or banding. Obliteration of varices in such a fashion has been shown to reduce the risk of subsequent bleeding (Terblanche, Burroughs, & Hobbs, 1989) and, in one study, to improve mortality (Westaby, MacDougall, & Williams, 1985). Variceal obliteration can be complemented by the use of β blocking agents, which reduce cardiac output and therefore decrease portal pressure (Hayes, Davis, Lewis, & Bouchier, 1990). These drugs should only be used in compliant patients. They may be of use in patients with known esophageal varices as a prophylactic measure, for example, to prevent the initial variceal bleed. The use of variceal obliteration as a prophylactic measure is controversial and is not commonly employed. Uncontrolled variceal bleeding presents a major problem for the clinician. Emergency surgery to decompress the portal venous system may be attempted, but such procedures have a very high mortality. More commonly, patients undergo a transjugular intrahepatic porto-systemic shunt. In this procedure, an expandable metal stent is placed, under radiological control, in the liver between the portal and systemic venous systems in order to decompress the portal system. This is a technically difficult procedure that should only be carried out in specialized centers and as a prelude to liver transplantation.

Patients with alcoholic cirrhosis and marked ascites are treated most efficiently by percutaneous drainage of the intra-abdominal fluid followed by prevention of its recurrence with the use of sodium restriction and diuretic therapy. A common complication of ascites in patients with alcoholic liver disease is spontaneous bacterial peritonitis (SBP). This condition results from translocation of intestinal bacteria into the ascitic fluid. Classic signs of peritonitis are often absent. A third-generation cephalosporin is the treatment of choice. SBP is associated with a grave prognosis, with 50% of patients dying during the hospital admission.

Patients with hepatic encephalopathy are best treated by lactulose, a drug that promotes an osmotic diarrhea, thereby purging the gut of nitrogenous substances that may give rise to the encephalopathy. Intractable, chronic cases may also require the use of neomycin—an antibiotic that alters bowel flora thereby reducing the production of encephalopathy-producing substances. Some degree of dietary protein restriction is mandatory in the encephalopathic patient. The degree of this restriction will depend on the patient's nutritional state.

Orthotopic liver transplantation is being increasingly used as a treatment modality for end-stage alcoholic liver disease, but its high cost raises many socioeconomic issues. Survival rates are comparable to those of patients with other liver diseases undergoing transplantation. Pretransplant abstinence and careful patient selection are essential.

PANCREATIC EFFECTS OF ALCOHOL

Alcoholic pancreatitis is an important complication of alcohol abuse occurring in up to 5% of heavy drinkers (Steinberg & Tenner, 1994). It is generally a chronic disorder resulting in significant mortality and morbidity, characterized by maldigestion, malnutrition, abdominal pain, diabetes, and the frequent need for surgery. Unemployment and narcotic addiction are frequent social sequelae. In severely affected patients, costs of health care have been estimated to approximate those of liver transplantation.

Pathogenesis

Pancreatitis is generally classified as either acute or chronic. The term acute implies a self-limiting episode with subsequent return to normal of pancreatic structure and function. The term chronic implies progressive loss of pancreatic structure and function.

Acute pancreatitis is characterized by edema, inflammatory cell infiltrate, and, in severe cases, necrosis and hemorrhage. Peripancreatic inflammation and fluid accumulation may also be present. With chronic pancreatitis, the gland appears fibrosed and atrophic. The main pancreatic duct and secondary ducts contain strictures with dilatation of the duct system proximally. Intraductal proteinaceous deposits are a characteristic (but not pathognomonic) finding.

The distinction between acute and chronic pancreatitis is often difficult in the initial stages: acute pancreatitis can recur, and chronic pancreatitis often presents initially as an acute episode. Alcoholic pancreatitis is usually classified as an example of chronic pancreatitis, which may present acutely. However, there is recent evidence to suggest that the so-called chronic pancreatitis of the alcoholic may result from repeated episodes of acute injury (Ammann & Muellhaupt, 1994).

Alcohol may cause chronic injury to the pancreas by inducing repeated episodes of autodigestion following contact between pancreatic digestive enzymes and lysosomal enzymes. Recent research has revealed a number of ethanol-induced alterations in pancreatic acinar cells that may predispose to autodigestion. These include an increased production of pancreatic digestive and lysosomal enzymes, increased fragility of lysosomes and increased fragility of pancreatic digestive enzymes (Wilson & Pirola, 1997). These changes, when taken together, would facilitate (in the presence of an appropriate trigger factor) contact between lysosomal hydrolases and digestive enzymes with subsequent activation of the latter.

Clinical Features

The majority of patients are males between 20 and 50 years of age. The predominance of males is probably a reflection of the increased incidence of ethanol abuse among men. Alcoholic pancreatitis rarely follows a single alcoholic debauch and usually requires between 5 to 15 years of heavy drinking before its first presentation.

The disease usually presents as acute pancreatitis. The major symptom of acute pancreatitis is constant, severe abdominal pain, usually epigastric or peri-umbilical, which may radiate to the back and into the chest or flanks. The pain is often relieved by sitting forward, and exacerbated by lying flat. Nausea and vomiting frequently occur.

Examination usually reveals abdominal tenderness and guarding, but these signs may be unimpressive when compared to the severity of the pain and the general condition of the patient. Fever, tachycardia, and signs of pulmonary decompensation may be present.

The major features of chronic pancreatitis are constant abdominal pain and pancreatic insufficiency (causing weight loss, steatorrhea, and diabetes). Jaundice may be present due to obstruction of the common bile duct by pancreatic fibrosis or because of concomitant alcoholic liver disease.

A diagnosis of an acute exacerbation of alcoholic pancreatitis should be suspected in any alcoholic with severe abdominal pain. Elevated serum levels of pancreatic enzymes (particularly amylase and lipase) are used to confirm the diagnosis. However, in the alcoholic, these tests may be normal during an acute exacerbation, and the diagnosis is often made clinically.

Chest and abdominal X rays are useful for excluding other diagnoses and may show pancreatic calcification, a hallmark of chronic pancreatitis. They may also show atelectasis and pulmonary effusions, which often complicate acute pancreatitis. CT scanning is the most sensitive radiological test for determining the size and the shape of the pancreas. All patients with acute pancreatitis or a suspected acute exacerbation of alcoholic pancreatitis should have a CT scan; this can help confirm the diagnosis (showing a swollen pancreas) and detect fluid collections and evidence of pancreatic necrosis. If the patient's condition does not improve as expected or deteriorates, a repeat scan should be performed to look for new complications. Abdominal ultrasonography is a less sensitive method for imaging the pancreas, but is the most reliable method for detecting gallbladder calculi, which can also cause acute pancreatitis.

The diagnosis of chronic pancreatitis should be suspected in any alcoholic patient with chronic abdominal pain, particularly if it is associated with steatorrhea or diabetes. A history of the passage of greasy stools is virtually pathognomonic of alcoholic pancreatitis in Western society, and represents a fecal fat excretion of more than 30–40 grams per day.

Diagnostic tests of chronic pancreatitis usually assess either pancreatic structure or pancreatic function. The most common test of pancreatic function, a 3-day fecal fat determination, may establish steatorrhea, but is difficult to carry out and is only positive in advanced cases when more than 90% of the exocrine pancreas has already been destroyed. A qualitative assessment of neutral fat in the stool using Sudan Black staining is usually adequate. The most sensitive test of pancreatic function is duodenal intubation and collection of pancreatic juice following administration of hormones, which can stimulate the pancreas (cholecystokinin and/or secretin). This test is time-

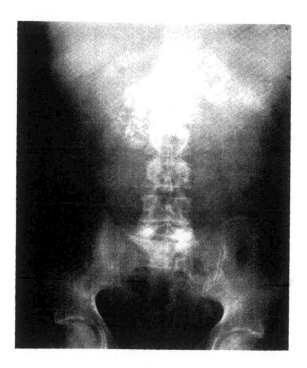

FIG. 5.1. Plain radiograph of the abdomen demonstrating pancreatic calcification. This finding is highly suggestive of chronic alcoholic pancreatitis.

consuming and uncomfortable for patients, and is rarely performed outside specialized units. For this reason, simpler tests of function have been devised using artificial pancreatic substrates administered orally followed by the measurement of metabolites in blood, urine (bentiromide and pancreolauryl tests), or breath (Korsten, Klapholz, Leaf, & Lieber, 1987). However, these tests lack adequate sensitivity and specificity to be clinically useful.

Tests of pancreatic structure are generally used to make the diagnosis of chronic pancreatitis. A simple abdominal X ray may reveal pancreatic calcification; this finding (in the appropriate clinical setting) will clinch the diagnosis, without the need for more extensive and expensive investigations. Pancreatic calcification is seen on abdominal films in 25 to 60% of patients with chronic pancreatitis. Abdominal CT scanning is more sensitive than plain abdominal X rays in detecting calcification, and is helpful in defining the size and shape of the pancreas. CT scanning may also detect fluid collections (i.e., pseudocysts) occurring as a result of pancreatic inflammation. Abdominal ultrasonography is patient- and operator-dependent, and is also useful for demonstrating the presence of pseudocysts.

If there is any doubt about the diagnosis, endoscopic retrograde cholangiopancreatography (ERCP) should be performed. The diagnosis of chronic pancreatitis can be made at ERCP by the finding of dilatation and distortion of the main pancreatic duct and the secondary ducts. This information may be useful if surgical decompression of the pancreatic duct is contemplated for pain relief.

Management

Bed rest, intravenous fluids, and narcotic analgesia are the cornerstones of treatment of acute episodes of pancreatitis in the person with alcoholism. The patient is kept fasting to avoid stimulation of pancreatic secretion. Although resting the pancreas is conceptually attractive, the pancreas probably secretes very little when it is acutely inflamed. Randomized prospective clinical trials of nasogastric suction, atropine, glucagon, calcitonin, cimetidine, and somatostatin (all of which may reduce pancreatic secretion) have uniformly failed to show benefit in acute exacerbations of pancreatitis (Leach, Gorelick, & Modlin, 1992). Nonetheless, refeeding a convalescent patient too early may cause a relapse of the disease. Despite the considerable evidence that acute pancreatitis is an autodigestive disease, trials of enzyme inhibitors (particularly anti-proteases) have been similarly disappointing (Leach et al., 1992).

Patients with clinical chronic pancreatitis require treatment for pancreatic insufficiency and chronic pain. Total abstinence from alcohol is paramount but is rarely achieved. Continued drinking indicates a poor prognosis and likely treatment failure.

Steatorrhea due to pancreatic insufficiency is treated with pancreatic enzyme supplements. Diabetes mellitus is treated in the standard manner, but patients can be extremely brittle with increased sensitivity to exogenous insulin.

The pathophysiology of pain in chronic pancreatitis is poorly understood, but it may be related to episodes of acute pancreatic inflammation, the presence of an intra-abdominal fluid collection, obstruction of the pancreatic duct, obstruction of the common bile duct, or perineural inflammation. Elevated pancreatic ductal and interstitial pressures are frequently found, and their reduction often correlates with the relief of pain.

In the evaluation of pancreatic pain, imaging by CT scan and ERCP is vital. CT scans will reveal the size and shape of the gland, and may show a dilated pancreatic duct, intraductal calculi, or fluid collection. ERCP is particularly valuable in delineating pancreatic duct size and may also reveal calculi, strictures, and fluid collections, as well as associated common bile duct strictures.

The presence of pancreatic proteases in the duodenum has been shown to inhibit pancreatic secretion via a negative feedback loop (Slaff, Wolfe, &

Toskes, 1985). The discovery of this phenomenon has led to the use of oral pancreatic enzyme replacement therapy (even in the absence of pancreatic insufficiency) in the treatment of pancreatic pain. Several small trials of this form of therapy have shown some benefit (Slaff, Jacobson, & Tillerman, 1984) but in the authors' experience, this treatment has been disappointing when applied to alcoholic pancreatitis. Octreotide, an analogue of somatostatin and a powerful inhibitor of pancreatic secretion, may have a role in the management of pancreatic pain, and is currently being studied in controlled trials. Pain can also be treated using endoscopic approaches. Encouraging early results have been reported using endoscopically placed stents and after clearing the pancreatic duct of stones.

Surgery can provide good pain relief in carefully selected patients. Those with fluid collections often benefit from surgical drainage. Patients with refractory pancreatic pain and a dilated main pancreatic duct often obtain relief of pain following pancreatico-jejunostomy to decompress the duct. Pancreatic duct strictures and isolated areas of pancreatitis may be treated by resection of the head of the pancreas (Whipple's procedure) or the tail of the gland; however, these operations are often unsuccessful because of undiagnosed disease in the remainder of the gland. Overall, some 80% of patients will obtain complete or partial relief from pancreatico-jejunostomy, although up to 20% will develop recurrence of pain during follow-up.

OTHER GASTROINTESTINAL EFFECTS OF ALCOHOL

Esophagus

Chronic heavy consumption of ethanol increases the risk of esophageal cancer (Breslow & Enstrom, 1974). Cigarette smoking, which frequently co-exists with heavy alcohol consumption, also increases the risk of esophageal cancer. These two factors, when coexistent, potentiate the risk of esophageal cancer. Esophageal cancer, when it develops in any individual, alcoholic or not, has a grave prognosis with an approximate 5% 5-year survival rate. Subjects commonly present with dysphagia (difficulty in swallowing), and may also present with gastrointestinal hemorrhage.

There is an increased incidence of gastro-esophageal reflux in alcoholics (Bucher, Lepsien, Sonnenberg, & Blum, 1978). Although the literature is somewhat confusing concerning the mechanisms behind this association, factors involved probably include a lowering of lower esophageal sphincter pressure, impairment of esophageal propulsive activity resulting in decreased clearance of refluxed acid (Hogan, Viegas De Andrade, & Winship, 1972), and possibly also stimulation by ethanol of gastric acid production

(Hirschowitz, Pollard, Hartwell, & London, 1956). Symptoms of esophagitis in the alcoholic include heartburn, gastrointestinal hemorrhage and dysphagia. Chronic reflux may lead to the development of Barrett's esophagus (which itself can lead to the development of esophageal cancer).

Abuse of ethanol is often associated with nausea and intractable vomiting. Vomiting can traumatize the mucosa overlying the junction of the esophagus and stomach resulting in a tear (Mallory-Weiss lesion) with subsequent gastrointestinal hemorrhage. The Mallory-Weiss tear is commonly encountered in clinical practice. It is diagnosed endoscopically and most often heals spontaneously following cessation of vomiting.

Stomach

Abuse of ethanol can lead to disruption of the surface epithelium of the stomach with the development of an erosive (and often hemorrhagic) inflammation (gastritis). The mechanism for this change is not completely clear but ethanol in high concentrations can be directly toxic to the gastric mucosa. It may disrupt the gastric mucosal barrier (a term used to describe a number of physiological features of the stomach that protect its lining against the acid that the gastric glands produce) (Davenport, 1967). This disruptive effect, in combination with a possible ethanol-induced stimulation of gastric acid production, may explain the gastric mucosal injury observed after heavy ethanol consumption. Consumption of large quantities of ethanol also appears to impair gastric emptying (Barboriak & Meade, 1970), and this effect may contribute to both the gastric and esophageal sequelae described above. The clinical features of ethanol-induced gastric damage include nausea, vomiting, abdominal pain, hematemesis, and melena.

Small Intestine

It appears as though alcohol also acts as a small intestinal mucosal toxin (Baraona, Pirola, & Lieber, 1974). These changes may lead to impaired absorption of nutrients (Roggin, Iber, Kaber, & Tabon, 1969) and contribute to the malnutrition commonly observed in the alcoholic. Malnutrition per se (especially folate and protein deficiency) appears to impair intestinal function and often contributes to the malabsorption abnormalities observed in alcoholics.

CARDIAC EFFECTS OF ALCOHOL

There is both good and bad news in terms of the effects of alcohol on the heart and circulation. The good news is that low to moderate intake of alcohol clearly decreases overall mortality compared to abstainers, an effect attributed largely to a decrease in coronary artery disease (CAD). The bad news is that alcohol abuse leads to an increase in cardiac morbidity and mortality. These dose-dependent effects of alcohol ingestion appear to explain the relationship that has been observed between mortality and alcohol consumption.

Effects of Low-Moderate Consumption of Alcohol

Numerous epidemiologic studies have established that, at least in men, low to moderate intake of alcohol (two drinks or about 30 grams), especially in the form of red wine, reduces the risk of CAD. A similar trend is seen in females but the phenomenon is most apparent in women with established coronary risk factors (Fuchs et al., 1995). A number of factors may explain this protective effect of alcohol: an increase in HDL (high density lipoprotein), a decrease in lipoprotein (a) (Sharpe, McGrath, McClean, Young, & Archbold, 1995), inhibition of platelet-mediated thrombus formation (Demrow, Slane, & Folts, 1995) and enhancement of t-PA (tissue plasminogen activator) mediated intravascular fibrinolysis (Ridker, Vaughan, Stampher, Glynn, & Hennekens, 1994). To what extent the protective effects of red wine are due to its alcohol content per se is an unanswered question. Indeed, it has been suggested that the salutory properties of red wine are, at least in part, related to congeners in the beverage (e.g., fungicides, tannins, anthocyanins, and flavanoids). This possibility is supported by the finding that unfermented (alcohol-free) grape juice has platelet inhibitory properties in dog models that are similar to that of red wine (Demrow et al., 1995).

Effects of Alcohol Abuse on the Cardiovascular System

The alcoholic is prone to a number of serious cardiovascular complications, including supraventricular arrhythmias (Holiday heart syndrome), myocardial infarction, hypertension (Klatsky, Friedman, Siegelaub, & Gerard, 1977), thrombotic and hemorrhagic stroke (Altura, Altura, & Carella, 1983; Donahue, Abbot, Reed, & Yano, 1986), and dilated cardiomyopathy. Typical presenting complaints are shortness of breath, palpitations, chest pain, fatigue, and swelling of the lower extremities. In patients with dilated cardiomyopathy, physical findings such as high systolic and diastolic pressures, cardiac gallops, displacement of the PMI (point of maximal impulse), systolic murmurs, jugular venous distension, and pitting edema are similar to those found in the nonalcoholic. Likewise, there are no pathognomonic findings on the ECG or in the results of imaging studies. Treatment of these complications of alcohol abuse involves total avoidance of alcohol. In patients with cardiomyopathy, preload (diuretics), afterload (ACE inhibitors) and anticoagulants are indicated. Digitalis must be used cautiously in patients with alcoholic cardiomyopathy given the increased possibility of toxicity (Friedman, Geller, & Lieber, 1982). Hypertension may be treated with antihypertensive medications or may resolve spontaneously in patients able to achieve sobriety. When hypertension recurs, it may indicate a relapse of alcoholism given the pressor effects of alcohol and the greater likelihood of poor compliance.

The relative roles of alcohol and nutrition in the pathogenesis of alcoholic cardiomyopathy remains unsettled although it now appears that cardiac damage can occur in the absence of nutritional deficiency. Thus, a number of cardiac indices including the ejection fraction and left ventricular mass can be shown to correlate with total lifetime dose of ethanol (Urbano-Marquez et al., 1989) and can be shown to be abnormal even when nutritional and smoking status are controlled (Dancey, Bland, Leech, & Gaitonde, 1985). Recent work at the subcellular level attempts to explain the pathogenesis of alcoholic cardiomyopathy. Of particular interest are studies that indicate that ethanol impairs the synthesis of myocardial contractile and mitochondrial proteins (Preedy & Richardson, 1994; Preedy, Salisbury, & Peters, 1994). There is also evidence indicating that this defect in protein synthesis may not be confined to cardiac muscle fibers. Indeed, patients with alcoholic cardiomyopathy are likely to have changes in skeletal muscle as well. In this respect, Fernandez-Sola et al. (1994) have shown that alcoholic patients with cardiomyopathy are very likely to have coexistent skeletal muscle fibrosis and weakness (alcoholic myopathy) and vice versa (vide infra).

In summary, the moderate consumption of alcohol may be helpful in protecting against CAD, whereas the abuse of alcohol is clearly associated with potentially adverse cardiac sequelae. Given the overall health hazards of alcohol and the difficulty that many might have in maintaining a moderate intake of alcohol, it would be unwise at this time to advise patients to increase their intake of alcohol to secure its cardioprotective effects.

HEMATOLOGIC EFFECTS OF ALCOHOL

The abuse of alcohol is a frequent cause of anemia, leukopenia, and thrombocytopenia. These complications of alcoholism arise as a result of 1) direct effects of alcohol on the bone marrow, 2) associated nutritional deficiencies especially of folic acid and pyridoxine, and 3) alcohol-induced liver injury.

Anemia

Megaloblastic anemia is frequently observed in the poorly nourished alcoholic. Almost always due to folate deficiency, megaloblastic anemia is characterized by an increased MCV (mean corpuscular volume) and hypersegmented neutrophils. When especially severe, folate deficiency may also account for leukopenia and thrombocytopenia. The diagnosis should be confirmed by assessing the level of folic acid in both red cells and serum prior to dietary replenishment. As red cell folate is a better measure of tissue stores, it may remain low longer than levels in the serum. It is also wise to assess B_{12} levels to exclude coexistent pernicious anemia. The cause of folate deficiency in the alcoholic is usually multifactorial: poor dietary intake, intestinal malabsorption (Halsted, Robles, & Mezey, 1973), increased urinary excretion (Russell et al., 1983), and abnormal utilization (Eichner & Hillman, 1983). In the absence of folate deficiency, it is also possible that the megaloblastic anemia is due to direct toxic effects of alcohol or acetaldehyde on marrow precursor cells (Savage & Lindenbaum, 1986).

Less frequently, other types of anemia, often related to defects in iron metabolism and ineffective erythropoesis, may complicate the hematologic status of the alcoholic. On the one hand, sideroblastic anemia may occur. It is characterized by the presence of ring sideroblasts, which are red cell precursors containing increased amounts of hemosiderin or ferritin. The accumulation of iron in red cells has been attributed to both pyridoxine deficiency and direct effects of alcohol on heme synthesis. Regardless of the pathogenesis, sideroblasts disappear rapidly from the bone marrow during abstinence. On the other hand, anemia due to iron deficiency may ensue in alcoholics that lose blood in the course of hemorrhage from the upper gastrointestinal tracts. Common sources of GI blood loss include variceal hemorrhage, Mallory-Weiss tears of the esophagus during retching, and erosive alcoholic gastritis. Routine tests of iron status may be unreliable in the alcoholic: RBC indices are misleading in the presence of megalocytes and iron stores may be falsely high in the presence of ineffective erythropoesis as noted above. Spur-cell anemia and hemolytic anemia (Zieve's syndrome) are interesting phenomena but beyond the scope of this general review.

Leukopenia

Chronic alcohol consumption depresses the number of leukocytes as well as their functional activity. Leukopenia per se probably is a result of a number of factors including direct toxicity of alcohol on the marrow, associated folate deficiency (vide supra), and splenic sequestration (i.e., hypersplenism). Abnormalities in the effector functions of both neutrophils (impaired adherence and chemotaxis) and lymphocytes (depressed delayed hypersensitivity) have been observed. Together, these immunosuppressive effects of alcohol appear to increase the risk of and the likelihood of a poor outcome in serious infections. Genetically engineered agents capable of reversing leukopenia such as recombinant G-CSF (granulocyte colony stimulating factor) may find a role in this clinical setting (Grimsley, 1995). Indeed, at least in the rat, this cytokine is an effective immunomodulator that reverses ethanol-induced defects in bacterial host defense (Lanng, Molina, & Abumrad, 1993).

Thrombocytopenia

Either by direct toxic effects (Lindenbaum & Lieber, 1969) or as a result of folate deficiency (see the preceding section on anemia), chronic intake of alcohol suppresses the number and functional integrity of platelets. Alcoholic thrombocytopenia is rarely a cause of complications and is rapidly reversible on withdrawal of alcohol. It is of interest that the cardioprotection afforded by low to moderate intake of alcohol could conceivably be due to a suppressive effect of ethanol on platelet aggregation and thrombus formation in the coronary circulation.

INFECTIOUS DISEASE AND ALCOHOL

As noted previously, alcohol is a potent immunosuppressant that effects a broad range of cells involved in both humoral and cellular immunity. In addition to immune dysfunction, other factors such as cigarette smoking and recurrent aspiration of pharyngeal contents predispose the alcoholic to infections, especially of the lung. The latter include bacterial pneumonia, lung abscess, pulmonary tuberculosis, and chronic bronchitis (Lyons, 1982). *Streptococcus pneumoniae* is a common pathogen in the alcoholic although other organisms such as *Klebsiella pneumoniae, Hemophilus influenzae, Staphylococcus aureus*, and anerobes may also be incriminated in the pathogenesis of pneumonia. Typical presenting features include shaking chills, cough, bloody sputum and pleuritic chest pain. Signs of lobar consolidation are usually present on physical examination and are confirmed on chest X ray. Although leukocytosis is usual, pneumonia may still be present in its absence given the immunosuppressive effects of chronic alcoholism (see hematologic section). Coexistent meningitis must be suspected in any alcoholic with pneumonia and altered sensorium. If there is any question regarding the cause of an altered mental status, a head CT scan should be performed followed by a lumbar puncture to obtain cerebrospinal fluid. Likewise, the onset of a cardiac murmur and/or positive blood cultures in a patient with pneumonia raise the possibility of endocarditis. In this setting, an echocardiogram may be useful for demonstrating vegetation on the heart valves. Pulmonary tuberculosis must be considered in the alcoholic complaining of cough, hemoptysis, weight loss, and night sweats. Tuberculosis usually involves the upper lobes of the lung and may be either fibronodular or cavitary. When suspected, a PPD should be planted and an acid fast stain of the sputum performed. Negative or equivocal PPD results are common in alcoholics with tuberculosis (Rooney, Crocco, Kramer, & Lyons, 1976) given their immunocompromised state and thus must be interpreted cautiously.

The development of alcoholic cirrhosis also increases the risk of certain infections. For example, spontaneous bacterial peritonitis (SBP) is common in alcoholics with ascites. The risk of SBP is especially pronounced when the protein content of the ascitic fluid is low or when the number of poly-morphonuclear cells in the fluid exceeds 250 per ml. *E. coli* is the most likely to be identified when the fluid is cultured but a variety of other organisms (*S. pneumoniae*, *Klebsiella*, and *S. fecalis*) may also be involved.

Recent data also indicate that alcoholism may increase the susceptibility to the Hepatitis B and C viruses and, perhaps, HIV as well. This susceptibility may result from the tendency of alcoholics to concurrently abuse drugs or engage in unsafe sexual behavior (Avins et al., 1994). Moreover, chronic consumption of alcohol may accelerate the progression to AIDS after HIV seroconversion (Balla, Lischner, Pomerantz, & Bagasra, 1994; Fong, Read, Wainberg, Chia, & Major, 1994). The role of alcoholism as a cofactor in the development of AIDS has been investigated in mice in which chronic alcohol exposure prior to retrovirus infection clearly altered immunoprotective cytokine production by thymocytes and splenocytes (Wang & Watson, 1994a, 1994b).

RESPIRATORY COMPLICATIONS OF ALCOHOL

Pulmonary infections (pneumonia, lung abscess, and tuberculosis), and hy-poxemia are common in the course of chronic alcoholism. A number of factors are probably involved in the alcoholics predisposition to respiratory infections. Among these, concomitant heavy smoking is probably the most important. However, poor dentition, recurrent aspiration, defective immune defenses, and homelessness are likely to further exacerbate the likelihood of lung disease. Hypoxemia often complicates pneumonia or chronic ob-structive pulmonary disease but may it patients with cirrhosis may also reflect the presence of pleural arteriovenous malformations. These shunts disturb the balance between pulmonary perfusion and ventilation resulting in venous admixture and oxygen desaturation (Berthelot, Walker, & Sher-lock, 1966). Another respiratory complication in cirrhosis is pulmonary hy-pertension, occurring in as many as 2% of patients with portal hypertension (Hadengue, Benhayoun, Lebrec, & Benhamou, 1991). Characteristic symp-toms and signs of pulmonary hypertension are exertional dyspnea and an accentuated P2, respectively. This poorly understood phenomenon has been linked to recurrent microemboli (Naeye, 1960), the actions of putative vasoconstrictive substances that bypass hepatic degradation (McDonnell, Toye, & Hutchins, 1983) and, conceivably, altered nitric oxide production in the pulmonary vasculature (Gaston, Drazen, Loscalzo, & Stamler, 1994). Finally, alcoholics exhibit a high incidence of lung cancer, but this may relate to high rates of smoking rather than the effects of alcohol per se.

RHEUMATIC AND MUSCULOSKELETAL EFFECTS OF ALCOHOL

The chronic intake of alcohol is associated with gouty arthropathy, osteoporosis, and myopathy.

Gout

For many years it has been recognized that gout can result from overindulgence in alcohol. It is clear from clinical studies that the chronic intake of alcohol raises serum uric acid levels, an effect that may be mediated by a redox change that favors the production of lactate from pyruvate (Lieber, Jones, Losowsky, & Davidson, 1962). Lactate, in turn, may decrease renal excretion of uric acid. However, despite the high prevalence of hyperuricemia in the alcoholic population, gout occurs in only about 1% of abusers (Olin, Devenyi, & Weldon, 1976). This suggests that alcoholism, rather than causing gout, may simply worsen it in those who are otherwise predisposed (Gordon & Lieber, 1992).

Osteoporosis

The male alcoholic is prone to a variety of fractures (especially of the ribs, hips, and wrists) after relatively trivial trauma. This tendency has been observed in the absence of cirrhosis, in abstinent as well as active drinkers and, at least in part, is related to the high incidence of osteoporosis after long-term alcohol consumption. The presence of osteoporosis has been established in premortem (Chappard, Plantard, Petitjean, & Riffat, 1991) and postmortem (Saville, 1965) biopsy studies, and radiographic surveys (Spencer, Rubio, Rubio, Indreika, & Seitan, 1986). Newer diagnostic modalities including computed tomography (Laitinen et al., 1990) and dual X-ray absorptiometry (Chon, Sartoris, Brown, & Clopton, 1992) have confirmed this high prevalence of osteoporosis. Interestingly, in the absence of cirrhosis or ovarian failure, alcoholism does not decrease bone mineral density in females (Laitinen et al., 1993). The mechanism of alcoholic osteopenia is complex and probably multifactorial. Disorders of vitamin D metabolism, altered calcium and magnesium homeostasis, and, more recently, reduced osteoblastic activity (Gonzalez-Calvin et al., 1993) have all been implicated.

Myopathy and Rhabdomyolysis

Acute alcoholic myopathy is characterized by pain and swelling of skeletal muscles in association with high serum levels of creatine kinase and myoglobinuria. In contrast, chronic myopathy presents with proximal muscle weakness and atrophy. The likelihood of myopathy appears to be independent of nutritional deficiency. Instead, these conditions appear to be direct inhibitory effects of alcohol on protein synthesis by Type II muscle fibers (Preedy, Siddiq, Why, & Richardson, 1994). Cardiac evaluation is indicated in alcoholic patients with myopathy because the inhibitory effects of alcohol on protein synthesis involve both cardiac as well as skeletal muscles. Accordingly, patients with alcoholic myopathy are likely to have echocardiographic, radionuclide, and endomyocardial biopsy findings suggestive of cardiomyopathy (Fernandez-Sola et al., 1994).

Additional Rheumatologic Effects

Septic arthritis is common in alcoholics and probably relates to unsafe sexual practices as well as immune deficiencies. Patients with peripheral neuropathy are likely to develop neuropathic arthropathy.

NEUROLOGIC EFFECTS OF ALCOHOL

A number of important neurologic problems develop in alcoholic patients—some of these are due to nutritional deficiencies that develop in active drinkers, whereas others arise in the course of alcohol withdrawal.

Alcohol Withdrawal Syndrome (AWS)

During the immediate withdrawal period, the person with alcoholism is likely to feel tremulous and exhibit tremor-like motor activity. These symptoms gradually abate over about 2 weeks, but neurophysiological indices such as evoked potentials may remain abnormal for much longer. This is the mildest form of withdrawal, occurring after overnight abstinence; the alcoholic often self-"treats" by consuming additional alcohol. Rapidly tapering doses of chlordiazepoxide or other minor tranquilizer (alprazolam, diazepam, or lorazepam) is typically employed in patients requesting detoxification. The shorter-acting benzodiazepines are probably preferable in the presence of liver dysfunction. However, the clinician must be aware of their side effects and the risk of dependency inherent in the use of these agents (Romach & Sellers, 1991). Hallucinations (both auditory and visual) and seizures ("rum fits") are other withdrawal manifestations during the early phase (first 24 hours) of abstinence. The latter are typically grand mal in quality; when focal seizures occur it may indicate a focal process such as a subdural hematoma or meningitis (Victor, 1992). Given the surgical potential in this setting, it is essential to further evaluate the nature of the seizure using computerized tomography. The concept that alcohol unmasks "latent epilepsy" has been discredited (Victor, 1992). As such, long-term treatment of alcohol withdrawal seizures is not indicated. However, short-term administration of benzodiazepines may prevent seizures in those who are known to be predisposed.

The most serious, though least common, component of AWS is delirium tremens (DTs). Occurring about 72 hours after termination of alcohol intake, delirium tremens may or may not be preceded by other AWS symptoms. It is characterized by marked confusion and autonomic instability (mydriasis, tachycardia, hypertension, drenching sweats). A medical emergency, patients with delirium tremens require supportive care in an intensive care unit. Principles of therapy include fluid resuscitation, correction of hypoglycemia and hypomagnesemia, pressors if necessary, judicious use of sedation, and overall nutritional repletion (especially B vitamins). Although the mortality in this condition is usually about 5% (Thompson, Johnson, & Maddrey, 1975), higher rates have been observed in patients with pneumonia or severe liver injury.

Neurologic Syndromes Related to Nutritional Deficiency

Wernicke-Korsakoff syndrome is characterized by nystagmus, ataxia, and conjugate gaze paresis in association with a certain degree of confusion and confabulation. This condition is likely due to thiamine deficiency and will respond to thiamine administration. A residual horizontal nystagmus is to be expected despite treatment. To avoid triggering the syndrome, it is recommended that thiamine be administered prior to glucose administration.

Cerebellar degeneration presents gradually over months or years and should be suspected in the presence of abnormal gait and ataxia. Like the Wernicke-Korsakoff syndrome, it probably results from thiamine deficiency and may resolve with thiamine repletion during early stages of the illness.

Alcoholic neuropathy causes weakness, paresthesias, and pain in the extremities, usually the legs, as a result of noninflammatory demyelination of peripheral nerves (Denny-Brown, 1958). In contrast to alcoholic myopathy, distal aspects of the extremities are more likely to be abnormal. As such, wrist drop and foot drop are typical findings. When sensory neurons are involved, there is usually a distal and symmetrical pattern (the "glove and stocking" distribution). No specific vitamin deficiency has been identified in this syndrome. However, empiric therapy with large doses of B vitamins may be useful.

Alcohol-related amblyopia is a degeneration of the optic nerve that is typically seen in malnourished alcoholics. The visual changes evolve gradually over time and are associated with a central scotoma in the visual fields. Although nutritional factors are strongly suspected, no specific vitamin deficiency has been identified (Victor, 1992).

METABOLIC EFFECTS OF ALCOHOL

In addition to alcoholic hyperuricemia, prolonged alcohol abuse results in a number of other metabolic derangements. Among these, hypoglycemia and ketoacidosis are the most clinically significant.

Alcoholic hypoglycemia, like other forms of hypoglycemia, is characterized by sweating, shakiness, anxiety, and hunger, all of which are a reflection of autonomic activation. Repeated episodes of hypoglycemia may result in permanent neurologic deficits and intellectual deterioration. Alcoholic hypoglycemia generally occurs in malnourished individuals after acute ingestion of alcohol. In this setting, the hypoglycemia is a likely consequence of redox changes that accompany alcohol breakdown and which, in turn, inhibit gluconeogenesis. Despite malnutrition, chronic alcoholics rarely exhibit hypoglycemia after an acute dose of alcohol. The problem drinker's resistance to alcoholic hypoglycemia support the experimental findings that redox changes during alcohol metabolism are blunted after chronic consumption of alcohol (Salaspuro, Shaw, Jayatilleke, Ross, & Lieber, 1981).

An alcoholic patient noted to have a metabolic acidosis (pH < 7.4, low serum bicarbonate) and an anion gap greater than 16 meq is a candidate for *alcoholic ketoacidosis*. Such ketosis may occur several days after the last drink of alcohol and following a period of fasting. In actively drinking alcoholics, in addition to an anion gap, there is an osmolal gap (the difference between the measured and calculated osmolality, which is an indication of unmeasured solutes such as ethanol). Fasting, however, is not a prerequisite for alcoholic ketoacidosis since administration of ethanol, in association with a calorically adequate fat-containing diet, still induces ketonemia (Lefevre, Adler, & Lieber, 1970). Alcoholic ketoacidosis responds rapidly to intravenous fluids and is rarely life threatening. β-hydroxybutyrate (rather than acetoacetate) must be measured in the blood if the condition is to be recognized (Gordon & Lieber, 1992).

DERMATOLOGIC EFFECTS OF ALCOHOL

A number of dermatologic problems are markers of alcohol abuse. These include facial edema, rosacea, and rhinophyma. Conditions that appear to exacerbated by alcohol include porphyria cutanea tarda (Tsukazaki et al., 1994), psoriasis, and discoid eczema (Higgins & duVivier, 1994). Alcoholics with liver dysfunction are likely to exhibit spider angiomata, palmar erythema, and altered hair distribution (in males). Additional dermatoses may arise from nutritional deficiencies. For example, pellagra may cause hyperkeratosis and desquamation, while zinc deficiency may give rise to desquamative or bullous lesions.

NUTRITIONAL EFFECTS OF ALCOHOL

Alcoholic beverages are practically devoid of nutritional value despite a theoretical caloric value of 7.1 kcal/g. In fact, experimental volunteers lost weight when alcohol was substituted isocalorically for dietary carbohydrate (Pirola & Lieber, 1972). In part, these results have suggested that the oxidation of a significant portion of alcohol-derived calories (via microsomal oxidizing systems) is not tightly coupled to energy conservation (i.e., ATP production). Thus, simply by displacing food with actual nutritional value, excessive use of alcohol can cause malnutrition. However, other less obvious effects may predispose the alcoholic to nutritional deficiencies. These include the nutritional consequences of alcohol-induced organ injury and effects of alcohol on the activation or inactivation of nutrients. Maldigestion (steatorrhea) as a result of chronic pancreatitis illustrates the former mechanism and decreased activation of pyridoxal-5-phosphate reflects the latter possibility.

Specific Nutritional Deficiencies

Folic acid deficiency, as discussed elsewhere (in the section on hematology), is extremely common in alcoholics and can cause megaloblastic anemia, thrombocytopenia, and granulocytopenia. Key factors in the development of folic acid deficiency are poor dietary intake, intestinal malabsorption, and abnormal utilization.

Pyridoxine deficiency has been implicated in the development of sideroblastic anemia. In addition to poor dietary intake, increased breakdown of pyridoxal-5-phosphate has been implicated by a number of investigators.

Thiamine deficiency probably plays a role in the pathogenesis of the Wernecke-Korsakoff syndrome. The deficiency has been traced to poor dietary intake, decreased absorption and, perhaps, defective activation. As noted elsewhere, thiamine repletion should precede administration of carbohydrate and the alcoholic should be provided 50 mg/day of this nutrient until adequate oral intake is resumed.

Iron deficiency may develop after gastrointestinal hemorrhage and may require replacement therapy. However, since iron absorption may be increased in some individuals (Chapman, Morgan, Boss, & Sherlock, 1983;

Charlton, Jacobs, Sefiel, & Bothwell, 1964), iron status must be carefully monitored (serum iron and iron bind capacity levels) to avoid iron overload.

Deficiencies of fat-soluble vitamins (ADK): In addition to poor intake, these vitamins are particularly prone to malabsorption in the presence of liver and/or pancreatic injury. Clinical sequelae include decreased night vision and hypogonadism (vitamin A), increased susceptibility to osteoporosis and fractures (vitamin D), and coagulopathy (vitamin K). As is the case with iron supplementation, caution must be exercised when replenishing fat-soluble vitamins given their potential toxicity.

REFERENCES

Altura, B. M., Altura B. T., & Carella, A. (1983). Ethanol produces coronary vasospasm: Evidence for a direct action of ethanol on vascular muscle. *British Journal of Pharmacology, 78*, 260–262.

Ammann, R. W., & Muellhaupt, B. (1994). Progression of alcoholic acute to chronic pancreatitis. *Gut, 35*, 552–556.

Avins, A. L., Woods, W. J., Lindan, C. P., Hudes, E. S., Clark, W., & Hulley, S. B. (1994). HIV infection and risk behaviors among heterosexuals in alcohol treatment programs. *Journal of the American Medical Association, 271*, 515–518.

Balla, A. K., Lischner, H. W., Pomerantz, R. J., & Bagasra, O. (1994). Human studies on alcohol and susceptibility to HIV infection. *Alcohol, 11*, 99–103.

Baraona, E., Pirola, R. C., & Lieber, C. S. (1974). Small intestinal damage and changes in cell population produced by ethanol ingestion in the rat. *Gastroenterology, 66*, 226–234.

Barboriak, J. J., & Meade, R. C. (1970). Effect of alcohol on gastric emptying in man. *American Journal of Clinical Nutrition, 23*, 1151–1153.

Berthelot, P., Walker, J. G., & Sherlock, S. (1966). Arterial changes in the lungs in cirrhosis of the liver-lung spider nevi. *New England Journal of Medicine, 274*, 291.

Breslow, N. E., & Enstrom, J. E. (1974). Geographic correlations between cancer mortality rates and alcohol-tobacco consumption in the United States. *Journal of the National Cancer Institute, 53*, 631–639.

Bucher, P., Lepsien, G., Sonnenberg, A., & Blum, A. L. (1978). Verlaufund prognose der Reflux-krankheit bei konservatier und chirurgischer Behandlung [Course and prognosis of reflux disease under conservative and surgical treatment]. *Schweizerische Medizinische Wochenschrift, 108*, 2072–2078.

Cabre, E., Gonzalez-Huix, F., Abad-Lacruz, A., Esteve, M., Acero, D., Fernandez-Banares, F., Xiol, X., & Gassull, M. A. (1990). Effect of total enteral nutrition on the short-term outcome of severely malnourished cirrhotics. *Gastroenterology, 98*, 715–720.

Chapman, R. W., Morgan, M. Y., Boss, A. M., & Sherlock, S. (1983). Acute and chronic effects of alcohol on iron absorption. *Digestive Diseases & Sciences, 28*, 321–327.

Chappard, D., Plantard, B., Petitjean, M., & Riffat, G. (1991). Alcoholic cirrhosis and osteoporosis in men: A light and scanning electron microscopy study. *Journal of Studies on Alcohol, 52*, 269–274.

Charlton, R. W., Jacobs, P., Sefiel, H., & Bothwell, T. H. (1964). Effect of alcohol on iron absorption. *British Medical Journal, 2*, 1427–1429.

Chon, K. S., Sartoris, D. J., Brown, S. A., & Clopton, P. (1992). Alcoholism-associated spinal and femoral bone loss in abstinent male alcoholics, as measured by dual x-ray absorptiometry. *Skeletal Radiology, 21*, 431–436.

Dancy, M., Bland, J. M., Leech, G., & Gaitonde, M. K. (1985). Preclinical left ventricular abnormalities in alcoholics are independent of nutritional status, cirrhosis and cigarette smoking. *Lancet, 1,* 1122–1125.

Davenport, H. W. (1967). Ethanol damage to canine oxyntic glandular mucosa. *Proceedings of the Society for Experimental Biology & Medicine, 126,* 657–667.

Demrow, H. S., Slane, P. R., & Folts, J. D. (1995). Administration of wine and grape juice inhibits in vivo platelet activity and thrombosis in stenosed canine coronary arteries. *Circulation, 91,* 1182–1188.

Denny-Brown, D. E. (1958). The neurological aspects of thiamine deficiency. *Federation Proceedings, 17* (supplement), 35.

DiPadova, C., Frezza, M., & Lieber, C. S. (1988). Gastric metabolism of ethanol: Implications for its bioavailability in men and women. In K. Kuriyam, A. Takada, & I. Ishi (Eds.), *Biomedical and social aspects of alcohol and alcoholism* (pp. 81–84). New York: Elsevier.

Donohue, R. P., Abbot, R. D., Reed, D. M., & Yano, K. (1986). Alcohol and hemorrhagic stroke. *Journal of the American Medical Association, 255,* 2311–2314.

Eichner, E. R., & Hillman, R. S. (1983). Effect of alcohol on serum folate level. *Journal of Clinical Investigation, 263,* 35–42.

Fernandez-Sola, J., Estruch, R., Grau, J. M., Pare, J. C., Rubin, E., & Urbano-Marquez, A. (1994). The relation of alcoholic myopathy to cardiomyopathy. *Annals of Internal Medicine, 129,* 529–536.

Fernandez-Sola, J., Scanella, E., Estruch, R., Nicolas, J. M., Grau, J. M., & Urbano-Marquez, A. (1995). Significance of type II fiber atrophy in chronic alcoholic myopathy. *Journal of the Neurological Sciences, 130,* 69–76.

Fong, I. W., Read, S., Wainberg, M. A., Chia, W. K., & Major, C. (1994). Alcoholism and rapid progression to AIDS after seroconversion. *Clinical Infectious Disease, 19,* 337–338.

Friedman, H. S., Geller, S. A., & Lieber, C. S. (1982). The effect of alcohol on the heart, skeletal and smooth muscle. In C. S. Lieber (Ed.), *Medical disorders of alcoholism-pathogenesis and treatment* (pp. 436–79). Philadelphia: Saunders.

Fuchs, C. S., Stampfer, M. J., Colditz, G. A., Giovannucci, E. L., Manson, J. E., & Kawachi, I. (1995). Alcohol consumption and mortality among women. *New England Journal of Medicine, 332,* 1245–1250.

Gaston, B., Drazen, J. M., Loscalzo, J., & Stamler, J. S. (1994). The biology of nitrogen oxides in the airways. *American Journal of Respiratory & Critical Care Medicine, 149,* 538–551.

Gonzalez-Calvin, J. L., Garcia-Sanchez, A., Bellot, V., Munoz-Torres, M. Raya-Alvarez, E., & Salvatierra-Rios, D. (1993). Mineral metabolism, osteoblastic function and bone mass in chronic alcoholism. *Alcohol & Alcoholism, 28,* 571–579.

Gordon, G. G., & Lieber, C. S. (1992). Alcohol, hormones, and metabolism. In C. S. Lieber (Ed.), *Medical and nutritional complications of alcoholism: Mechanisms and management* (pp. 55–90). New York: Plenum.

Grimsley, E. W. (1995). Granulocyte colony stimulating factor in the treatment of alcohol abuse, leukopenia, and pneumococcal sepsis. *Southern Medical Journal, 88,* 220–221.

Hadengue, A., Benhayoun, M. K., Lebrec, D., & Benhamou, J. P. (1991). Pulmonary hypertension complicating portal hypertension: Prevalence and relation to splanchnic hemodynamics. *Gastroenterology, 100,* 520–528.

Halsted, C. H., Robles, E. A., & Mezey, E. (1973). Intestinal malabsorption in folate-deficient alcoholics. *Gastroenterology, 64,* 526–532.

Hayes, P. C., Davis, J. M., Lewis, J. A., & Bouchier, I. A. D. (1990). Meta-analysis of value of propranolol in prevention of variceal hemorrhage. *Lancet, 336,* 153–156.

Higgins, E. M., & du Vivier, A. W. (1994). Cutaneous disease and alcohol misuse. *British Medical Bulletin, 50,* 85–98.

Hirschowitz, B. I., Pollard, H. M., Hartwell, S. W., & London, J. (1956). The action of ethylalcohol on gastric acid secretion. *Gastroenterology, 30,* 244–253.

Hoerner, M., Beh, U. J., Worner, T. M., Blacksberg, I., Braly, L. F., Schaffner, F., & Lieber, C. S. (1988). The role of alcoholism and liver disease in the appearance of serum antibodies against acetaldehyde adducts. *Hepatology, 8,* 569–574.

Hogan, W. J., Viegas De Andrade, S. R., & Winship, D. H. (1972). Ethanol-induced acute esophageal motor dysfunction. *Journal of Applied Physiology, 32,* 755–760.

Imperiale, T. F., & McCullogh, A. J. (1990). Do corticosteroids reduce mortality from alcoholic hepatitis? *Annals of Internal Medicine, 113,* 299–307.

Klatsky, A. L., Friedman, G. D., Siegelaub, A. B., & Gerard, M. J. (1977). Alcohol consumption and blood pressure: Kaiser-Permanente multiphasic health examination data. *New England Journal of Medicine, 296,* 1194–200.

Korsten, M. A., Klapholz, M. B., Leaf, M. A., & Lieber, C. S. (1987). Use of the triolein breath test in alcoholics with liver damage. *Journal of Laboratory & Clinical Medicine, 109,* 62–66.

Laitinen, K., Karkkainen, M., Lalla, M., Lamberg-Allardt, C., Tunninen, R., Tahtela, R., & Valimaki, M. (1993). Is alcohol an osteoporosis-inducing agent for young and middle-aged women? *Metabolism, 42,* 875–881.

Laitinen, K., Valimaki, M., Lamberg-Allardt, C., Kivisaar, L., Lalla, M., & Karkkainen, M. (1990). Deranged vitamin D metabolism but normal bone mineral density in Finnish noncirrhotic male alcoholics. *Alcoholism: Clinical & Experimental Research, 14,* 551–556.

Lanng, C. H., Molina, P. E., & Abumrad, N. N. (1993). Granulocyte colony-stimulating factor prevents ethanol-induced impairment in host defense in septic rats. *Alcoholism: Clinical & Experimental Research, 17,* 1268–1274.

Leach, S. D., Gorelick, F. S., & Modlin, I. M. (1992). New perspectives on acute pancreatitis. *Scandinavian Journal of Gastroenterology, 27* (supplement 192), 29–38.

Lefever, A., Adler, H., & Lieber, C. S. (1970). Effect of ethanol on ketone metabolism. *Journal of Clinical Investigations, 49,* 1775–1782.

Lelbach, W. K. (1976). Epidemiology of alcoholic liver disease. *Progress in Liver Diseases, 5,* 494–515.

Lieber, C. S. (1995). The metabolism of alcohol and its implications for the pathogenesis of disease. In V. R. Preedie, & R. R. Watson (Eds.), *Alcohol and the gastrointestinal tract* (pp. 19–39). New York and London: CRC Press.

Lieber, C. S., Jones, D. P., Losowsky, M. S., & Davidson, C. S. (1962). Interrelation of uric acid and ethanol metabolism in man. *Journal of Clinical Investigation, 41,* 1863–1870.

Lindenbaum, J., & Lieber, C. S. (1969). Hematologic effects of alcohol in man in the absence of nutritional deficiency. *New England Journal of Medicine, 281,* 333–338.

Lyons, H. A. (1982). The respiratory system and specifics of alcoholism. In E. M. Patison & E. Kaufman (Eds.), *Encyclopedic handbook of alcoholism* (pp. 325–331). New York: Gardner.

McDonnell, P. J., Toye, P. A., & Hutchins, G. M. (1983). Primary pulmonary hypertension and cirrhosis: are they related? *American Review of Respiratory Disease, 127,* 437–441.

Mezey, E., Caballeria, J., & Mitchell, M. C. (1991). Effect of parenteral amino acid supplementation on short-term and long-term outcomes in severe alcoholic hepatitis: a randomized controlled trial. *Hepatology, 14,* 1090–1096.

Naeye, R. L. (1960). Primary pulmonary hypertension with coexisting portal hypertension. A retrospective study of six cases. *Circulation, 22,* 376–384.

Olin, J. S., Devenyi, P., & Weldon, K. L. (1976). Uric acid in alcoholics. *Quarterly Journal of Studies on Alcohol, 34,* 1202–1207.

Pirola, R. C., & Lieber, C. S. (1972). The energy cost of the metabolism in drugs, including ethanol. *Pharmacology, 7,* 185–196.

Powell, W. J., & Klatskin, G. (1968). Duration of survival in patients in Laennec's cirrhosis. *American Journal of Medicine, 44,* 406–420.

Preedy, V. R., & Richardson, P. J. (1994). Ethanol induced cardiovascular disease. *British Medical Bulletin, 50,* 152–63.

Preedy, V. R., Salisbury, J. R., & Peters, T. J. (1994). Alcoholic muscle disease: Features and mechanisms. *Journal of Pathology, 173*, 309–315.

Preedy, V. R., Siddiq, T., Why, H., & Richardson, P. J. (1994). The deleterious effects of alcohol on the heart: Involvement of protein turnover. *Alcohol & Alcoholism, 29*, 141–147.

Ridker, P. M., Vaughan, D. E., Stampher, M. J., Glynn, R. J., & Hennekens, C. H. (1994). Association of moderate alcohol consumption and plasma concentration of endogenous tissue-type plasminogen activator. *Journal of the American Medical Association, 272*, 929–933.

Roggin, C. M., Iber, F. L., Kaber, R. M. H., & Tabon, F. (1969). Malabsorption in the chronic alcoholic. *Johns Hopkins Medical Journal, 125*, 321–330.

Romach, M. K., & Sellers, E. M. (1991). Management of the alcohol withdrawal syndrome. *Annual Review of Medicine, 42*, 323–340.

Rooney, J. J., Crocco, J. A., Kramer, S., & Lyons, H. A. (1976). Further observations on tuberculin reactions in active tuberculosis. *American Journal of Medicine, 60*, 517–522.

Rosman, A. S., & Lieber, C. S. (1992). Biological markers of alcoholism. In C. S. Lieber (Ed.), *Medical and nutritional complications of alcoholism: Mechanisms and management* (pp. 531–563). New York and London: Plenum.

Russell, R. M., Rosenberg, I. H., Wilson, P. D., Iber, F. L., Oaks, E. B., & Giovetti, A. (1983). Increased urinary excretion and prolonged turnover time of folic acid during ethanol ingestion. *American Journal of Clinical Nutrition, 38*, 64–70.

Salaspuro, M. P., Shaw, S., Jayatilleke, E., Ross, W. A., & Lieber, C. S. (1981). Attenuation of the ethanol induced hepatic redox change after chronic alcohol consumption in baboons: Metabolic consequences in vivo and in vitro. *Hepatology, 1*, 33–38.

Savage, D. S., & Lindenbaum, J. (1986). Anemia in alcoholics. *Medicine, 65*, 322–338.

Saville, P. D. (1965). Changes in bone mass with age and alcoholism. *Journal of Bone and Joint Surgery, 47A*, 492–499.

Sharpe, P. C., McGrath, L. T., McClean, E., Young, I. S., & Archbold, G. P. (1995). Effect of red wine consumption on lipoprotein (a) and other risk factors for atherosclerosis. *Quarterly Journal of Medicine, 88*, 101–108.

Slaff, J., Jacobson, D., & Tillerman, R. C. (1984). Protease-specific suppression of pancreatic exocrine secretion. *Gastroenterology, 87*, 44–52.

Slaff, J. I., Wolfe, M. M., & Toskes, P. P. (1985). Elevated fasting cholecystokinin levels in pancreatic exocrine impairment: Evidence to support feedback regulation. *Journal of Laboratory & Clinical Medicine, 105*, 282–285.

Spencer, H., Rubio, N., Rubio E., Indreika, M., & Seitan, A. (1986). Chronic alcoholism: Frequently overlooked cause of osteoporosis in men. *American Journal of Medicine, 80*, 393–397.

Steinberg, W., & Tenner, S. (1994). Acute pancreatitis. *New England Journal of Medicine, 330*, 1198–1210.

Terblanche, J., Burroughs, A. K., & Hobbs, K. E. F. (1989). Controversies in the management of bleeding esophageal varices Part II. *New England Journal of Medicine, 320*, 1469–1475.

Thompson, W. L., Johnson, A. D., & Maddrey, W. L. (1975). Diazepam and paraldehyde for treatment of severe delirium tremens. *Annals of Internal Medicine, 82*, 175–180.

Tsukazaki, N., Tanaka, K., Irifune, H., Yoshida, H., Wantanabe, M., Ohgami, T., & Nonaka, S. (1994). Relationship between porphyria cutanea tarda (PCT) and viral hepatitis. *Journal of Dermatology, 21*, 411–414.

Urbano-Marquez, A., Estruch, R., Navarro-Lopez, F., Gran, J. M., Mont, L., & Rubin, E. (1989). The effects of alcoholism on skeletal and cardiac muscle. *New England Journal of Medicine, 320*, 409–415.

Victor, M. (1992). The effects of alcohol on the nervous system. Clinical features, pathogenesis, and treatment. In C. S. Lieber (Ed.), *Medical and nutritional complications of alcoholism: Mechanisms and management* (pp. 413–457). New York: Plenum.

Wang, Y., & Watson, R. R. (1994a). Chronic ethanol consumption before retrovirus infection is a cofactor in the development of immune dysfunction during murine AIDS. *Alcoholism: Clinical & Experimental Research, 18*, 976–981.

Wang, Y., & Watson, R. R. (1994b). Chronic ethanol consumption prior to retrovirus infection alters cytokine production by thymocytes during murine AIDS. *Alcohol, 11*, 361–365.

Westaby, D., MacDougall, B. R., & Williams, R. (1985). Improved survival following injection sclerotherapy for esophageal varices: Final analysis of a controlled trial. *Hepatology, 5*, 827–830.

Wilkinson, P., Santamaria, J. N., & Rankin, J. G. (1969). Epidemiology of alcoholic cirrhosis. *Australasian Annals of Medicine, 18*, 222–226.

Wilson, J. S., & Pirola, R. C. (1997). The drinker's pancreas: Molecular mechanisms begin to emerge (Editorial). *Gastroenterology, 113*, 355–358.

6

Health Effects of Tobacco

Reginald V. Fant
Pinney Associates

Wallace B. Pickworth
National Institute on Drug Abuse

Jack E. Henningfield
Johns Hopkins University School of Medicine
and Pinney Associates

MORBIDITY AND MORTALITY

It has been estimated that during the second half of this century, 60 million premature deaths in developed countries will have been caused by smoking and that worldwide annual mortality attributable to smoking will increase from 2 million a year to 10 million a year by 2010 (Peto, Lopez, Boreham, Thun, & Heath, 1994). Peto et al. estimated that 40 million of these 60 million deaths will have occurred in people under the age of 70. This analysis can be extended to smokers in the United States. In 1990, it was estimated that over 418,000 premature deaths (approximately 20% of all deaths) in the United States were attributable to smoking primarily from cardiovascular diseases, cancers, and respiratory diseases (Centers for Disease Control [CDC], 1993). This was approximately 4 times the number of deaths caused by alcohol (100,000) and 20 times the number attributable to illicit drug use (20,000) (McGinnis & Foege, 1993). Even with advances in the medical treatment of tobacco-caused disease, these data suggest that more than 12 million of the 46 million current tobacco users in the United States will prematurely die. This assumes 1) a continuation of the trend whereby 2.5% of smokers quit per year, and 2) that risk on quitting falls to the never-smoker level.

There is a prevailing belief that smoking-related mortality occurs only in the older sector of the population—a group in which nonsmoking related mortality is quite high. Data from the CDC tend to contradict this notion (CDC, 1993). Although the rates of smoking-related death and disease increase with age, over 120,000 of the deaths caused by smoking in 1990 occurred in people younger than 65 years of age. By our estimates, approximately one-third of the 12 million deaths among current smokers will occur in those under the age of 65.

Along with the mortality produced by smoking, general quality of life decreases as well. One study that examined the general health status of ever-smokers and never-smokers found that ever-smokers reported worse health in four of the eight parameters measured (Lyons, Lo, & Littlepage, 1994). The four measures on which ever-smokers fared worse were physical functioning, bodily pain, general health perceptions, and vitality. No differences were found on measures of physical problems, social functioning, emotional problems, or mental health.

CANCER

In 1990, approximately 505,000 Americans died of cancer, making it the second leading cause of death in the United States after heart disease (National Center for Health Statistics, 1993). It has been reported that tobacco causes between 11% and 30% of all cancer deaths (McGinnis & Foege, 1993). Lung cancer is a disease of smokers and it has been estimated that over 85% of all lung cancer may be avoided by not smoking (U.S. Department of Heath and Human Services [USDHHS], 1989). In 1990, 119,920 premature lung cancer deaths were attributable to smoking (CDC, 1993). An estimated 35,741 (30%) of these cancer deaths were among females and approximately 41,574 (35%) of these deaths occurred in people younger than 65 years of age.

It has been reported that the age at smoking initiation may play a role in the development of lung cancer (Hegmann et al., 1993). After controlling for demographic and amount of tobacco exposure, men who began to smoke before the age of 20 had a chance of developing lung cancer twice as high as those who started smoking after age 20. The odds ratio for those who started before age 20 was 12.7 and for those who started after age 20 was 6.0 relative to never smokers. For women, the odds ratio for those who started before age 25 was 10.0; for women who started at age 26 or older, the ratio was 2.6. Similarly, lung cancer mortality ratios have also been shown to be related to age of initiation (Kahn, 1966).

Associations have also been shown between smoking and other forms of cancer (USDHHS, 1989). In the United States in 1990, an estimated 31,402 premature deaths were attributable to smoking-induced cancers of the lip and oral cavity (6,475), esophagus (7,284), pancreas (6,114), larynx (2,990), uterine cervix (1,294), bladder (4,026), and kidney (3,219) (CDC, 1993).

Cigarette smoking has been shown to have a strong interaction with alcohol intake in the development of oral and pharyngeal cancers (Blot et al., 1988), as well as esophageal cancer (Gao et al., 1994). For example, Blot et al. found that the risks of oral and pharyngeal cancers were increased for both smokers and users of alcohol compared to nonusers of either substance. However, for users of both alcohol and tobacco, the combined effect was dramatic—the risk ratios increased to more than 35 times the risks to nonusers (Blot et al., 1988). Likewise, the study by Gao et al. (1994) on the effects of alcohol and cigarette smoking on esophageal cancer found that the risk of developing esophageal cancer was doubled for smokers and increased by 40% for alcohol drinkers over nonusers of either substance. However, the risk increased by 12-fold for users of both substances compared to nonusers.

Cigarette smoke is known to contain more than 4,000 compounds including at least 43 carcinogens that include polyaromatic hydrocarbons, heterocyclic hydrocarbons, N-nitrosamines, aromatic amines, aldehydes, volatile carcinogens, inorganic compounds, and radioactive elements (USDHHS, 1989). Because of the wide diversity of these compounds, there is some ambiguity about the relative contributions of each to cancer development (USDHHS, 1989). Carcinogenesis may be divided into two phases: initiation, in which DNA is damaged by the bonding of the carcinogen, and promotion, in which initiated cells become malignant. The polyaromatic hydrocarbons contained in the particulate matter ("tar") of cigarette smoke have been shown to be major tumor initiators in animal studies (International Agency for Research on Cancer, 1986). However, the identities of the promoters (in cigarette smoke or elsewhere) that accelerate the action of the initiators are unknown.

Of the cancers in which there is a change in the relative risk of disease development due to smoking, endometrial cancer is the only one in which smoking seems to have a protective effect (USDHHS, 1990). A review of the literature in the 1990 Surgeon General's Report (USDHHS, 1990) suggests that risk is approximately 30% lower in smokers than never smokers. Relative risks reported ranged from 0.5 to 0.8 for smokers compared to nonsmokers. However, it should be noted that in terms of a risk/benefit ratio, the increases in risks of other forms of cancer due to smoking far outweigh the benefits of smoking for the protective effects against endometrial cancer.

CARDIOVASCULAR DISEASE

The relationship between smoking and cardiovascular disease was first reported in 1940 (English, Willius, & Berkson, 1940). Since then, smoking has been firmly linked to increased risks of cardiovascular diseases including coronary heart disease, arteriosclerotic peripheral vascular disease, and stroke (USHDDS, 1989). Cardiovascular disease is the leading cause of death in the United States and cigarette smoking is considered one of the three major risk factors for development of cardiovascular disease along with hypertension and cholesterol disorders. In the United States in 1990, 179,820 premature cardiovascular deaths were attributed to smoking (CDC, 1993), which included 98,921 deaths from ischemic heart disease and 23,281 deaths from cerebrovascular diseases. Of these cardiovascular deaths due to smoking, 61,216 (34%) occurred among women and 55,455 (31%) occurred in people less than 65 years of age.

Krupski (1991) reviewed the literature and found a number of mechanisms by which smoking may increase the risk of cardiovascular disease. The author found that nicotine and carbon monoxide acutely affect myocardial performance and cause tachycardia, hypertension, and vasoconstriction. Components of cigarette smoke injure the walls of blood vessels by destroying endothial cells. Smoking produces metabolic and biochemical changes including elevations in plasma, free fatty acids, and vasopressin. Smoking causes an inhibition of cyclo-oxygenase, which decreases levels of prostacyclin and increases levels of thromboxane A2. Chronic smoking leads to atherosclerosis by increasing serum cholesterol and reducing high density lipoprotein. In addition, smokers have increased platelet adhesiveness and aggregability that may lead to an increased risk of thrombosis.

NONMALIGNANT RESPIRATORY DISEASE

Smoking is the leading cause of pulmonary disease and death in the United States (USDHHS, 1989). It is estimated that in 1990 over 84,000 deaths due to smoking were caused by such pulmonary problems as chronic obstructive pulmonary disease (COPD), asthma, pneumonia, influenza, bronchitis, and emphysema (CDC, 1993). Of these deaths, 32,597 (39%) occurred in females and 12,112 (14%) occurred in smokers below the age of 65 years. In 1990, chronic obstructive pulmonary disease was the fifth leading cause of death in the United States accounting for approximately 87,000 deaths (CDC, 1993). The 1989 Surgeon General's Report (USDHHS, 1989) attributed smoking to 84% of COPD deaths among men and 79% among women. In 1990, chronic bronchitis and emphysema accounted for 14,865 smoking-related premature deaths, and asthma accounted for 1,095 deaths.

Reviews of the literature cite several mechanisms by which smoking may contribute to the development of respiratory diseases (Sherman, 1992; USDHHS, 1984). These include smoking-induced alterations of central and peripheral airways, alveoli and capillaries, and immune function. Changes in the central airways include loss of cilia, mucus gland hyperplasia, increased number of goblet cells, and histologic changes. These histologic changes include regression of normal pseudostratified ciliated epithelium to squamous metaplasia, carcinoma in situ, and eventually invasive bronchogenic permeability. Changes in peripheral airways include inflammation and atrophy of the airways, goblet cell metaplasia, squamous metaplasia, mucus plugging, smooth muscle hypertrophy, and peribronchiolar fibrosis. Changes in alveoli and capillaries include destruction of peribronchiolar alveoli, reduction in the number of small arteries, bronchoalveolar lavage fluid abnormalities, elevated levels of IgA and IgG, and increased percentages of activated macrophages and neutophils. A number of effects of smoking have been implicated in the development of lung diseases that deal with the immune function. Smoking produces higher peripheral leukocyte cell counts, elevations in peripheral eosinophils, increased levels of serum IgE, lower allergy skin test reactivity, and reduced immune response to inhaled antigens.

REPRODUCTIVE EFFECTS

There are at least three known effects of smoking on reproduction including reduced fertility, spontaneous abortion, and reduced birthweight (USDHHS, 1990). Studies have indicated that smokers have lower fertility than nonsmokers (USDHHS, 1989). For example, Howe, Westhoff, Vessey, and Yeates (1985) found that women who smoked a pack of cigarettes or more per day were twice as likely than nonsmoking women to have not conceived after 5 years of actively attempting pregnancy. The reduction in the fertility of smokers may be caused by a number of effects of smoking (USDHHS, 1990). Smoking produces a disturbance of hypothalamic-pituitary function, which may decrease ovulation. Smoking also impairs tubal motility and implantation of the embryo. Each of these effects of smoking on fertility has been shown to be reversible soon after smoking cessation. However, there is an increase in oocyte depletion in smokers due to direct toxicity, which may be irreversible.

Spontaneous abortions occur more in smokers than in nonsmokers. For example, Stein, Kline, Levin, Susser, and Warburton (1981) found that the odds of spontaneous abortion were 61% higher for women who smoked 20 or more cigarettes per day than for nonsmoking women. However, the mechanism for this effect remains unclear, but may be the result of direct toxicity from smoke constituents (USDHHS, 1990).

Babies born to smokers weigh less than those born to nonsmokers, and studies have shown that women who smoke during pregnancy have a 90% higher chance of having a low-birthweight baby (<2,500 g) than women who do not smoke (USDHHS, 1990). Low-birthweight infants have much higher mortality rates than normal-weight infants (McCormick, 1985). A review of the literature in the 1990 Surgeon General's Report (USDHHS, 1990) explains that the primary mechanism through which cigarette smoking affects birthweight is intrauterine hypoxia. Cigarette smoking during pregnancy reduces the availability of oxygen to the fetus by two mechanisms. First, carbon monoxide crosses the placenta and binds with hemoglobin to produce carboxyhemoglobin, which reduces the ability of blood to carry oxygen. Second, smoking causes vasoconstriction of the umbilical arteries, which may also impair the oxygen availability to the fetus.

OTHER NONMALIGNANT DISEASES

HIV/AIDS

The prevalence of smoking is very high in some groups who are also at high risk for HIV infection (i.e., gay men and drug abusers). One unpublished study reported that 37.3% of gay men in 1991 smoked (Santa Barbara Gay & Lesbian Resource Center, 1991). Rounsaville, Kosten, Weissman, and Kleber (1985) reported that 97% of their sample of opiate addicts in treatment were cigarette smokers. Because of the prevalence of smoking among these high HIV high-risk groups, the negative effects of smoking on HIV and AIDS is of particular importance.

Cigarette smoking may increase the risk of progression to AIDS in HIV-positive individuals. For example, one study found that the median progression time to AIDS among HIV-seropositive smokers was 8.2 months and 14.5 months for HIV-seropositive nonsmokers (Nieman, Fleming, Coker, Harris, & Mitchell, 1993). Data from the San Francisco Men's Health Study indicated that CD4+ T-lymphocyte cell counts fell faster in HIV-seroconverters who smoked than among those who did not smoke (Royce & Winkelstein, 1990). Cigarette smoking increased the susceptibility of alveolar macrophages to infection with HIV-1 and may have enhanced the rate of progression to AIDS in seropositive smokers (Abbud, Finegan, Guay, & Rich, 1995). Among HIV-seropositive patients undergoing investigation for respiratory symptoms or abnormal chest radiograph, patients who smoked were more likely to have HIV-related infection of the lung which was, in turn, associated with increased mortality (Clarke et al., 1993).

Some studies, however, have found no interaction between smoking and the progression of HIV-seropositive patients to AIDS. For example, after controlling for a number of other variables, Eskild and Petersen (1994) found no positive association between cigarette smoking and progression to AIDS in HIV-infected gay men. Another study found no difference between CD4 and CD8 cell counts in smoking and nonsmoking HIV-seropositive gay men, no difference in rate of progression to AIDS, and no difference in development of Pneumocystis carinii pneumonia (Craib et al., 1992).

Persons with HIV infection are at increased risk for bacterial pneumonia and other opportunistic infections. Nieman et al. (1993) found that HIV-positive smokers developed *Pneumocystis carinii* pneumonia more rapidly (median = 9 months) than nonsmokers (median = 16 months). Seropositive smokers with CD4 lymphocyte counts of fewer than 200 cells per cubic mm. have a greater chance of developing bacterial pneumonia than similarly immunocompromised nonsmokers (Hirschtick et al., 1995). Among HIV-positive intravenous drug users, cigarette smokers were twice as likely to develop pneumonia (Caiaffa et al., 1994). *Pseudomonas aeruginosa*, another pathogen of the respiratory system in seropositive persons, has also been found with greater frequency in smokers than in nonsmokers (Doyle, Doherty, & Zimmerman, 1995). HIV-seropositive homosexual men who smoke have an increased risk of developing oral lesions than homosexual men who do not smoke (Lamster et al., 1994). A positive association has also been found between smoking and development of anal human papillomavirus infection and precancerous anal disease among HIV-positive homosexual men (Palefsky, Shiboski, & Moss, 1994). The studies cited above suggest that cigarette smoking in HIV-positive men increases the risk of several opportunistic AIDS-related diseases.

Cigarette smoking may increase the risk of maternal transmission of HIV. One study found that groups of mothers with low CD4+ levels and groups of mothers who developed premature rupture of membranes both had increased risks of maternal transmission. In both studies, risks were increased among mothers who smoked cigarettes after the first trimester (Burns et al., 1994).

Because a large percentage of gay men and illicit drug users are smokers and are both groups at high risk for development of HIV/AIDS, definitive data is clearly needed on the risks posed by cigarette smoking. Because HIV/AIDS is a disease of the immune system and smoking has been shown to affect the immune system, it seems quite likely that smoking might enhance the effects of HIV on immunity. More research is needed to clarify this issue.

Peptic Ulcer Disease

A review of the literature in the 1990 Surgeon General's Report (USDHHS, 1990) found that cigarette smokers are approximately twice as likely to develop peptic ulcer disease than nonsmokers. The review also found that the increased risk of morbidity or mortality from peptic ulcer disease attributable to smoking is decreased upon cessation of smoking.

Reviews of the literature cite several effects of smoking on gastrointestinal physiology that may increase the risks of peptic ulcer diseases. Some of these actions are rapidly reversed by abstinence from smoking (Kikendall,

Evaul, & Johnson, 1984; USDHHS, 1990). The primary mechanism by which smoking increases the risk of peptic ulcer disease development is that chronic smokers have higher gastric acid output than nonsmokers (Kikendall et al., 1984; USDHHS, 1990). Smokers have higher pentagastrin-stimulated acid secretion and higher basal serum pepsinogen-1 levels (Parente, Lazzaroni, Sangaletti, Baroni, & Bianchi Porro, 1985). The higher maximal gastric acid secretory rates in smokers may be linked to the increased risk of peptic ulcer disease. Other effects of smoking that may increase risk of peptic ulcer disease include: decreased gastric emptying time, decreased synthesis of prostaglandin, decreased alkaline secretions from the pancreas, increased duodenogastric reflux, and decreased gastric mucosal blood flow (Kikendall et al., 1984; USDHHS, 1990).

Osteoporosis

Osteoporosis is a reduction in bone mass that increases the risk of fractures in postmenopausal women and older persons in general (Consensus Conference, 1984). Smoking may increase the risk osteoporosis development and the risk of fracture through several mechanisms (USDHHS, 1990). Women who smoke undergo menopause 1 to 2 years earlier than never-smokers; because bone loss accelerates at menopause, women who smoke may develop osteoporosis earlier than women who do not smoke. The risk of osteoporotic fracture is greater among persons with a small body frame; because smokers generally weigh less than nonsmokers, the risk of fracture may be higher. Finally, smoking has been shown to reduce the production of, and increase the metabolism of, endogenous estrogen, which may play a role in the development of the disease.

PASSIVE SMOKING

It has been estimated that environmental tobacco smoke (ETS) in nonsmokers contributes to 53,000 deaths per year (Glantz & Parmley, 1991), making passive smoking the third leading preventable cause of death after active smoking and alcohol. Of these deaths due to ETS, 37,000 were caused by heart disease (Glantz & Parmley, 1991). Glantz and Parmley (1995) reviewed the literature on mechanisms by which ETS might cause heart disease. Passive smoking reduces the blood's ability to deliver oxygen to the myocardium and reduces the ability of the myocardium to use the oxygen it receives effectively. ETS activates blood platelets increasing the likelihood of thrombus formation, which can damage the lining of the coronary arteries and can lead to the development of atherosclerotic lesions. There is biochemical evidence that components of cigarette smoke may accelerate the development of atherosclerosis. Constituents of passive smoke worsen the outcome of an ischemic event in the heart through the activity of free radicals during reperfusion injury. Finally, there are animal data that suggest that ETS promotes more tissue damage following myocardial infarction.

It has been estimated that ETS causes about 3,000 lung cancer deaths per year among nonsmokers (U.S. Environmental Protection Agency, 1992). It is interesting to note that ETS-related lung cancer mortality is quite low relative to cardiovascular mortality. This may be due to the fact that the polyaromatic hydrocarbons, major tumor initiators, are contained in the particulate matter of cigarette smoke. This particulate matter may not be as readily transmitted from passive smoking as it is in active smoking. Thus, cardiovascular diseases, which are often linked directly to toxins such as carbon monoxide, are seen more often as a result of ETS.

THERAPEUTIC EFFECTS OF NICOTINE

There are a number of potential therapeutic uses of nicotine. It is important to note that available data indicate that nicotine, and not other tobacco constituents, is the source of these therapeutic benefits. In fact, it would seem to be a misnomer to discuss the therapeutic or beneficial effects of smoking in light of the morbidity and mortality related to tobacco-delivered nicotine. Additionally, further research on the use of nicotine or nicotine analogs is needed to assess the value of nicotine medications over known medications.

Weight Control

There is a great deal of evidence that chronic smoking may reduce body weight (USDHHS, 1988). About four out of five persons who quit smoking gain weight; the average weight gain is about 2.3 kg (USDHHS, 1990). Leischow and Stitzer (1991) reviewed the literature and found two probable causes for this weight gain following cessation: decreased energy expenditure and metabolism, and increased caloric intake.

The effects of smoking on weight have been cited as a reason for both initiation continuation of smoking (Klesges, Meyers, Klesges, & La Vasque, 1989). However, any health benefits in the form of weight loss gained by tobacco use are clearly superseded by the many negative effects of tobacco use. Nicotine replacement therapies may obtund the weight gain attributed to smoking cessation (Gross, Stitzer, & Maldonado, 1989). The strength and persistence of these effects of nicotine and tobacco have not been compared to those produced by medications proven to be effective in weight control.

Tourette's Disorder

Studies have examined the effects of nicotine on symptoms of Tourette's disorder. For example, a study by McConville et al. (1992) found that chewing nicotine gum, but not placebo gum, reduced tic severity and potentiated the beneficial effects of haloperidol. Although we have found no reports on the effects of tobacco on Tourette's symptoms (as opposed to nicotine in gum or patch), it is likely that similar effects could be observed. However, because beneficial effects may be seen with nicotine alone, the use of tobacco products in the treatment of Tourette's disorder should not be encouraged.

Ulcerative Colitis

There is ample evidence that smoking is protective against the development of ulcerative colitis (Harries, Baird, & Rhodes, 1982). Because of the negative association between smoking and development of ulcerative colitis, studies have been conducted that have examined the ability of transdermal nicotine to alleviate symptoms of the disease. For example, Pullan et al. (1994) treated 72 patients with either transdermal nicotine or placebo patches and found that twice as many patients in the transdermal nicotine group achieved complete remission than in the placebo group. The nicotine group was also found to have greater improvement in the global clinical and histologic grades of colitis, lower stool frequency, less abdominal pain, and less fecal urgency. Whereas transdermal nicotine may be useful in the treatment of active ulcerative colitis, it may not be efficacious as a maintenance therapy for patients in remission. Thomas et al. (1995) found no difference between transdermal nicotine- and placebo-treated groups of patients in remission for colitis. The authors suggested that noncompliance due to side effects of the nicotine therapy may have reduced the efficacy of the transdermal nicotine therapy.

Possibility of Alzheimer's Prevention

Alzheimer's disease is characterized by large reductions in nicotinic cholinergic binding sites in the brain (Coyle, Price, & DeLong, 1983). Lee (1994) reviewed the literature and conducted a meta-analysis of 19 case-control studies of the association between Alzheimer's disease and smoking. The author found a highly significant negative association between development of the disease and ever-smoking. A risk ratio of 0.60 was found for ever-smokers compared to never-smokers.

Because of the neural effects of nicotine and the epidemiological negative association between disease development and smoking, it has been suggested that nicotine may be used to reduce the cognitive deficits associated with Alzheimer's through cholinergic stimulation (Newhouse et al., 1988). A number of studies support this notion. For example, Jones, Sahakian, Levy, Warburton, and Gray (1992) administered subcutaneous doses of nicotine or placebo to Alzheimer's patients and measured the effects on a variety of cognitive tasks. They found that nicotine significantly improved sustained visual attention, reaction time, and perception, but did not affect visual or auditory short-term memory. Wilson et al. (1995) conducted a double-blind study in which Alzheimer's patients were exposed to transdermal nicotine or placebo. They found that learning significantly improved during the nicotine condition. Memory, behavior, and global cognition, however, were not significantly affected. Thus it seems that nicotine may be used to lessen some of the symptoms of Alzheimer's disease.

CONCLUSION

The 1964 Report of the Surgeon General's Advisory Committee on Smoking and Health concluded that "cigarette smoking is a health hazard of sufficient importance in the United States to warrant appropriate remedial action" (U.S. Public Health Service, 1964). This conclusion was reached after a review of the literature implicating cigarette smoking as a causal determinant of lung cancer and as a major risk factor for other diseases. Over the past three decades, the role of tobacco use has been implicated in many major forms of disease development. The harmful effects of smoking have drastic personal and public health consequences. The morbidity and mortality associated with smoking has led the AMA, ADA, and other professional organizations and governmental bodies to urge health care professionals to actively promote smoking cessation. Additionally, the impact of tobacco-caused diseases with respect to health care expenditures and reduced worker productivity may soon exceed 100 billion dollars in the United States (CDC, 1994; Henningfield et al., 1994). Because the risk of most diseases can be substantially reduced by smoking cessation, stronger efforts are clearly warranted to develop more effective smoking cessation treatments and to make effective treatments as widely available as possible.

REFERENCES

Abbud, R. A., Finegan, C. K., Guay, L. A., & Rich, E. A. (1995). Enhanced production of human immunodeficiency virus type 1 by in vitro-infected alveolar macrophages from otherwise healthy cigarette smokers. *Journal of Infectious Diseases, 172,* 859–863.

Blot, W. J., McLaughlin, J. K., Winn, D. M., Austin, D. F., Greenberg, R. S., Preston-Martin, S., Bernstein, L., Schoenberg, J. B., Stemhagen, A., & Fraumeni, J. F. (1988). Smoking and drinking in relation to oral and pharyngeal cancer. *Cancer Research, 48,* 3282–3287.

Burns, D. N., Landesman, S., Muenz, L. R., Nugent, R. P., Goedert, J. J., Minkoff, H., Walsh, J. H., Mendez, H., Rubinstein, A., & Willoughby, A. (1994). Cigarette smoking, premature rupture of membranes, and vertical transmission of HIV-1 among women with low CD4+ levels. *Journal of Acquired Immune Deficiency Syndromes, 7,* 718–726.

Caiaffa, W. T., Vlahov, D., Graham, N. M., Astemborski, J., Solomon, L., Nelson, K. E., & Munoz, A. (1994). Drug smoking, Pneumocystis carinii pneumonia, and immunosuppression increase risk of bacterial pneumonia in human immunodeficiency virus-seropositive injection drug users. *American Journal of Respiratory Critical Care Medicine, 150,* 1493–1498.

Centers for Disease Control. (1993). Cigarette smoking–attributable mortality and years of potential life lost–United States, 1990. *Morbidity and Mortality Weekly Report, 42,* 645–649.

Centers for Disease Control. (1994). Medical-care expenditures attributable to cigarette smoking–United States, 1993. *Morbidity and Mortality Weekly Report, 43,* 469–472.

Clarke, J. R., Taylor, I. K., Fleming, J., Nukuna, A., Williamson, J. D., & Mitchell, D. M. (1993). The epidemiology of HIV-1 infection of the lung in AIDS patients. *AIDS, 7,* 555–560.

Consensus Conference. (1984). Osteoporosis. *Journal of the American Medical Association, 252,* 799–802.

Coyle, J. T., Price, D. L., & DeLong M. R. (1983). Alzheimer's disease: a disorder of cortical cholinergic innervation. *Science, 219,* 1184–1190.

Craib, K. J., Schechter, M. T., Montaner, J. S., Le, T. N., Sestak, P., Willoughby, B., Voigt, R., Haley, L., & O'Shaughnessy, M. V. (1992). The effects of cigarette smoking on lymphocyte subsets and progression to AIDS in a cohort of homosexual men. *Clinical & Investigative Medicine, 15,* 301–308.

Doyle, R. L., Doherty, J. J., & Zimmerman, L. H. (1995). Recovery of Pseudomonas aeruginosa in respiratory specimens from HIV positive patients being evaluated for Pneumocystis carinii pneumonia. *Thorax, 50,* 548–550.

English J. P., Willius, F. A., & Berkson, J. (1940). Tobacco and coronary disease. *Journal of the American Medical Association, 115,* 1327–1329.

Eskild, A., & Petersen, G. (1994). Cigarette smoking and drinking of alcohol are not associated with rapid progression to acquired immunodeficiency syndrome among homosexual men in Norway. *Scandinavian Journal of Social Medicine, 22,* 209–212.

Gao, Y. T., McLaughlin, J. K., Blot, W. J., Ji, B. T., Benichou, J., Dai, Q., & Fraumeni, J. F. (1994). Risk factors for esophageal cancer in Shanghai, China. I. Role of cigarette smoking and alcohol drinking. *International Journal of Cancer, 58,* 192–196.

Glantz, S. A., & Parmley, W. W. (1991). Passive smoking and heart disease: Epidemiology, physiology, and biochemistry. *Circulation, 83,* 1–12.

Glantz, S. A., & Parmley, W. W. (1995). Passive smoking and heart disease: Mechanisms and risk. *Journal of the American Medical Association, 273,* 1047–1053.

Gross, J., Stitzer, M. L., & Maldonado, J. (1989). Nicotine replacement: Effects on post cessation weight gain. *Journal of Consulting and Clinical Psychology, 57,* 87–92.

Harries, A. D., Baird, A., & Rhodes, J. (1982). Non-smoking: A feature of ulcerative colitis. *British Medical Journal, 284,* 706.

Hegmann, K. T., Fraser, A. M., Keaney, R. P., Moser, S. E., Nilasena, D. S., Higham-Gren, L., & Lyon, J. L. (1993). The effect of age at smoking initiation on lung cancer risk. *Epidemiology, 4,* 444–448.

Henningfield, J. E., Ramström, L. M., Husten, C. G., Giovino, G. A., Zhu, B. P., Barling, J., Weber, C., Kelloway, E. K., Strecher, V. J., Jarvis, M. J., & Weiss, J. (1994). Smoking and the workplace: Realities and solutions. *Journal of Smoking-Related Disease, 5,* 261–270.

Hirschtick, R. E., Glassroth, J., Jordan, M. C., Wilcosky, T. C., Wallace, J. M., Kvale, P. A., Markowitz, N., Rosen, M. J., Mangura, B. T., & Hopewell, P. C. (1995). Bacterial infection in persons infected with the human immunodeficiency virus: Pulmonary complications of HIV infection study group. *New England Journal of Medicine, 333,* 845–851.

Howe, G., Westhoff, C., Vessey, M., & Yeates, D. (1985). Effects of age, cigarette smoking, and other factors on fertility: Findings in a large prospective study. *British Medical Journal, 290,* 1697–1700.

International Agency for Research on Cancer: Tobacco Smoking. (1986). *IARC monographs on the carcinogenic risk of chemicals to humans: Volume 38.* Lyon: International Agency for Research on Cancer.

Jones, G. M., Sahakian, B. J., Levy, R., Warburton, D. M., & Gray, J. A. (1992). Effects of acute subcutaneous nicotine on attention, information processing and short-term memory in Alzheimer's disease. *Psychopharmacology (Berlin), 108,* 485–494.

Kahn, H. A. (1966). The Dorn study of smoking and mortality among US veterans: Report on eight and one-half years of observation. In W. Haenzel (Ed.), *Epidemiological approaches to the study of cancer and other chronic diseases* (NCI Monograph 19, pp. 1–125). Washington, DC: Department of Health, Education, and Welfare, U.S. Public Health Service, National Cancer Institute.

Kikendall, J. W., Evaul, J., & Johnson, L. F. (1984). Effect of cigarette smoking on gastro-intestinal physiology and non-neoplastic digestive disease. *Journal of Clinical Gastroenterology, 6,* 65–79.

Klesges, R. C., Meyers, A. W., Klesges, L. M., & La Vasque, M. E. (1989). Smoking, body weight, and their effects on smoking behavior: A comprehensive review of the literature. *Psychological Bulletin, 106,* 204–230.

Krupski, W. C. (1991). The peripheral vascular consequences of smoking. *Annals of Vascular Surgery, 5,* 291–304.

Lamster, I. B., Begg, M. D., Mitchell-Lewis, D., Fine, J. B., Grbic, J. T., Todak, G. G., el-Sadr, W., Gorman, J. M., Zambon, J. J., & Phelan, J. A. (1994). Oral manifestations of HIV infection in homosexual men and intravenous drug users: Study design and relationship of epidemiologic, clinical, and immunologic parameters to oral lesions. *Oral Surgery, Oral Medicine, and Oral Pathology, 78,* 163–174.

Lee, P. N. (1994). Smoking and Alzheimer's disease: A review of the epidemiological evidence. *Neuroepidemiology, 13,* 131–144.

Leischow, S. J., & Stitzer, M. L. (1991). Smoking cessation and weight gain. *British Journal of Addiction, 86,* 577–581.

Lyons, R. A., Lo, S. V., & Littlepage, B. N. C. (1994). Perceptions of health amongst ever-smokers and never-smokers: A comparison using the SF-36 Health Survey Questionnaire. *Tobacco Control, 3,* 213–215.

McConville, B. J., Sanberg, P. R., Fogelson, M. H., King, J., Cirino, P., Parker, K. W., & Norman, A. B. (1992). The effects of nicotine plus haloperidol compared to nicotine only and placebo nicotine only in reducing tic severity and frequency in Tourette's disorder. *Biological Psychiatry, 31,* 832–840.

McCormick, M. C. (1985). The contribution of low birth weight to infant mortality and childhood morbidity. *New England Journal of Medicine, 312,* 82–90.

McGinnis, J. M., & Foege, W. H. (1993). Actual causes of death in the United States. *Journal of the American Medical Association, 270,* 2207–2212.

National Center for Health Statistics. (1993). *Advance report of final mortality statistics, 1990. Monthly vital statistics report, 41.* Hyattsville, MD: U.S. Department of Health and Human Services.

Newhouse, P. A., Sunderland, T., Tariot, P. N., Blumhardt, C. L., Weingartner, H., Mellow, A., & Murphy, D. L. (1988). Intravenous nicotine in Alzheimer's disease: A pilot study. *Psychopharmacology, 95,* 171–175.

Nieman, R. B., Fleming, J. Coker, R. J., Harris J. R., & Mitchell, D. M. (1993). The effects of cigarette smoking on the development of AIDS in HIV-1-seropositive individuals. *AIDS, 7,* 705–710.

Palefsky, J. M., Shiboski, S., & Moss, A. (1994). Risk factors for anal papillomavirus infection and anal cytologic abnormalities in HIV-positive and HIV-negative homosexual men. *Journal of Acquired Immune Deficiency Syndromes, 7,* 599–606.

Parente, F., Lazzaroni, M., Sangaletti, O., Baroni, S., & Bianchi Porro, G. (1985). Cigarette smoking, gastric acid secretion, and serum pepsinogen I concentrations in duodenal ulcer patients. *Gut, 26*, 1327–1332.

Peto, R., Lopez, A. D., Boreham, J., Thun, M., & Heath, C. (1994). *Mortality from smoking in developed countries 1950–2000.* Oxford: Oxford University Press.

Pullan, R. D., Rhodes, J., Ganesh, S., Mani, V., Morris, J. S., Williams, G. T., Newcombe, R. G., Russell, M. A. H., Feyerabend, C., Thomas, G. A. O., & Säwe, U. (1994). Transdermal nicotine for active ulcerative colitis. *New England Journal of Medicine, 330*, 811–815.

Rounsaville, B. J., Kosten, T. R., Weissman, M. M., & Kleber, H. D. (1985). *Evaluating and treating depressive disorders in opiate addicts* (DHHS Publication No. ADM 85-1406). Washington, DC: U.S. Government Printing Office.

Royce, R. A., & Winkelstein, W. (1990). HIV infection, cigarette smoking and CD4+ T-lymphocyte counts: Preliminary results from the San Francisco Men's Health Study. *AIDS, 4*, 327–333.

Santa Barbara Gay & Lesbian Resource Center. (1991). *Gay and lesbian smoking and health survey.* Santa Barbara, CA: Author.

Sherman, C. B. (1992). The health consequences of smoking: Pulmonary diseases. *Medical Clinics of North America, 76*, 355–375.

Stein, Z., Kline, J., Levin, B., Susser, M., & Warburton, D. (1981). Epidemiologic studies of environmental exposures in human reproduction. In G. G. Berg & H. D. Maillie (Eds.), *Measurement of risks* (pp. 163–183). New York: Plenum.

Thomas, G. A. O., Rhodes, J., Mani, V., Williams, G. T., Newcombe, R. G., Russell, M. A. H., & Feyerabend, C. (1995). Transdermal nicotine as maintenance therapy for ulcerative colitis. *New England Journal of Medicine, 332*, 988–992.

U.S. Department of Health and Human Services. (1984). *The health consequences of smoking: Chronic obstructive lung disease. A report of the Surgeon General* (DHHS Publication No. PHS 84-50205). Rockville, MD: U.S. Department of Health and Human Services, Public Health Service, Center for Disease Control, Center for Chronic Disease Prevention and Health Promotion, Office on Smoking and Health.

U.S. Department of Health and Human Services. (1988). *The health consequences of smoking: Nicotine addiction: A report of the Surgeon General* (DHHS Publication No. CDC 88-8406). Rockville, MD: U.S. Department of Health and Human Services, Public Health Service, Center for Disease Control, Center for Chronic Disease Prevention and Health Promotion, Office on Smoking and Health.

U.S. Department of Health and Human Services. (1989). *Reducing the health consequences of smoking: 25 years of progress. A report of the Surgeon General* (DHHS Publication No. CDC 89-8411). Rockville, MD: U.S. Department of Health and Human Services, Public Health Service, Center for Disease Control, Center for Chronic Disease Prevention and Health Promotion, Office on Smoking and Health.

U.S. Department of Health and Human Services. (1990). *The health benefits of smoking cessation. A report of the Surgeon General* (DHHS Publication No. CDC 90-8416). Rockville, MD: U.S. Department of Health and Human Services, Public Health Service, Center for Disease Control, Center for Chronic Disease Prevention and Health Promotion, Office on Smoking and Health.

U.S. Environmental Protection Agency. (1992). *Respiratory health effects of passive smoking: Lung cancer and other disorders* (EPA Publication No. EPA 600/6-90/006F). Washington, DC: U.S. Environmental Protection Agency.

U.S. Public Health Service. (1964). *Smoking and health: Report of the Advisory Committee to the Surgeon General of the Public Health Service* (PHS Publication No. 1103, p. 33). Rockville, MD: U.S. Department of Health, Education and Welfare, Public Health Service, Center for Disease Control.

Wilson, A. L., Langley, L. K., Monley, J., Bauer, T., Rottunda, S., McFalls, E., Kovera, C., & McCarten, J. R. (1995). Nicotine patches in Alzheimer's disease: Pilot study on learning, memory, and safety. *Pharmacology, Biochemistry, and Behavior, 51*, 509–514.

SOCIETAL IMPACT
AND RESPONSE

7

Driving Under the Influence

Herbert Moskowitz
Southern California Research Institute
and
University of California—Los Angeles

For a scientist, driving under the influence of alcohol or drugs is a problem that suggests inquiries into the character of the impairment of skilled performance produced by different drug dose levels. Data from epidemiological and experimental studies and from human factors analysis of driving requirements all contribute to the analysis of the issues involved.

Driving under the influence is also a legal term in all 50 states. What defines the term is written into law by state legislatures and is utilized by law enforcement personnel. Throughout the world, including the United States, the legal definition of driving under the influence of either alcohol or drug is determined primarily by political considerations and public opinion, and only secondarily by the current state of scientific information.

A scientific examination of the effects of alcohol on automobile driving has a relatively short history. Although a 1904 editorial in the *Quarterly Journal of Inebriety* (as cited in U.S. Department of Transportation, 1968) noted reports of an association between alcohol consumption and automobile accidents, there was little public or legal recognition of a safety issue. Few police officers reported the presence of alcohol in traffic accidents. The assumption at that time, and one still held by some today, associates impaired driving with drunken intoxicated behavior. Even if one accepts the assumption that driving under the influence requires the condition of intoxication, it remains difficult for officers to recognize intoxication by behavioral observations. Questioning the assumption that intoxication is required for impaired driving requires an analysis of the levels of alcohol in accident-involved individuals compared to non-accident-involved individuals. This requires the availability of inexpensive, sensitive, and reliable methods for measuring alcohol levels in drivers, and such techniques were not available at the turn of the century.

DIFFICULTY IN OBSERVING ALCOHOL INTOXICATION

The difficulties confronting police officers in recognizing intoxication can be seen in several studies. Compton (1985) performed a study in which police officers attempted to discriminate between impaired and sober drivers at a sobriety checkpoint. In this experimental situation, the drivers were actually administered alcohol, and the officers anticipated the presence of alcohol. Nevertheless, only drivers at the range of .10% blood alcohol concentration (BAC) and above were recognized as impaired by a majority of officers. In a study of more than 9,000 drivers who volunteered BACs after completion of their stop at 156 sobriety check points in North Carolina, police officers failed to detect 62% of the drivers above the BAC legal limit (.08%) (Wells, Greene, Foss, Ferguson, & Williams, in press).

The problem of perceiving impairment and intoxication by observation is not confined to police officers. Urso, Gavaler, and Van Theil (1981) had physicians evaluate subjects who reported drinking alcohol prior to admission at a hospital emergency room. Seventy-six patients who were deemed nonintoxicated by physicians had BAC levels ranging from .12% to .54% with a mean of .27%. A study by Perper, Ywerski, and Weinand (1986) included 57 alcoholics who were alcohol-positive on admission to a recovery program. After examination on a six-item test battery by two physicians, 35% were evaluated as normal and nonintoxicated. These included 24% of the 54 subjects with BACs of .20% or higher.

In an extensive study of almost 7,000 arrested drivers in Finland (Penttilä, Tenhu, & Kataja, 1971), specialist police physicians administered a 13-item behavioral test battery. In most case, only arrestees above .10% BAC were evaluated as intoxicated and some arrestees with BACs as high as .24% were reported as nonintoxicated.

The difficulty of observing intoxication in drivers is undoubtedly one of the reasons that the probability of being arrested for driving under the influence, when the driver is above the legal limit, has been variously estimated, depending on the legal jurisdiction, as ranging between 1 in 200 to 1 in 1,000. The role of alcohol in raising the probability of driving accidents and increasing their severity remained unappreciated for many decades. The assumption that accidents require observable intoxication is still the basis for the underappreciation of alcohol's influence by some individuals.

ALCOHOL INVOLVEMENT IN ACCIDENTS

Perhaps the earliest systematic scientific investigation of the role of alcohol in driving occurred under the direction of Erik Widmark in Sweden (Andréasson & Jones, 1995). He undertook research to develop sensitive and reliable laboratory techniques for analysis of BACs in the 1920s. These methods were then made available for use in studying the relation between alcohol and driving accidents.

The 1920s produced more voices of concern regarding the role of alcohol in traffic accidents, but estimates, based on police reports, remained low. In response to a claim by the Pennsylvania Deputy Commissioner of Motor Vehicles that fewer than 1% of 2,038 fatally injured drivers were drunk, Heise and Halporn (as cited in Borkenstein, 1985) tested urine from 15 injured drivers and found alcohol present in 9, or 60%. However, the few studies of alcohol-related traffic accidents coupled with the lack of comparison studies of alcohol in non-accident-involved drivers failed to convince the judicial system or the general public. Obtaining the cooperation of drivers for such studies was unlikely to occur if drivers were requested to supply blood or urine samples for analysis. Comparative epidemiological studies with both accident and non-accident-involved drivers had to await the development of breath alcohol sampling devices. The late 1930s saw the first practical alcohol breath sampling devices.

Thus, it was not until 1938 that the first case control study was published. It compared the alcohol level in drivers involved in 270 injury crashes with the alcohol level in 1,760 randomly sampled drivers (Holcomb, 1938). Holcomb reported alcohol present in 12% of the randomly selected drivers, but in 46% of the injury crash drivers. Although earlier studies had suggested the over-representation of alcohol in traffic accidents, the Holcomb study was the first with a comparative baseline of alcohol in non-accident-involved drivers. Since 1938, only about a dozen such case control studies have been performed worldwide. The relative infrequency of such studies is due to their complexity and cost. The largest case control study compared the alcohol level in some 6,000 crash-involved drivers, with 7,600 non-accident-involved drivers in Grand Rapids, Michigan (Borkenstein, Crowther, Shumate, Ziel, & Zylman, 1964). This study required research personnel to rush to the site of traffic accidents and persuade the drivers to provide a breath specimen and complete a questionnaire. The alcohol levels in the accident-involved drivers were compared with alcohol levels in control drivers. The latter were drivers stopped by police officers and asked to provide breath specimens and fill out questionnaires when they passed the accident sites at the same time of day and day of week as the accident time. Data collection involved 24-hour-per-day availability of research crews for an entire year. It is understandable why there are few such studies.

Much of the results produced by the above studies and other epidemiological investigations were summarized in an influential report to the U.S. Congress from the Secretary of Transportation (U.S. Department of Transportation, 1968). This report raised public and legislators' awareness of the dangers of alcohol in driving. Further, it stimulated interest in providing additional funds for further scientific research. The report to Congress noted that 70% of drivers involved in fatal single vehicle accidents had alcohol in their bodies. Roughly 55% of fatally injured drivers in multiple car crashes, where other vehicles were not believed to be at fault, had alcohol present. Overall, alcohol was present in more than 50% of fatally injured drivers in all types of crashes.

Evans (1990) noted that these data could be subjected to further statistical and analytical analysis to determine the percentage of fatal injuries due to alcohol. For example, the analysis should include drivers killed in accidents caused by drivers under the influence of alcohol who were not themselves killed. These and other factors led Evans to conclude that even in 1987 when alcohol-related fatal accidents had decreased by 12%, almost half of traffic fatalities remained attributable to alcohol.

The 1968 Department of Transportation (DOT) compilation of studies reported that between 25% and 45% of drivers involved in serious injury automobile crashes had alcohol present in their blood. The studies also noted a concentration of alcohol-related fatal accidents between 9:00 p.m. and 6:00 a.m., primarily on weekends. This finding is consistent with epidemiological studies indicating the times of maximum use of alcoholic beverages.

During the decades since the report to Congress there have been massive efforts by local, state and federal authorities, as well as volunteer groups such as Mothers Against Drunk Driving, to reduce the alcohol-related traffic toll. The last two decades have seen a 15% reduction in alcohol-related fatalities. More significantly, random roadside surveys have shown an even greater reduction in the presence of alcohol in drivers. This indicates a growing appreciation of the alcohol driving problem by the public and a modification of their behavior (Lund & Wolfe, 1991).

Nevertheless, the U.S. Department of Transportation reported that more than 1.5 million drivers were arrested in 1993 for driving under the influence of alcohol, an astonishing figure when one considers the low probability of being arrested for driving above the legal limit. In 1994 there were still 16,589 alcohol-related motor vehicle fatalities and roughly 297,000 persons injured in crashes where police reported alcohol present (U.S. Department of Transportation, 1994). Even these numbers have to be considered underestimations because, as recent studies document, the police investigations frequently fail to uncover the presence of alcohol, which is subsequently documented by hospital emergency rooms and medical examiners (Öström, Huelke, & Waller, 1992).

One scientific question considered by the case control studies was the relationship between the probability of a driver being involved or being at fault in a motor vehicle accident versus BAC. Such analyses have been particularly important in their influence on the level at which legislatures establish alcohol BAC limits for driving. In the Grand Rapids Study (Borkenstein et al., 1964), which had the largest sample size of all case control studies, the relationship between accident causation and BAC was an exponential function, increasing 600% and 2500% at BACs of .10% and .15%, respectively. Below .04% the report failed to show an increase in accident probability.

Analysis of the Grand Rapids data, however, was criticized by Allsop (1966), Hurst (1973), and others for its failure to take into account that alcohol and non-alcohol drivers differed in many factors important for accident involvement probability. The relationship between accident probability and BAC is obtained by comparing the percentage of accidents in zero alcohol drivers with the percentage of accidents among the drivers at various positive alcohol levels. Such a comparison carries the implicit assumption that the drivers in both groups are essentially the same in the propensity to be involved in an accident, assuming no alcohol were present. Unfortunately, this was not true either in the Grand Rapids study nor in nearly all the other case control studies. For example, in the Grand Rapids study, the zero alcohol group had a preponderance of very young (16- and 17-year olds) and elderly drivers. These groups have much higher accident rates per mile than drivers in the age category of 25 to 55 years. On the other hand, the positive alcohol drivers were predominantly 25 to 55 years old. Similar disparity in characteristics of the alcohol and nonalcohol groups occurred in drinking frequency, education, yearly miles driven, and other factors. Consider whether a 30-year-old driver who drives 20,000 miles annually, drinks daily, and is at a .02% BAC is more likely to be involved in an accident than a sober 16-year-old who has driven 500 miles with a license issued 3 months ago. Extracting the role of alcohol in such comparisons requires sophisticated statistical techniques, such as logistic regression analysis. The methodological error in analysis of the Grand Rapids data is identified in the statistical literature as either Yule's Reversal Paradox or Simpson's Paradox (Mittal, 1991).

As Allsop (1966) and Hurst (1973) pointed out, their analysis of the Grand Rapids Study demonstrated the importance of age, education, drinking frequency, mileage driven, etc., in determining accident rate. Several factors exhibited a significant interaction with the presence of alcohol, such that there is increased accident probability in the presence of alcohol. For example, the accident probability of 16- and 17-year-old drivers increased more than 500% from imbibing the equivalent of a single beer, which might produce between .01% to .04% BAC. The frequency and quantity of drinking also interacted with the presence of alcohol. Drivers who might drink as infrequently as yearly exhibited a 760% increase in accident probability at BACs of .05% to .079%, the accident probability of daily drinkers at that BAC level increased only 60%. Nonetheless, both Allsop and Hurst demonstrated that when alcohol groups were compared to nonalcohol groups with similar characteristics (age, drinking practices, education, etc.) that the presence of *any* alcohol increased the probability of an accident.

Their analysis showed that more frequent consumption of alcohol was associated with a smaller increase in accident probability with BAC, indicating increased tolerance to alcohol for more frequent drinkers. Of greater significance, however, was the demonstration that the increased tolerance was not associated with an increased threshold or BAC at which increased accident probability occurred. The tolerance effect was on the slope, or rate of increase in accidents with increasing BAC. The threshold of increase in accident probability was the same for both the novice infrequent drinker and the heavy daily drinker.

It is of further interest to note that both epidemiological and experimental data demonstrate that, contrary to popular myth, the presence of alcohol in a driver increases the probability of death and severity of injury should an accident occur. That is, alcohol contributes not only to accident causation, but to the resulting injury (Evans, 1993).

As with epidemiological studies, the 1930s saw the beginning of an expansion of experimental studies on the effects on alcohol on driving. It is, of course, possible to perform such studies with less expense than epidemiological studies, and hundreds have been performed. Concern about the increasing use of alcohol and increasing social problems, which followed the end of Prohibition, stimulated research into many behaviors influenced by alcohol, not all of which are relevant for driving. For example, there is an extensive literature reporting the effects of alcohol on memory, which is of great importance in flying and in military activity. Research on human factors important to motor vehicle operation, however, has failed to demonstrate that recalling where you want to exit a freeway is a major factor in driving accidents. For that reason, the following section does not report on all behaviors under alcohol, such as memory, but concentrates on those skills which are important in accident causation.

In this regard, the movies typically present automobile accidents as a consequence of wild, out-of-control driving. In fact, multidisciplinary accident investigation studies, such as the 5-year study at Indiana University (Treat, 1980), found that only 8% of human failure accidents are due to motor performance failure. Forty-eight percent of human errors, which accounted for between 85% to 90% of all causes, were recognition or information processing errors. Drivers either totally failed to see or had unusually long delays in recognition of important factors that produced the accident.

Thirty-six percent of the errors were decision errors, such as excessive speed. Similar findings have been obtained from studies in England, Switzerland, and Germany.

A recent large review of the literature on alcohol effects on skills important for driving reveal that, with the exception of simple reaction time (as noted below), nearly any behavioral variable of importance to driving is impaired by alcohol (Moskowitz & Robinson, 1988). There are, of course, differences between variables both in the BAC at which impairment was first detected and in the rate of increase in impairment with increasing BACs.

All studies on reaction time other than those involving simple reaction time reported impairment. In simple reaction time the subject knows the single stimulus, the single response, and the likelihood of the stimulus appearance, but when reaction time requires selection among different stimuli, selection of different responses, or uncertainty in appearance of the stimuli, alcohol produced impairment.

ALCOHOL EFFECTS IN TRACKING

Studies of tracking, which is the analogue of the car-control aspects of driving, were among the early studies of alcohol effects. Newman and Fletcher (1940) examined pursuit tracking, in combination with a visual search and recognition task, and reported impairment near .10%. Newman (1949) utilized a compensatory tracking task and failed to find impairment until .18% BAC. Studies from the period of the 1940s to the 1970s exhibited great variability in the BACs at which impairment occurred and in the magnitude of that impairment.

However, under the influence of the increasing attention to performance research, with emphasis on information processing and time-sharing in machine control systems, the laboratory simulation of man-machine tasks improved. The improvement led to greater sensitivity of the laboratory tasks to the effects of alcohol.

A study by Chiles and Jennings (1970) examined performance in a compensatory tracking task while simultaneously, but intermittently, performing a series of subsidiary tasks. Peak BACs were near .10%. Tracking, in the presence and not in the presence of the subsidiary task, was analyzed separately. None of the tracking measures were significantly affected by alcohol except in the presence of the subsidiary task. The authors suggested that, in fact, the more important area of alcohol impairment might be time-sharing information, with motor performance less easily affected. Similarly, Moskowitz (1971) examining performance in a driving simulator, with and without a subsidiary task, demonstrated the insensitivity of car control measures alone to .10% BAC. The car control measures demonstrated impairment under alcohol only in the presence of the subsidiary task.

ALCOHOL AND DRIVING-RELATED SKILLS

Beginning in 1968 (e.g., Moskowitz & DePry, 1968), Moskowitz performed studies of the effects of alcohol on information processing and time-sharing, as divided attention. These studies demonstrated both the relevance of divided attention to man-machine tasks, such as driving, and its sensitivity. Moskowitz, Burns, and Williams (1985) used a battery of information processing and divided attention tasks and found all subjects impaired at .015%.

In the Moskowitz and Robinson (1988) review, studies of divided attention showed the lowest threshold for alcohol effects. For man-machine activities, time-sharing performance is critical and may well underlie the susceptibility of driving at low BACs.

Among skills examined by Moskowitz and Robinson (1988) were information processing rate capabilities. This is a measure of the brain's capacity to process the information necessary to organize a response. This ability underlies all reaction time studies, because unless one can process information rapidly, responses will be delayed.

Other skills impaired by alcohol are ocular and optometric functions, such as the ability to control the movement of the eyes, perception (which involves the ability to interpret what information is being presented to the sensory system), and psychomotor performance (which deals with the quality of motor output for vehicle control). Each of these areas exhibited impairment at most BACs tested. The 177 reviewed studies all met rigorous criteria for information about subject alcohol dosing and performance measures.

The review also examined performance measures in studies of driving in closed tracks and in simulators. The reviewed studies reported impairment by .05% in nearly all response areas and in many areas by .02% to .03%. Thirty-five studies reported impairment at or below .04% BAC. The review found no evidence for a threshold for alcohol effects on driving skills. There is no lower limit that would scientifically assure that a driver would not be impaired in one or more areas of driving skills.

At least two factors delayed the realization of how little alcohol is required to impair skills performance. One factor was the emphasis in the earlier studies on the motor aspect of car control. This behavioral area is less sensitive to alcohol effects than the cognitive areas of visual detection and perception of potential dangers, information processing, and division of attention. The other factor was that most studies of driving-related behaviors under alcohol tested no more than one or two BACs. The BACs typically were those currently in use as a legal limit for driving. The few studies, which employed a range of BACs with suitable behavioral measures, did note that impairment occurred at the lowest BACs tested. One such drug-dose study by Drew, Colquhoun, and Long (1959), used a driving simulator and demonstrated impairment beginning at .02% BAC. Note that the simulator required division of attention.

An additional advantage of experimental studies is that variables, which are hard to examine in epidemiological studies, can be examined accurately in the laboratory. For example, Moskowitz and Burns (1976) studied the effects of the rate of drinking on skilled performance. In their study with five groups, four groups received alcohol treatment and one received a placebo. The alcohol groups received alcohol sufficient to produce a .10% BAC after drinking either 15 minutes, 30 minutes, 60 minutes, or 4 hours. All subjects were impaired in comparison to the placebo group, and impairment was greater the more rapidly the alcohol was consumed. Note that with a longer time to get to a given BAC, more alcohol had to be consumed because the body was metabolizing part of the consumption. Thus, the group that showed the least impairment, the group that drank the alcohol over a 4-hour period, actually drank considerably more than the other groups.

In another study, Burns and Moskowitz (1978) dosed men and women to the same BAC level given their gender, height, and weight. With subjects at the same BAC there were no significant differences by gender in impairment on driving-related skills. This corrects several studies that have found differences after giving equal dosages to subjects without taking into account the different body water content of male and females and the differences in BAC reached.

Another issue difficult to study epidemiologically, but which has been examined by Roth, Roehrs, and Merlotti (1989), is the interaction between alcohol and sleep-related variables such as number of hours of sleep, time of day when alcohol is consumed, and time of day when a task is performed. Evidence suggests that alcohol has an increasing impairment effect on vigilance and divided attention tasks in individuals who have had insufficient sleep or are functioning outside of their normal circadian awake period.

As noted above, decision or judgment errors are an important factor in accident causation. Although often described in police reports, such behavior is difficult to model in an experimental situation. In such a study, Cohen, Dearnaley, and Hansel (1958) examined the effect of alcohol on the skills involved in maneuvering a bus through a narrow gap between two upright posts. These were English bus drivers skilled in driving through narrow streets. In the study, the smallest gap through which the drivers could reliably drive a bus was only 6/10 of an inch wider after consumption of 6 ounces of whiskey. However, there was a large increase in the frequency at which drivers attempted to drive their bus through two posts that were closer together than the width of the bus. Cohen suggests that, rather than a perceptual or motor impairment, the effect of alcohol was on the risk-taking of the drivers.

The scientific data from both epidemiological and experimental studies indicate there is no threshold for alcohol impairment of skills performance and an increase in accident probability. At low BACs, such as .015%, .02%, and .03%, terms such as intoxication or drunkenness or inebriation are inappropriate. From a pharmacological point of view, the term "intoxication" refers to the effect of any psychoactive substance in the body. For the general public, police officers, and judges, intoxication is associated with images of grossly deviant and easily observed behavioral changes.

BAC LIMITS

To improve the ability of officers in detecting and evaluating alcohol-impaired drivers, the National Highway Traffic Safety Administration of the U.S. Department of Transportation sponsored studies to develop a sobriety test battery (Burns & Moskowitz, 1979). The battery includes alcohol gaze nystagmus, which will reliably evaluate alcohol effects in more than 85% of drivers at .08%, given that the officer is trained and skilled. The current development of small inexpensive hand-held alcohol breath testers are even more capable of providing officers conclusive evidence of the presence and level of alcohol in drivers.

Despite the growing body of evidence demonstrating the impairment of driving at low BACs, "driving under the influence" laws in most states set legal BAC limits at .10%, or at best .08%. In many states, however, this level has been reduced to as low as .02% for drivers under the age of 21. Both the National Safety Council and the American Medical Association have called for reducing the level to .05%, as in some European countries, and many groups are in favor of even further reductions.

There clearly remains a lag between the evaluations of scientists as to the BACs of driving under the influence and the perceptions and willingness of legislators to accept the scientific findings. Meanwhile, other countries, such as Sweden, have adopted a universal .02% limit.

DRUGS

Analogous to the laws in the United States prohibiting driving under the influence of alcohol are a parallel set of laws prohibiting driving under the influence of drugs. Unlike the laws limiting the level of alcohol permitted for driving, the laws for drugs do not stipulate a level either in blood or urine beyond which driving is prohibited. There is a good reason for this.

Alcohol is a drug with the unique faculty of moving rapidly throughout the body to an equilibrium level wherever there is water. Determining the alcohol level in the water of the blood, the urine, or the breath is an excellent measure of the alcohol level in the water of the brain. It is, of course, the presence of alcohol in the brain that produces the change in behavior that leads to driving impairment. Unfortunately, nearly all other drugs lack this faculty. As a result, the level of drug in blood samples have a complex relationship to the level of drugs at any other site in the body.

Some drugs remain fairly tightly compartmentalized in the areas into which the body admits them. For that reason, obtaining a drug blood level is rarely sufficient, except at very high levels, for predicting whether or not an individual is impaired by that drug. The metabolites of some drugs appear in the blood and urine for weeks beyond the point at which there is any behavioral impairment. On the other hand, there are other drugs that vanish from the blood into other body compartments while the subjects continue to exhibit behavioral impairment.

This characteristic of drugs, and of course the great variability between drugs, leads to considerable difficulty in performing epidemiological studies. It is perhaps why most epidemiological studies of drugs in driving utilize the presence or absence of the drug rather than attempt any analysis based on the quantitative level of the drug.

Another difficulty for performing epidemiological studies is the difficulty of finding control subjects willing to give blood or urine samples to establish a baseline presence of the drug in a group comparable to the accident involved drivers. As noted earlier, it was the development of alcohol breath testing devices that permitted case controlled alcohol epidemiological studies.

Before prosecuting an individual for being under the influence of a drug, it is necessary to establish in court, via scientific studies, that the drug in question actually produces an increase in driving accidents. Given the difficulty of obtaining adequate control groups from volunteer subjects near an accident site, some investigators have resorted to correlating the presence or absence of the drug with the assignment of responsibility for causing an accident in accident-involved drivers. The ability to perform such studies, of course, rests on the reliability of the judgments made primarily by police officers in assigning responsibility for crashes. This is a task for which most police officers are scarcely qualified (Shinar, Treat, & McDonald, 1983).

A major study in this area was performed by Terhune et al. (1992) using blood specimens from 1,882 fatally injured drivers. Drugs were found in 18% of the fatalities spread across several categories of drugs. In general, it was found that drug users were more likely to be ascribed as responsible for crashes than nondrug users. The analysis of the data was complicated by the fact that many of the drug users simultaneously consumed several drugs, including (by more than half) alcohol. There have, of course, been other epidemiological studies that have simply reported on the relative presence of drugs, primarily in fatally injured drivers. While inconclusive without a comparative control group, the frequency of the appearance of drugs in such accidents suggests that, in fact, a correlation exists between the use of some drugs and the probability of accident involvement (Stoduto et al., 1991).

Much of the information regarding specific drugs has been obtained from experimental studies examining that specific drug. In these cases, behavioral impairment on tasks, ranging from simple laboratory tests to driving simulators, has been correlated with the size of the administered dose, the time since administration, and the blood level of the drug. As noted before, the correlations between drug levels over time and impairment have often been difficult to interpret. However, there have been unambiguous results in many studies when the measure is the dose administered and the time from the dose. See for example, Moskowitz (1985) for several reviews dealing with specific drug categories and driving.

Although the epidemiological studies suggest that tranquilizers, antihistamines, and antidepressants are over-represented among injured drivers in epidemiological studies, the experimental studies report impairment by many more drugs.

Complicating a simple description of the impairment likely in a drug category is the change in medicinal drugs over time. Drug regulatory agencies throughout the world have paid increasing attention to the behavioral effects of drugs. In turn, this has stimulated pharmaceutical companies to develop alternate drugs that lack the negative behavioral effects. Recently introduced tranquilizers and antihistamines produce only a fraction of the impairments associated with older drugs in those categories.

Given the complexity of demonstrating that an individual is under the influence of a drug in driving situations, there are few arrests in comparison to the large number of arrests for driving under the influence of alcohol. The emphasis of enforcement of these laws has been concentrated on the illicit drugs. The federal government and local agencies have sponsored specific programs to train officers to recognize the signs and symptoms of drug categories. Compared to alcohol, such drug judgments are not easily made. Thus, the typical arrest and conviction—driving under the influence of a drug—involves an illicit drug at a fairly high level where overt behavioral effects are more likely to be seen. Moreover, securing a conviction after a blood or urine sample has been taken often requires the interpretation of both the behavioral evidence and the pharmacological evidence by an expert in toxicology or psychopharmacology.

The most frequently prosecuted drug influence cases involve marijuana, a drug for which epidemiological studies show high prevalence among drivers. Except for alcohol, marijuana is the most frequently studied illicit drug in laboratory, driving simulator, and over-the-road studies. Nearly all of these studies have produced evidence of impairment in coordination, perception, vigilance, and attention as well as other behavioral areas.

Marijuana is a drug that disappears from the blood within a few hours after ingestion. Metabolites of marijuana, however, can be found in urine for 3 weeks or more. The problem then is that if there is no auxiliary information, the urine specimen provides only ambiguous information about when ingestion occurred and about the likelihood of behavioral impairment. Reliance has to be placed on the behavioral judgments of the arresting officers.

Several conclusions can be drawn from this brief discussion of driving under the influence of drugs. First, that there is only a limited scientific base, and that restricts our ability to determine whether and to what degree most drugs impair the ability to drive safely. There are unlimited opportunities for research on the effects of drugs on performance as a function of dose and time of administration. Second, given the complex relation between blood or urine levels and the effects of most drugs, it is unlikely that the relation between drugs and accident probability will be fully understood in the short term. The best source likely for that knowledge would be from experimental studies, where the relation between dose, time, and effect are unambiguous. Until a broader scientific base has been created, scientists' ability to assist in the development of public policy concerning drugs and driving will be limited. For the present, few of the many drivers who are using drugs, either licit or illicit, will be apprehended and convicted of DUI drugs.

There is a contrary situation with regard to alcohol. An extensive rigorous scientific base of knowledge exists indicating the extent of the problems associated with alcohol and driving, the nature of alcohol-induced impairments, the magnitude of performance deficits as a function of BAC, and the common use patterns and the variation in impairment by numerous demographic features. The encyclopedic fund of knowledge about alcohol, however, has had limited influence on public policy as exemplified by the actions of legislatures, judiciary and police agencies. Only to the extent that the scientific knowledge has been taken up by public advocacy groups, or has influenced the U.S. Department of Transportation, has scientific knowledge contributed to the legal system's concepts of driving under the influence. However, as with tobacco, the public's view of the acceptability of driving with alcohol has been changing. Perhaps the next decades will see a definition of driving under the influence by legal authorities that will be more in concert with the scientific data.

REFERENCES

Allsop, R. E. (1966). *Alcohol and road accidents: A discussion of the Grand Rapids Study* (RRL Report No. 6). Harmondsworth, Great Britain: Ministry of Transport, Road Research Laboratory.
Andréasson, R., & Jones, A. W. (1995). Erik M. P. Widmark (1889–1945): Swedish pioneer in forensic alcohol toxicology. *Forensic Sciences International, 72,* 1–14.

Borkenstein, R. F. (1985). Historical perspectives: North American traditional and experimental response. *Journal of Studies on Alcohol* (Suppl. 10), 3–18.

Borkenstein, R. F., Crowther, R. F., Shumate, R. P., Ziel, W. B., & Zylman, R. (1964). *The role of the drinking driver in traffic accidents: [The Grand Rapids Study]*. Bloomington, IN: Department of the Police Administration, Indiana University. (Revised version in *Blutalcohol, 11*, 1974.)

Burns, M., & Moskowitz, H. (1978). Gender-related differences in impairment of performance by alcohol. In F. Seixas (Ed.), *Currents in alcoholism* (Vol. 3, pp. 479–492). New York: Grune & Stratton.

Burns, M., & Moskowitz, H. (1979). Alcohol impairment tests for DWI arrests. *Transportation Research Record #739*. Washington, DC: Transportation Research Board, National Academy of Sciences.

Chiles, W. D., & Jennings, A. E. (1970). Effects of alcohol on complex performance. *Human Factors, 12*, 605–612.

Cohen, J., Dearnaley, E. J., & Hansel, C. E. M. (1958, June 21). The risk taken in driving under the influence of alcohol. *British Medical Journal*, 1438–1442.

Compton, R. P. (1985). *Pilot test of selected DWI detection procedures for use at sobriety checkpoints* (Report No. DOT HS 806 724). Springfield, VA: National Highway Traffic Safety Association.

Drew, G. C., Colquhoun, W. P., & Long, H. A. (1959). *Effect of small doses of alcohol on a skill resembling driving*. London: HMSO, Medical Research Counsel.

Evans, L. (1990). The fraction of traffic fatalities attributable to alcohol. *Accident, Analysis and Prevention, 22*, 587–602.

Evans, L. (1993). Alcohol's effect on fatality risk from physical insult. *Journal of Studies on Alcohol, 54*, 441–449.

Holcomb, R. L. (1938). Alcohol in relation to traffic accidents. *Journal of the American Medical Association, 3*, 1076–1085.

Hurst, P. M. (1973). Epidemiological aspects of alcohol in driver crashes and citations. *Journal of Safety Research, 5*, 130–148.

Lund, A. K., & Wolfe, A. C. (1991). Changes in the incidence of alcohol-impaired driving in the United States, 1973–1986. *Journal of Studies on Alcohol, 52*, 293–301.

Mittal, Y. (1991). Homogeneity of subpopulations and Simpson's Paradox. *Journal of the American Statistical Association, 86*, 167–172.

Moskowitz, H. (1971). *The effects of alcohol on performance in a driving simulator of alcoholics and social drinkers* (Report No. UCLA-ENG-7205). Los Angeles: University of California at Los Angeles, School of Engineering (Also issued as Report No. DOT HS-800-570). Washington, DC: U.S. Department of Transportation, National Highway Traffic Safety Administration.

Moskowitz, H. (Ed). (1985). Special issue on drugs and driving. *Accident Analysis and Prevention, 17*.

Moskowitz, H., & Burns, M. (1976). Effects of rate of drinking on human performance. *Journal of Studies on Alcohol, 37*, 598–605.

Moskowitz, H., Burns, M., & Williams, A. (1985). Skills performance at low blood alcohol levels. *Journal of Studies on Alcohol, 46*, 482–485.

Moskowitz, H., & DePry, D. (1968). Differential effect of alcohol on auditory vigilance and divided-attention tasks. *Quarterly Journal of Studies on Alcohol, 29*, 54–63.

Moskowitz, H., & Robinson, C. D. (1988). *Effect of low doses of alcohol on driving-related skills: A review of the evidence* (Report No. DOT HS-807-280). Washington, DC: U.S. Department of Transportation.

Newman, H. W. (1949). The effect of altitude on alcohol tolerance. *Quarterly Journal of Studies on Alcohol, 10*, 398–403.

Newman, H., & Fletcher, E. (1940). The effect of alcohol on driving. *Journal of the American Medical Association, 115*, 1600–1602.

Öström, M., Huelke, D. F., & Waller, P. F. (1992). Some biases in the Alcohol Investigative Process in Traffic Fatalities. *Accident Analysis and Prevention, 24*, 539–545.

Penttilä, A., Tenhu, M., & Kataja, M. (1971). *Clinical examination for intoxication in cases of suspected drunken driving: An evaluation of the Finnish system on the basis of 6,839 cases* (pp. 1–43). Helsinki, Finland: Statistical and Research Bureau of Talja.

Perper, J. A., Ywerski, A., & Weinand, J. W. (1986). Tolerance at high blood alcohol concentrations: A study of 110 cases and review of the literature. *Journal of Forensic Sciences, 31*, 212–221.

Roth, T., Roehrs, T., & Merlotti, L. (1989). Ethanol and daytime sleepiness. *Alcohol, Drugs and Driving, 5 & 6*, 357–362.

Shinar, D., Treat, J. R., & McDonald, S. T. (1983). The validity of police reported accident data. *Accident Analysis and Prevention, 15*, 175–191.

Stoduto, G., Vingilis, E., Kapur, B. M., Sheu, W. J., McLeelan, B. A., & Liban, C. B. (1991). Alcohol and drugs in motor vehicle collision admissions to a regional trauma unit: Demographic, injury and crash characteristics. *35th Annual Proceedings, Association for the Advancement of Automotive Medicine* (pp. 235–247). Toronto: n.p.

Terhune, K. W., Ippolito, C. A., Hendricks, D. L., Michalovic, J. G., Bogema, S. C., Santinga, P., Blomberg, R., & Preusser, D. F. (1992). *The incidence and role of drugs in fatally injured drivers* (Report No. DOT HS-808-065). Washington, DC: U.S. Department of Transportation, National Highway Traffic Safety Administration.

Treat, J. R. (1980). A study of precrash factors involved in traffic accidents. *The HSRI Research Review, 10 & 11*, 1–35.

Urso, T., Gavaler, J. S., & Van Theil, D. H. (1981). Blood ethanol levels in sober alcohol users seen in an emergency room. *Life Sciences, 28*, 1053–1056.

U.S. Department of Transportation. (1968). *Alcohol and highway safety: A report to the congress from the secretary of transportation*. Washington, DC: Author.

U.S. Department of Transportation. (1994). *Traffic safety facts: alcohol*. Washington, DC: National Highway Traffic Safety Administration, National Center for Statistics and Analysis, Research and Development.

Wells, J. K., Greene, M. A., Foss, R. D., Ferguson, S. A., & Williams, A. F. (1997). Drivers with high BACs missed at sobriety checkpoints. *Journal of Studies on Alcohol, 58*, 513–517.

8

Drug Abuse and Infectious Disease

Richard H. Needle
Elizabeth Y. Lambert
Susan Coyle
National Institutes of Health
National Institute on Drug Abuse

Harry W. Haverkos
Food and Drug Administration
Division of Antiviral Drug Products

DRUG ABUSE AND INFECTIOUS DISEASE

Drug injection and the spread of infectious diseases were recognized more than 50 years ago when unexplained outbreaks of malaria occurred in New York, San Francisco, and Chicago. The malaria epidemic, eventually attributed to multiperson reuse of syringes by injection drug users (IDUs), is of historical relevance because it foretells our current concerns about emerging and re-emerging infections and the risk behaviors that underlie transmission of blood-borne diseases. Before World War II, most drug users in the United States injected subcutaneously, mainly risking tetanus or cutaneous abscesses. Later, as drug users began to inject intravenously, infectious complications such as malaria and endocarditis became more prevalent.[1]

Today, there are co-occurring epidemics of human immunodeficiency virus (HIV), hepatitis B virus (HBV), and hepatitis C virus (HCV) among IDUs, largely spread through multiperson use of contaminated injection equipment such as syringes and through unprotected sexual intercourse with infected individuals. Between July 1995 and June 1996, over 70,000 new cases of Acquired Immunodeficiency Syndrome (AIDS) were reported in the United States, raising the cumulative total to 548,102 cases (Centers for Disease Control and Prevention [CDC], 1996a). Each year, an estimated 41,000 new HIV infections occur in the United States (Holmberg, 1996), and at least 140,000 HBV infections and 35,000 HCV infections are estimated to occur (CDC, 1996b). In the year ending 1995, more than a third of all new AIDS cases in the United States were attributable, directly or indirectly, to injection drug use (CDC, 1996a). As of July 1996, the Joint United Nations Programme on HIV/AIDS (UNAIDS) estimates that 21.8 million adults and children were living with HIV/AIDS worldwide (UNAIDS, 1996). Although 75% to 85% of the global burden of adult HIV infections is attributable to unprotected sexual intercourse, injection drug use is a major mode of transmission in many areas of the world. Injection drug use has been reported in 118 countries, and AIDS cases attributed to injection drug use have been reported in over 80 of these countries (Des Jarlais et al., 1995).

This chapter examines the drug use practices of chronic drug users that increase the likelihood of acquiring or transmitting infections. Our discussion will center primarily on chronic use of heroin, powdered cocaine, crack cocaine, and methamphetamine, as well as on three parenterally and sexually transmitted blood-borne pathogens (HIV, HBV, HCV), other sexually transmitted diseases (STDs), and tuberculosis (TB).[2] Other STDs (e.g., gonorrhea, syphilis, and chlamydia) are prevalent among drug users and are closely linked to unprotected sexual activity and sex-for-drug exchanges. TB is also widespread among drug users. A number of other infectious diseases in addition to those discussed here pose major risks to drug users, and to others who are immunosuppressed. These include human T-lymphotropic viruses (HTLV), endocarditis, and sepsis. Risks for these infections are high among IDUs, particularly those who engage in multiperson use of injecting equipment and who "register," "boot," and "backload" drugs or drug solutions (see Shah et al., 1996).

Epidemiology of Drug Abuse

In the United States, there are an estimated 2.7 million chronic drug users, 78% of whom are estimated to be injecting and noninjecting users of cocaine, and 22% of whom are estimated to be injecting and noninjecting users of heroin (Office of National Drug Control Policy [ONDCP], 1996a). Holmberg (1996) estimates that there are 1.5 million IDUs in the 96 largest metropolitan areas of the United States. Table 8.1 provides information from various reporting systems on the nature, extent, and trends of drug use in the United States, including data from national surveys of household and high risk populations, unpublished survey data from not-in-treatment drug users, and information from community-based ethnographers who study drug abuse and emerging drug use patterns in the field.

National data provide point prevalence estimates about drug abuse, which are helpful for understanding the magnitude of the problem and its general trends. However, these data are less informative about regional and local drug use patterns. Throughout the United States, there are consider-

TABLE 8.1
National Drug Use Indicator Data, 1995 and 1996

Indicator	Population/Sources	Type of Drug			
		Heroin	Cocaine	Crack	Amphetamine
No. of past week "hardcore" users	U.S. population ≥ 12 years old, estimated 1995	586,000[a]	2,100,000[b]	420,000[b]	n/a
No. of past year users	U.S. population ≥ 12 years old, estimated 1995[b]	428,000	3,700,000	1,000,000	760,000–1,000,000
No. of lifetime users	U.S. population ≥ 12 years old, estimated 1995[b]	1,400,000	21,700,000	3,900,000	4,700,000
No. of drug-related ER episodes in last 6 months	Emergency room patients, January–June 1995[c]	38,100	76,800	n/a	10,600
Rate of use by arrestees	Arrestee sample, 1995[d]	0.7%	36%	n/a	0.6%
Incidence pattern	Selected U.S. cities[e]	Increasing, young users	Stable, young users	Stable, "older" users	Increasing, whites age 26–34
Injecting trends	Selected U.S. cities[e]	Increasing	Increasing	n/a	Increasing
Snorting/smoking trends	Selected U.S. cities[e]	Increasing	Stable	Stable	Increasing
Purity of drug (%) range	Selected U.S. cities[e]	16–71% per mg	25–94% per gm	50–95% per gm	30–98% per gm
Price of drug (range)	Selected U.S. cities[e]	$.36–2.19 per mg	$33–150 per gm	$10–50 per rock $100–2,600 per oz	$27–200 per gm

[a]ONDCP (1996a), "hardcore" users are individuals who use illicit drugs at least weekly and exhibit behavioral problems stemming from their drug use.
[b]SAMHSA (1996a), National Household Survey on Drug Abuse.
[c]SAMHSA (1996b), Drug Abuse Warning Network (numbers of drug-related emergency room episodes in 21 major U.S. metropolitan areas).
[d]NIJ (1996), Drug Use Forecasting (DUF) program (urine tests and interviews of adult/juvenile booked arrestees in up to 23 DUF sites).
[e]NIDA/CEWG (June 1996), ethnographic observations in 20 metropolitan areas; also, ONDCP (Spring 1996), Pulse Check of 17 urban areas/4 regions.

able local and regional variations in drug use prevalence and incidence, supply of and demand for different drug types and forms, prices and purities, and routes of drug use administration. An important source of national data is the National Household Survey on Drug Abuse (NHSDA), an ongoing survey of the civilian noninstitutionalized population of the United States aged 12 years and older (see Substance Abuse and Mental Health Services Administration [SAMHSA], 1996a). In spite of its importance, however, the NHSDA has limitations because it underrepresents hidden, hard-to-reach, and nonhousehold populations, such as the homeless, the institutionalized, and the incarcerated, whose rates of drug abuse tend to be higher. Because a disproportionate share of chronic drug users are represented in these population subgroups, estimates from the NHSDA are conservative (National Institute on Drug Abuse [NIDA], 1994). Other data sources, however, help to characterize the patterns of drug use in these subgroups. ONDCP has developed a strategy to estimate drug use at the national level by combining data from the NHSDA and the Drug Use Forecasting (DUF) system, a federally sponsored data system that monitors trends and patterns of drug use among arrestees.[3] The Drug Abuse Warning Network (DAWN), a SAMHSA-sponsored project that collects information on drug-related hospital emergency room episodes,[4] and NIDA's community-based studies of drug users, such as the Cooperative Agreement for AIDS Community-Based Outreach/Intervention Research Program (CA) and the Community Epidemiology Work Group (CEWG),[5] are other informational sources on the epidemiology and ethnography of drug abuse. Although estimates from each of these data sources are imperfect, they are the best and most current estimates available. In the following section, we refer directly or indirectly to these multiple data sources to describe patterns and trends in heroin, cocaine, crack, and methamphetamine use.

Heroin

Musto characterizes the history of heroin use in the United States, from the time of its original synthesis in 1874 to the 1990s, as one of cyclic patterns and trends. Heroin is a narcotic drug that can be injected subcutaneously and intravenously, smoked or inhaled (sometimes known as "chasing the dragon" [see Friedman et al., 1996; Kaplan, Janse, & Thuyns, 1986]), and snorted or sniffed. Changes in route of administration have been linked to a number of factors, including interpersonal group and peer pressures, prior injecting history, duration and intensity of noninjected use, knowledge of and attitudes towards injecting and the risk of AIDS, and price, purity, and availability (Friedman et al., 1996). For example, when heroin supply and purity are up, and costs are down, it is relatively easy to acquire for noninjecting use (i.e., by snorting and inhaling) (Friedman et al., 1996). These qualities may appeal to persons who are uncomfortable with use of needles and fearful of AIDS (Friedman et al., 1996). Heroin sniffers and snorters in New York City report that, by not injecting, they can enjoy the drug without losing control, hold down a job, and maintain social relationships with their friends (Friedman et al., 1996). Other noninjecting heroin users who also smoke crack cocaine indicate they fear needles and are concerned about AIDS, but find that snorting or smoking heroin helps them to ease down from a crack high. As Friedman et al. (1996) point out, "to the extent that noninjected use is a stage in a progression of noninjectors to injection, then the large pool of noninjecting heroin users presents a high probability of future HIV infections among those who begin to inject" (p. 49). The availability of high purity heroin is cited as one reason why noninjecting use has become a preferred mode of administration. However, if supply and purity decline while prices increase, noninjecting users—particularly those who have sniffed or snorted heroin intensively over a long period of time and have developed dependency—may "start to inject because of the increased efficiency of injecting" (p. 50).

Users report an immediate "rush" or pleasurable sensation from heroin that, at least initially, provides relief from symptoms of agitation and depression (Freitas, 1985; NIDA, 1997). Intensified and chronic use develops as the user becomes progressively more dependent on the drug, both psychologically and physically (Freitas, 1985; NIDA, 1997). As duration of use lengthens, addiction develops, and the user becomes increasingly preoccupied with drug-taking and seeking relief from "dope sickness" or the symptoms and signs of drug withdrawal. Withdrawal from heroin may begin within a few hours after the last dose was taken, beginning with relatively mild experiences of restlessness, insomnia, and yawning. Major withdrawal symptoms, including abdominal pain, nausea, fever, dehydration, hyperglycemia, diarrhea, and "fetal" posturing (Freitas, 1985), peak between 24 and 48 hours later. Although withdrawal symptoms usually subside within a week, some people have shown persistent signs for as long or longer than six months (Freitas, 1985; NIDA, 1997). In addition to the sickness of withdrawal, adverse health consequences may occur from consuming the drug itself—for example, by overdosing on high-purity heroin, by experiencing a toxic reaction to adulterants, or by using heroin in combination with other substances, such as alcohol, which magnifies its depressant effects. Unsafe injection practices, notably sharing syringes and ancillary equipment with persons who may themselves be infected, are critical risk factors for HIV. Sexual partners who begin to inject, peer groups, and other social and interpersonal relationships have been identified as risk factors for transitioning from noninjecting to injecting heroin use (Friedman et al., 1996). In addition, Neaigus et al. (1996) found that new injectors who share syringes and who have a high-frequency injector in their personal risk network also have a significant likelihood of becoming infected with HIV. The risk of HIV infection is substantial within the first year of injection, and for some injectors, increases with the duration of the user's injecting career.

Of the estimated 2.7 million chronic drug users currently in the United States, about 586,000 (22%) are users of heroin (ONDCP, 1996a). During the 1992–1995 period, the majority (73%) of out-of-treatment IDUs recruited to NIDA's CA Research Program were injecting heroin. Data collected from over 10,000 heroin IDUs participating in the research program show that they injected heroin an average of 56.4 times (a median of 40) in the past 30 days (see Table 8.2). Many are also polydrug users, often reporting the injection of cocaine or "speedball" (a mixture of heroin and cocaine) and thus increasing the number of occasions when they risk being exposed to or transmitting disease. In addition, two-thirds of the heroin injectors report smoking crack cocaine in the past 30 days, a drug that may seriously harm the health of the user, as discussed in a later section.

In the United States today, there are indications that the numbers of new and younger heroin users are increasing. Historically, heroin has been associated with older, injection drug users. Recent data indicate that this pattern is changing, however, with an increasing incidence in heroin use by younger persons who begin by snorting or smoking the drug (ONDCP, 1996a). In addition, many older users appear to be changing their patterns from heroin injection to heroin snorting and smoking. These changes have been partly attributed to the ready availability of high-grade heroin at low retail cost that is purer today than any recent time in history. For example, the National Narcotics Intelligence Consumers Committee (NNICC) Report on the supply of illicit drugs to the United States stated that the average nationwide purity of heroin in 1992 was 37%, compared to 26.6% in 1991 and to only 7.0% in the early 1980s (Drug Enforcement Administration [DEA], 1993). In New York City, a major hub for traffickers who smuggle heroin in from Southeast Asia (DEA, 1993), the purity of retail heroin has generally exceeded 60% since 1992, and averaged as high as 79.5% in mid-1995 (Frank & Galea, 1996). Although new heroin smokers and snorters have reported using the drug by these routes because of concerns about acquiring HIV and other infections from contaminated needles, many are at risk of transitioning to injected use as addiction develops or as the price and purity of heroin fluctuate (Friedman et al., 1996).

A critical factor in predicting the spread of infectious diseases is the extent to which mixing and interacting occur among persons who are unexposed and persons who are infected. If new injectors mix with partners, groups, or networks in which infectious diseases are endemic, the spread of blood-borne diseases will continue. Indeed, the risk of acquiring viral infections is extremely high in the first year after initiating injection drug use. A recent study of IDUs who had initiated injection within the last 6

TABLE 8.2

Past 30-Day Drug Use Patterns of Injection Drug Users (IDUs) and Crack Cocaine Users (CCUs) Enrolled in NIDA's Cooperative Agreement Program, 1992–1995

Type of Drug Injected or Smoked	All Drug Users Responding to Questions on This Drug	IDUs Using This Drug ≥ 1 Time in Past 30 Days	CCUs Injecting This Drug ≥ 1 Time in Past 30 Days	CCUs Not Injecting Any Drug Past 30 Days
Heroin	13,931	10,136	4,550	n/a
Mean no. of injections	41.1	56.4	52.4	
Median no. of injections	20	40	30	
Cocaine	13,690	8,123	4,343	n/a
Mean no. of injections	27.2	45.8	38.0	
Median no. of injections	20	40	11	
Speedball	13,962	6,739	3,171	n/a
Mean no. of injections	24.2	50.0	44.8	
Median no. of injections	0	20	15	
Amphetamines	13,707	888	339	n/a
Mean no. of injections	1.4	21.4	16.4	
Median no. of injections	0	9	5	
Crack	15,977	6,862	n/a	9,072
Mean no. of times smoked	74.8	57.2		88.1
Median no. of times smoked	30	20		30

years included a subsample of IDUs who had been injecting for less than one year. The prevalence of disease infection within the entire group was 65.7% for HBV, 76.9% for HCV, 20.5% for HIV, and 1.8% for HTLV. In comparison, prevalence among the group injecting for less than a year was 49.8% for HBV, 64.7% for HCV, 13.9% for HIV, and 0.5% for HTLV (Garfein, Vlahov, Galai, Doherty, & Nelson, 1996). This research underscores the potential for widespread transmission of blood-borne infections directly among IDUs and indirectly between IDUs and their noninjecting drug use and sexual partners.

Cocaine

Cocaine was first introduced in the United States during the 1880s (Musto, 1989). Like heroin, the patterns and trends of cocaine use in this country have been cyclic. In the United States today, cocaine hydrochloride (powdered cocaine) is injected, snorted, or smoked (by "freebasing" or converting the drug into crack cocaine). The NHSDA estimates that there were 1.4 million current (past month) users of cocaine in the United States in 1995 (SAMHSA, 1996a). By combining data from multiple sources, the ONDCP estimates that there were 2.1 million heavy (defined as "use at least weekly") cocaine users in the United States in 1993, accounting for over two-thirds of the nation's current cocaine consumption (ONDCP, 1996a). Many chronic cocaine injectors also inject other drugs, such as heroin, methamphetamine, and illegally diverted pharmaceutical agents (e.g., Dilaudid or hydromorphone), singly or in combination with cocaine, as in a "speedball" mixture.

Cocaine is a psychomotor stimulant that produces its most intense euphoric effects 3 to 5 minutes after injection, which then subside within 30 to 45 minutes. By contrast, heroin is a narcotic/analgesic whose effects begin to dissipate between four to six hours following the prior dose (Freitas et al., 1985). As a result, the two drugs are associated with different and unique injecting practices and risks of acquiring or transmitting infections. Cumulative data from cocaine injectors enrolled in NIDA's CA program between 1992–1995 are shown in Table 8.2. The data suggest that long-time cocaine injectors inject on fewer occasions over time than heroin injectors—that is, on an average of 12 days a month for a mean of 45.8 injections (median of 40) in the last 30 days. However, because cocaine provides a relatively short duration of euphoria, compulsive high-dose injectors are likely to binge, repeatedly injecting cocaine over a brief period of time (Gawin & Ellinwood, 1988). This characteristic pattern of frequent cocaine injection, often in a group of both new and experienced drug injectors, provides the context in which multiperson reuse of syringes and drug paraphernalia occurs. When new injectors mix with older, experienced injectors in such a high-risk context, particularly in areas with high levels of HIV/AIDS seroprevalence, their chances of being exposed to disease from contaminated blood increase substantially (Alcabes & Friedland, 1995).

Crack

In the mid-1980s, a new form of cocaine known as crack cocaine or "freebase" emerged and its use became widespread throughout the United States National surveys may not always make clear distinctions between crack cocaine use and powdered cocaine use. Estimates from the NHSDA, however, suggest there were over 400,000 current users of crack cocaine in the United States in 1995 (SAMHSA, 1996a), an estimate that has not changed significantly since 1988. In addition, many drug users only smoke crack, whereas others smoke crack and use injection drugs. For example, of 15,977 total crack smokers who participated in the NIDA Cooperative Agreement between 1992 and 1995, 6,862 (43%) also injected drugs in the past 30 days. This group smoked crack an average of 57.2 times (median of 20) and injected one or more other drugs 76.3 times in the last 30 days. The remaining 9,072 crack smokers were noninjectors who reported using crack a mean of 88.1 times in the past 30 days (median = 30) (see Table 8.2).

Crack cocaine is relatively cheap and easy to manufacture, transport, and sell. Because it is smoked, crack provides the user with a nearly instant, concentrated high that lasts for about 5 minutes and is highly addictive. Gawin and Ellinwood (1988) characterize the euphoric effects of cocaine as having a nearly immediate onset and a brief duration of less than 45 minutes, followed by rapid dissipation (often referred to as the "crash" of coming down from the high). They also describe addicted or compulsive use as resulting from either greater access to the drug and a marked escalation in dose, or when the user makes the transition from a more indirect or slower route of drug administration to one which is direct and immediate, such as from sniffing or snorting to smoking or injecting (Gawin & Ellinwood, 1988).

Crack use and unprotected sexual contact between multiple and anonymous partners over short periods of time are common occurrences in crack houses, where the drug is sold, bought, and used.[6] Just as a shooting gallery is the high-risk environment for infectious disease transmission among IDUs, a crack house is the context for high-risk sex-for-drug exchanges and for rapid spread of HIV and other STDs among its customers (Inciardi, 1993). But sex-for-drug exchanges also occur outside the crack house environment. For example, a study of young crack smokers and nonsmokers in New York, San Francisco, and Miami found that regular crack users (i.e., who used the drug at least 3 days a week over the past 30 days) were significantly more likely than nonsmokers to have engaged in high-risk sexual practices, including, for women, unprotected sexual work and, for men, anal intercourse, and, for both men and women, sex with a partner believed to be an IDU (Edlin et al., 1994). Crack smokers were also more likely than nonsmokers to have had multiple (in some instances, more than 50) sexual partners. The prevalence of HIV was highest among crack-smoking women (16.3%), followed by crack-smoking men (13.1%), nonsmoking men (9.7%), and nonsmoking women (7.3%).[7]

Although the epidemic of powdered and crack cocaine use may now be leveling off, there are indications that use of a strong, longer-lasting, and less expensive substitute for cocaine—methamphetamine—is becoming more prevalent. As discussed in the next section, many subgroups of the drug using population, as well as the communities in which they live, are experiencing significant increases in the use of methamphetamine, and in the health and social consequences associated with its use (ONDCP, 1996b, 1997).

Methamphetamine

Methamphetamine first emerged as a legal stimulant in the United States during the 1930s. Its prevalence of use was high during the 1960s and, after a period of relative quiescence, is again increasing, as are methamphetamine-related health and social consequences. A psychomotor stimulant, methamphetamine is referred to as "speed," "crystal," "crank," and "ice," and can be injected, snorted, smoked, or ingested in pill form. From the NHSDA, it is estimated that 4.1 million persons in the United States household population have tried the drug (SAMHSA, 1996a) and that between 760,000 to 1 million persons used methamphetamine in the past year (Greenblatt, personal communication, 1996). Estimates of current methamphetamine use are less precise than those for cocaine and heroin, partly because cocaine and heroin use have been at epidemic levels for more than a decade. By contrast, since the 1960s, methamphetamine has been associated with relatively small groups and geographical areas, such as motorcycle gangs in the Western United States (ONDCP, 1996b).

There are indications that patterns of methamphetamine use, however, are rapidly changing. ONDCP's *Pulse Check* (1996b), a compilation of reporting systems from treatment providers, police sources, and ethnographers, points to a significant methamphetamine problem on the West Coast. For example, treatment providers in several Western States have reported substantial increases in the numbers of clients entering drug treatment with methamphetamine problems. Ethnographers provide similar accounts, noting that many of the methamphetamine users today appear to be "converts" from cocaine, some of whom are also speedball users who are now mixing heroin with speed rather than with cocaine. Ethnographers and police sources in several parts of the country have observed that methamphetamine is gaining popularity in demographic groups that are generally viewed as naive to the hard drug scene, such as young clubgoers, suburbanites, high school students, and college or university students (ONDCP, 1996b). In addition, recent DUF drug test data from adult and juvenile arrestees in 23 cities show increases in methamphetamine use across the country, with 6% of all arrestees from all sites testing positive for the drug in 1995. In particular, eight cities in the West, Southwest, and Midwest reported significant increases in rates of methamphetamine use by arrestees in 1995, including San Diego, Phoenix, San Jose, Portland, Omaha, Los Angeles, Denver, and Dallas (ONDCP, 1997).

The ready availability of methamphetamine, along with its relatively low and stable price and ease of manufacture and transport, may account for its increased prevalence of use. In addition, Gorman, Morgan, and Lambert (1995) describe the very high-risk sexual practices of methamphetamine users, many of which involve anonymous sex with multiple partners over prolonged periods of time. Health departments in 11 cities and states between 1990 and 1993 reported that 16% of HIV-infected drug injectors had used methamphetamine as their drug of choice. Moreover, HIV-infected male IDUs who had sex with men were significantly more likely than heterosexual male IDUs to cite methamphetamine as their primary drug of choice (Diaz et al., 1994). The relationship between frequent methamphetamine use/injection and sexual risk behavior is an important bridge for the transmission of HIV and other serious infectious diseases between methamphetamine users and their sexual partners.

Thus far, we have discussed patterns of use of four major illicit drugs that are closely linked to the transmission of HIV and other infectious diseases. We will now describe the drug injection behaviors associated with transmission of blood-borne viruses.

INJECTION PRACTICES THAT RISK DISEASE TRANSMISSION

It is widely known from both epidemiologic and ethnographic studies that serial use of drug injection equipment such as needles and syringes exposes IDUs to the risk of HIV transmission (Alcabes & Friedland, 1995). Risks of disease transmission also result from indirect sharing practices (Clatts, Davis, Deren, Goldsmith, & Tortu, 1994; Koester, 1994; McCoy et al., 1994; Neaigus et al., 1996; Needle et al., 1997), including multiperson use of cookers (bottle caps or spoons that are used to dissolve drugs in water before injection), cottons (bits of cotton or cigarette filters to screen out insoluble adulterants when the drug is drawn into a syringe), and water (to mix drugs or to rinse and unclog a used syringe). A recent study by Shah et al. (1996) demonstrated the risks of HIV transmission from indirect sharing practices. They determined from laboratory analysis that HIV-1 DNA was present in visibly contaminated syringes as well as in paraphernalia and rinse water collected from shooting galleries in Miami. What is more, serial use of drug preparation paraphernalia may be a more common practice among IDUs than serial use of syringes, yet the extent to which IDUs are aware of the risks associated with indirect sharing is unclear (Koester & Hoffer, 1994).

Alcabes and Friedland (1995) review the epidemiology and natural history of HIV in drug injectors and the impact injection drug use has had on the course of the HIV/AIDS epidemic. They describe how, as long ago as the mid-1970s, HIV may have entered the IDU population in New York City—which was largely comprised of heroin injectors who began injecting during the 1960s. In the early 1980s, at roughly the time when AIDS was first recognized in homosexual men, powdered cocaine became widely available at relatively low cost. The authors posit that older heroin IDUs began to inject cocaine at about the same time as many of the new cocaine injectors; however, syringes were scarce because of highly restricted access at pharmacies and punitive syringe possession laws and policies. Consequently, many IDUs began to frequent "shooting galleries" to rent syringes and have a relatively secure place for injecting. This convergence of factors became pivotal in the subsequent and rapid dissemination of the HIV infection through the drug injector population and their sexual partners. As Alcabes and Friedland (1995) point out, "One could hardly imagine a better vehicle for dissemination of bloodborne infection[s]—sequential, anonymous sharing of needles and syringes contaminated with infected blood" coupled with the "effective mixing of individuals from different social groups and even geographic areas" (p. 1469).

EPIDEMICS OF INFECTIOUS DISEASES AMONG IDUs

This section addresses the co-occurring epidemics of infectious diseases that have so widely affected injection drug users, their sexual partners, and the infants of infected mothers. Table 8.3 presents the estimated incidence and prevalence of HIV, HBV, and HCV in IDUs. Current estimates indicate that approximately half of all IDUs are infected with one or both of the hepatitis viruses and 14% are infected with HIV (CDC, 1996a, 1996b; Holmberg, 1996; Hagan, Des Jarlais, Friedman, Purchase, & Alter, 1995; Levine, Vlahov, & Nelson, 1994; Murphy et al., 1996).

Human Immunodeficiency Virus (HIV)

HIV is a viral infection that reduces immune function and leads to opportunistic infections, wasting syndrome, neurologic disease, and other AIDS-related illnesses (see Table 8.4). It is transmitted by exposure to infected blood. HIV transmission among adults is primarily through multiperson use

TABLE 8.3
Estimated Cases of Selected Infectious Diseases in the U.S.

Infectious Disease[i]	Cumulative Cases: Reported (R) or Estimated (E)	Most Recent Year Cases: Reported (R) or Estimated (E)	Prevalence in IDU (Estimated)	Mortality Rates[a] and Other Comments
AIDS	Years: 1985–Jun 1996[c]	Jul 1995–Jun 1996[c]	n/a	Mortality: see data for HIV, below. 193,278 cases (36%) were attributed to IDU alone or combined with sexual contact (in persons > 13 years).
Total	548,102 (R)	72,416 (R)		
IDUs	140,467 (R)	18,587 (R)		
MSM and IDU[b]	35,218 (R)	3,198 (R)		
Heterosex w/ IDU	21,535 (R)	3,042 (R)		
HIV	Years: 1991–Jun 1996[d]	Jul 1995–Jun 1996[d]	14%[d]	Mortality: 16.2 per 100,000 in 1994. Multiple exposure risks include MSM and IDU, other sexual contact with IDU and/or crack users.
Total	80,476 (R)	14,799 (R)		
IDUs	14,857 (R)	2,517 (R)		
MSM and IDU	3,944 (R)	509 (R)		
Heterosex w/ IDU	3,438 (R)	631 (R)		
Hepatitis B Virus (HBV)	Through: 1994[e] 1,000,000–1,250,000 (E)	Year: 1994[f] 12,517 (R) 140,000 (E)	70–90%[f]	Mortality: 0.9 per 100,000 in 1994. Prevalence in IDU varies with injection history, geography, sexual orientation.
Hepatitis C Virus (HCV)	Through: 1994[f] 3,900,000 (E)	Year: 1994[f] 4,470 (R) 35,000 (E)	50–83%[g]	Mortality: 0.9 per 100,000 in 1994. Parenteral transmission is primary; sexual transmission is inefficient.
Tuberculosis (TB)	n/a	Year: 1994[h] 24,361 (R)	n/a	Mortality: 0.6 per 100,000 in 1994.

[a]CDC, 1996c.
[b]"MSM and IDU" refers to men who have sex with men and who inject drugs.
[c]CDC, 1996a.
[d]Holmberg, 1996 (assumes 204,000 cases in 1.5 million IDUs).
[e]CDC, 1996b.
[f]Levine et al., 1994.
[g]Hagan et al., 1995 (estimating 50–80%); Murphy et al., 1996 (estimating 65–83%).
[h]CDC, 1996d.
[i]Case reports meet the criteria for a laboratory confirmed case definition. Note: HIV, HBV, and HCV infections are likely underreported due to incomplete case information, asymptomatic or unreported infections, or different clinical and vital status surveillance practices among states.

TABLE 8.4
Characteristics of Infectious Diseases Common Among Drug Users

Disease	Agent	Classic Presentation	Diagnosis	Treatment	Prevention
HIV/AIDS	RNA Virus	Opportunistic infections, lymphadenopathy, neurologic disease	Serology	Antiretrovirals, antibiotics for opportunistic infections	Use of sterile injection equipment; use of condoms; safe sex practices; drug treatment
HBV	DNA Virus	Acute/chronic hepatitis	Serology	Supportive care	Use of sterile injection equipment; use of condoms; safe sex practices; vaccine; drug treatment
HCV	RNA Virus	Acute/chronic hepatitis	Serology	Supportive care; Interferon	Use of sterile injection equipment; no needle sharing; drug treatment; safe sex practices
TB	Bacterium *Mycobacterium tuberculosis*	Chronic upper lobe pneumonia	Culture, X ray, skin test, special stains	Multiple antibiotics	Avoid crowding; air filtration and circulation; infected persons must complete full antibiotic regimen
Gonorrhea	Bacterium *Neisseria gonorrhoeae*	Urethritis (males), cervicitis (females)	Culture, gram stain (males)	Ceftriaxone	Avoid unsafe sex practices with multiple partners; use of condoms
Syphilis	Bacterium *Treponema pallidum*	3 stages: 1-chancre, 2-rash and fever, 3-neurosyphilis, cardiovascular disease	Serology, CSF exam, Darkfield exam	Penicillin by injection	Avoid unsafe sex practices with multiple partners; use of condoms
Chlamydia	*Chlamydia trachomatis*	Urethritis (males), cervicitis (females)	Tissue culture, enzyme immunoassay, fluorescent antibody	Doxycycline	Avoid unsafe sex practices with multiple partners; use of condoms

of contaminated syringes and other drug injection equipment or through unprotected sexual contact with an infected partner. Pediatric AIDS occurs most frequently as a result of vertical transmission, when an infant is exposed to the infection from an HIV seropositive mother.

Between 1981 and mid-1996, a cumulative total of 540,806 AIDS cases in adults aged 13 and over in the United States had been reported to the Centers for Disease Control and Prevention. Although 51% of the cases (274,192 cases) were attributed to men having sex with men, a substantial proportion (36%, or 193,278 cases) were directly related to injection drug use or to unprotected sexual contact with an IDU.[8] In addition, over half the cases (54%, or 3,942 cases) in children under age 13 were linked to a mother who injected drugs or to a mother's IDU sexual partner (CDC, 1996a). The dynamics of HIV/AIDS epidemiology in the United States have shifted since the first cases were reported in 1981. An apparent stabilization in seroincidence among such high-risk populations as men who have sex with men is now partly offset by what Holmberg (1996) refers to as "troublesome subepidemics" now appearing in metropolitan statistical areas between Boston and Washington, D.C., in Miami, and in San Juan, Puerto Rico. These areas are experiencing relatively high HIV seroincidence rates among IDUs compared to areas like New York City and Los Angeles that previously had record numbers of incident cases and are now experiencing declines, or at least a stabilization (Holmberg, 1996). The size of at-risk IDU populations in the "subepidemic" cities is not currently known, but the estimate will likely increase if the new heroin smokers and snorters of today become the heroin injectors of tomorrow (Friedman et al., 1996).[9]

It is now estimated that there are 700,000 prevalent and 41,000 new HIV infections occurring yearly in the United States. Although geographic variation in serostatus is considerable, Holmberg (1996) estimates that nationally, the HIV seroincidence rate among IDUs is now almost twice that of men who have sex with men, or roughly 1.5 infections per 100 person years, for an annual total of 19,000 new infections. As Holmberg points out, the "HIV epidemic is now clearly driven by infections occurring among injection drug users, their sex partners, and their offspring" (Holmberg, 1996, p. 649). For example, 80% of the estimated 9,300 new infections that occur each year in persons whose exposure category is heterosexual activity have occurred among the heterosexual, non-IDU partners of HIV-positive IDUs. Moreover, 70% to 80% of persons infected through heterosexual contact are women, many of whom are the sexual partners of IDUs.[10] More specifically, the profile of the at-risk heterosexual today is emerging as a young, lower income, minority female who smokes crack, exchanges sex for drugs with multiple partners, and is or has been infected with other STDs such as syphilis and herpes (Holmberg, 1996).

Hepatitis: HBV and HCV

Hepatitis B and hepatitis C (HBV and HCV) are widespread viral infections among IDUs that may progress to chronic hepatitis, cirrhosis, or liver cancer. Persons with parenteral exposures (i.e., IDUs, transfusion recipients, and hemophiliacs) constitute one of the highest risk groups for both types of viral hepatitis (Hagan, Des Jarlais, Friedman, Purchase, & Alter, 1995). Among IDUs, many if not most infections are contracted soon after drug injection is initiated (Garfein et al., 1996). As Table 8.3 shows, HBV seroprevalence in IDUs is estimated at 70 to 90% or more, depending on the personal injecting history, geographical location, and sexual orientation of the IDU. The seroprevalence of HCV in IDUs varies by these same factors, and is currently estimated to range between 50% to 83% of IDUs in the United States (Hagan et al., 1995). In the general population, an estimated 3.9 million Americans are currently infected with HCV, and an estimated 8,000 to 10,000 deaths each year result from HCV-associated chronic liver disease (Alter 1997; CDC 1996b).

HBV is readily transmitted from exposure to contaminated blood or blood products, which makes injection drug use a principal risk behavior for the disease. In a review of 25 national and international studies on the prevalence of HBV seromarkers in IDUs between 1989 and 1991, Levine and others (1994) found that IDU exposure to HBV was more common than not, especially if the IDUs were not in treatment. Of the 9,566 IDUs tested in the studies, an estimated 74% were HBV seropositive; the prevalence of HBV ranged between 38% to 99% among IDUs in drug treatment, and between 81% to 87% among not-in-treatment IDUs. In a study of 2,558 IDUs in Baltimore (Levine et al., 1995), a similar proportion—80%—of those who were not in treatment tested seropositive for HBV. In that study, predictors of HBV were related to IDU practices such as duration of injecting, injecting at least once daily, sharing needles, and using shooting galleries. Moreover, HBV infection was found to be strongly associated with HCV and HIV infections, but not to high-risk sexual activity or previous infection with other STDs. Similarly, the study by Garfein and colleagues (1996) identified unsafe IDU practices such as frequent injecting, injecting cocaine, injecting for more than 6 months, and not using needles packaged in sterile wrappers as significant risk variables associated with HBV and HCV, but not sexual risks such as men having sex with men.

Although injection drug-related transmission of HBV appears to be more efficient in IDUs than sexual transmission, the virus also spreads with efficiency through sexual contact (Alter et al., 1986). Since chronic HBV carriers are efficient reservoirs of infectivity, HBV seropositive individuals are bridges for rapid disease transmission to others exposed to their blood, semen, and saliva (Heathcote, Cameron, & Dane, 1974). Thus, IDUs who share drug injection syringes and paraphernalia, or who have unprotected sexual contact with their partners, are at high risk for acquiring and transmitting the infection. Moreover, a woman infected with HBV, whether an IDU herself or the sexual partner of an IDU, is very likely to transmit the HBV infection perinatally to her developing fetus or newborn infant (Chen et al., 1996).

HBV vaccines were introduced in the United States in the early 1980s and are among the safest and most efficacious vaccines available (Lemon & Thomas, 1997). HBV immunization is also widely recommended as one of the routine vaccinations for children, particularly in areas with endemic levels of HBV (Kane, 1995). The average wholesale costs per single-unit adult dose of HBV vaccine (excluding dialysis patients) is $57 (Lemon & Thomas, 1997), which is dwarfed by the social and medical costs for treating persons with chronic liver disease, hepatocellular carcinoma, and other HBV-related health consequences.

Other Sexually Transmitted Diseases

Other STDs, such as gonorrhea, syphilis, herpes virus, soft sore (chancroid), genital warts, and chlamydia, are common among drug users. STDs have serious health consequences in and of themselves, including sterility, cardiovascular damage, and genital sores or inflammation (cervicitis, urethritis). While some STDs are viral infections (e.g., HBV and HIV), others, like gonorrhea and syphilis, are bacterial, and are associated with diverse symptomatology and health outcomes. The incidence of gonorrhea is much higher than that of syphilis: in 1994, there were 418,068 new cases of gonorrhea reported to the CDC, versus 20,627 cases of primary and secondary syphilis (if the multiple stages of syphilis cases and congenital syphilis cases are combined, the total number was 81,696) (CDC, 1995; see also Table 8.3).

Recent patterns of gonorrhea and syphilis in urban areas appear as geographical clusters in relative proportion to the epidemic use of crack cocaine and its associated high-risk sexual behaviors (including unprotected sex with multiple partners, inconsistent use of condoms, and sex-for-crack exchanges; see also Fullilove & Fullilove, 1989). Factors related to gonorrhea rates in rural areas are similar to those in urban areas (e.g., sex-for-crack exchanges), but reinfection rates tend to be more common among men in rural areas and more variable between the genders in urban settings. The relatively higher rates of reinfection in rural communities have also been linked to fewer health care resources and a lack of anonymity, which may inhibit treatment seeking and willingness to admit having engaged in high risk sexual practices (Thomas, Schoenbach, Weiner, Parker, & Earp, 1996).

Nationally, gonorrhea and syphilis incidence rates have been on the decline since the mid-1970s. Nonetheless, there has been an increase in numbers of cases among females and younger age groups. While incidence rates in males continued to decrease in 1994, they rose among females, particularly in the younger age groups (10- to 14-year-olds and 15- to 19-year-olds). That these increases are associated with drug use is suggested by several studies in areas with high STD rates, which have identified positive serologies for STDs in young women as markers for crack cocaine and other illicit drug use as well as for high-risk sexual behavior, including sex-for-drug exchanges (Booth, Watters, & Chitwood, 1993; Edlin et al., 1994; Fullilove, Fullilove, Bowser, & Gross, 1990).

Tuberculosis

In the United States, infectious tuberculosis (TB) case rates had steadily declined since the 1950s, from a high of 53 per 100,000 population (84,304 cases) in 1953 to a low of 9.3 per 100,000 population (22,201 cases) in 1985 (CDC, 1996d). After 1985, however, along with the increased incidence and prevalence of HIV and AIDS, TB re-emerged as a national public health concern, with as many as 10.5 new cases per 100,000 population reported to CDC in 1992 (26,673 cases). The disturbing trend in new TB cases has since subsided, largely as the result of aggressive prevention, control, and disease surveillance strategies, including community-based outreach, directly observed therapy, and intensive follow-up. A mycobacterial infection (see Table 8.4), TB is commonly transmitted in airborne droplets from the sputum of infected persons. Susceptibility to TB is general, with increased risk to persons who are immunosuppressed, such as people who are HIV seropositive. For example, Selwyn and colleagues (1992) found that HIV-infected IDUs with cutaneous anergy (i.e., who were not responsive to the skin test for TB) were at high risk of TB. Antonucci, Girardi, Raviglione, and Ippolito (1995) report that persons dually infected with HIV and TB are most likely to develop clinically active disease.

The incidence of multidrug-resistant TB cases began to rise shortly after the emergence of HIV and the increased prevalence of AIDS, particularly affecting persons who are impoverished, immunosuppressed, and living in crowded conditions. Thus, because of their confined quarters and often poor ventilation, jails and prisons have been identified as potential reservoirs for TB. For example, Pelletier and colleagues (1993) reported that, in an outbreak of TB in a Nassau County (New York) jail, 58% of inmates who developed TB had a history of injecting drugs and 35% were HIV seropositive. Moreover, TB "clusters" or outbreaks have been reported among noninjecting drug users and their children and extended family members, such as the cluster of TB infections among 89 persons who resided in or frequented two crack houses in San Mateo County, California (Leonhardt, Gentile, Gilbert, & Aiken, 1994).

Previous sections of this chapter have focused on the epidemiology of drug abuse, injection drug practices associated with disease transmission, and epidemics of infectious disease among IDUs. The final section addresses prospects for prevention of drug abuse, as well as of the drug injecting behaviors that transmit serious infections to other drug users, their sexual partners, and their children.

PROSPECTS FOR PREVENTION

A number of research studies (Booth, Crowley, & Zhang, 1996; Chitwood et al. 1991; Rhodes & Malotte, 1996; Stephens, Simpson, Coyle, McCoy, & National AIDS Research Consortium, 1993; Wiebel et al., 1996) have shown that transmission of HIV and other infectious diseases can be prevented among drug users and their sexual partners by reducing drug use, unsafe needle use, and sexual risk-taking behaviors. Combinations of behavioral change interventions, including community-based outreach and risk reduction interventions, needle exchange programs, substance abuse treatment, interventions to reduce sexual risk behavior, and HBV vaccination programs, have been shown to provide an effective and multifaceted approach for reducing risk behaviors and preventing the spread of HIV, HBV, and other STDs (NIH, 1997).

Needle and Coyle (1997) describe the model for community-based outreach and HIV testing and counseling and summarize findings from a review of 36 publications on the efficacy of this approach for reducing HIV risk-taking and increasing the protective behaviors of IDUs. Community-based outreach, first developed and implemented as a drug treatment intervention strategy in Chicago in the mid-1960s, provided the basis for an adaptation of the street-based outreach model in the 1980s (Coyle, 1993; Wiebel, 1993) in response to the rapid spread of HIV among IDUs. Needle and Coyle (1997) report that community-based outreach interventions are effective in facilitating behavior change among many IDUs: For example, some IDUs will stop using drugs altogether, while many who continue to use will decrease their injection frequency, reduce or stop multiperson reuse of needles and other injection equipment, stop visiting shooting galleries, and routinely practice needle disinfection procedures.

Vlahov (1997) examined published research studies on the effectiveness of needle exchange programs (NEPs) for limiting the spread of blood-borne infections. Based on his review, Vlahov concludes that there is positive benefit from NEPs. Specifically, IDUs who participate in NEPs will change their drug-injecting behaviors (i.e., sharing and reusing contaminated syringes) and thus reduce their risks for HIV and other infections. Importantly, NEPs do not increase drug use among participants or the recruitment of new injectors (Vlahov, 1997). An in-depth analysis of NEPs in New York City by Des Jarlais et al. (1996) also found that IDU participation in NEPs leads to individual-level protection against incident HIV infection.

Metzger (1997) reviewed the research findings from numerous studies on the relation between substance abuse treatment and reduction in drug use–related risk behaviors among drug users. He concluded that drug treatment serves the goals of primary prevention by significantly lowering the rates of risk behaviors of in-treatment drug users, which in turn reduces the likelihood that they will transmit or acquire HIV and other infectious diseases. In particular, he observed that the results of different types of studies converged, including those that compare the behavioral risk patterns of IDUs in and out of treatment, before and during treatment, and during and after treatment, and those that use serologic data from cohorts of drug users to evaluate the role of treatment on HIV seroincidence and prevalence (Metzger, 1997). Moreover, treatment programs have great "prevention potential" (p. 95). That is, "as one of the few organized social institutions with access to drug users at risk of HIV infection, treatment programs have in many ways become the 'staging areas' for risk reduction interventions directed at IDUs" because drug users "who are in treatment provide access to a much larger community of drug users who are not in treatment" (p. 96).

In conclusion, this chapter has addressed the epidemiology of drug abuse, injection drug practices associated with disease transmission, epidemics of infectious disease among IDUs, and prospects for preventing the spread of new infections. While there has been considerable progress in controlling the spread of infections in drug users as well as in the general population, there is still a long way to go. Future challenges include the need to improve intervention approaches to reach chronic and "hidden" IDUs who, for whatever reason, continue to practice high-risk injection behaviors, to strengthen effective interventions so that IDUs who have modified their risks are given periodic reinforcement of their behavioral change, and, if they have not entered drug treatment, encouragement to do so, and finally, to enhance community-based outreach efforts aimed at intense users of noninjecting drugs so that they fully appreciate the risks of noninjecting drug use and are discouraged from ever starting to use injection drugs.

NOTES

1. Brecher (1941) provides details on drug injection practices of heroin addicts in Cairo; Crane (1991) also posits that intravenous injection methods originated in Egypt, where merchant seamen learned the procedures and exported them to the United States.

2. While this chapter focuses on high-risk and chronic drug users, infections such as HIV, the hepatitis viruses, TB, and other STDs can occur in all populations—drug users, however infrequent the use, as well as nonusers—who may interact with infected people. The probability of becoming infected from exposure to a pathogen is largely a function of unsafe

interpersonal mixing patterns, whether drug-related or sexual, with transmission probabilities increasing with the numbers of partners (Blower & Boe, 1993).

3. Under the aegis of the National Institute of Justice (1996), the DUF system administers interviews and collects/screens anonymous, voluntarily provided urine samples from adult male booked arrestees in 23 United States sites, adult female booked arrestees in 21 sites, and juvenile male arrestees/detainees in 12 sites.

4. DAWN is an ongoing, voluntary, and confidential survey of a probability sample of non-federal, short-stay general hospitals with 24-hour emergency departments in the United States. In five metropolitan statistical areas, all eligible hospitals have been selected for the sample; in 16 MSAs, a sample of hospitals has been selected; and in areas outside these 21 MSAs, hospitals have been assigned to a National Panel and sampled. Of 634 eligible hospitals, 489 (77%) participated in DAWN in the first half of 1995 (data are collected and released semiannually).

5. The CA Research Program monitors HIV serostatus and risk behaviors and delivers/evaluates risk reduction interventions targeted to not-in-treatment drug users recruited through street outreach in 23 communities across the United States, Puerto Rico, and Brazil. Data collection began in January 1992; as of December 1995, the database contained detailed behavioral and demographic information on nearly 23,500 multiethnic male and female IDUs and crack users. CEWG is a network of researchers from 20 sentinel metropolitan areas of the United States and selected foreign countries who meet semiannually to provide ongoing community-level public health surveillance of drug abuse from analysis and discussion of quantitative and qualitative research data.

6. Recommended reading on this topic is *Crack Pipe as Pimp* (Ratner, 1993), a compendium of findings from an eight-city ethnographic study of crack cocaine smoking and its role in making sex-for-drug exchanges a common practice of crack addicts who have no other resources for acquiring the drug.

7. Compounding the health and behavioral consequences of crack abuse, the implements or paraphernalia used for smoking may themselves be associated with an increased risk for HIV transmission, as they may cause burns and ulcerations that are open to infection if users share smoking paraphernalia or engage in unprotected oral sexual activity. For example, Porter (1993) identified the use of metal tubes and car antennae as a popular way to smoke crack in Philadelphia, although the heated metal produced blisters and burns on the users' lips. Similarly, glass pipes used to smoke crack often chip and cut users' lips.

8. Specifically, 32% (161,891) of AIDS cases were attributed to IDU and 4% (18,710) were attributed to unprotected heterosexual contact with an IDU.

9. As noted earlier, research by Garfein and colleagues (1996) indicates that the period of greatest risk for transmission of infectious diseases in IDUs occurs immediately after they initiate injection as a route of drug administration.

10. Among heterosexuals who have contact with IDUs or with bisexual men, the estimated HIV seroincidence rate is 0.5 per 100 person years (Holmberg, 1996).

REFERENCES

Alcabes, P., & Friedland, G. (1995). Injection drug use and human immunodeficiency virus infection. *Clinical Infectious Diseases, 20,* 1467–1479.

Alter, M. J. (1997). Epidemiology of hepatitis C. In *Management of hepatitis C* (pp. 67–74). NIH Consensus Development Conference (Programs & Abstracts). NIH/OMAR.

Alter, M. J., Ahlone, J., Weisfuse, I., Starko, K., Vacalis, T. D., & Maynard, J. E. (1986). Hepatitis B virus transmission between heterosexuals. *Journal of the American Medical Association 256*, 1307–1310.

Antonucci, G., Girardi, E., Raviglione, M. C., & Ippolito, G. (1995). Risk factors for tuberculosis in HIV-infected persons; A prospective cohort study. *Journal of the American Medical Association, 274*, 143–148.

Blower, S. M., & Boe, C. (1993). Sex acts, sex partners, and sex budgets: Implications for risk factor analysis and estimation of HIV transmission probabilities. *Journal of Acquired Immune Deficiency Syndromes, 6*, 1347–1352.

Booth, R., Crowley, T. J., & Zhang, Y. (1996). Substance abuse treatment entry, retention, and effectiveness: Out-of-treatment opiate injection drug users. *Drug and Alcohol Dependence, 42*, 11–20.

Booth, R. E., Watters, J. K., & Chitwood, D. D. (1993). HIV risk-related sex behaviors among injection drug users, crack smokers, and injection drug users who smoke crack. *American Journal of Public Health, 83*, 1144–1148.

Brecher, E. M. (1941, February). The case of the missing mosquitoes. *Reader's Digest, 56*.

Centers for Disease Control and Prevention. Division of STD Prevention. (1995). *Sexually Transmitted Disease Surveillance, 1994*. U.S. Department of Health and Human Services, Public Health Service. Atlanta: Author.

Centers for Disease Control and Prevention. (1996a). *HIV/AIDS Surveillance Report* (midyear edition, 8, no. 1). U.S. Department of Health and Human Services, Public Health Service. Atlanta: Author.

Centers for Disease Control and Prevention. Hepatitis Branch. (1996b). *Tabular published and unpublished data on disease burden from viral hepatitis A, B, and C in the United States*. Atlanta: Author.

Centers for Disease Control and Prevention. National Center for Health Statistics. (1996c). *Advanced report of final mortality statistics, 45*, supplement. Atlanta: Author.

Centers for Disease Control and Prevention. Division of TB Elimination. (1996d). *Tuberculosis cases and death rate data: United States, 1953–1994*. U.S. Department of Health and Human Services, Public Health Service. Atlanta: Author.

Centers for Disease Control and Prevention. (1997). *MMWR, 46*, 165–173.

Chen, H., Chang, M., Ni, Y., Hsu, H., Lee, P., Lee, C., & Chen, D. (1996). Seroepidemiology of hepatitis B virus infection in children: Ten years of mass vaccination in Taiwan. *Journal of the American Medical Association 276*, 906–908.

Chitwood, D. D., Inciardi, J. A., McBride, D. C., McCoy, C. B., McCoy, H. V., & Trapido, E. J. (1991). *A community approach to AIDS intervention: Exploring the Miami Outreach Project for injecting drug users and other high risk groups*. Westport, CT: Greenwood.

Clatts, M. C., Davis, W. R., Deren, S., Goldsmith, D., & Tortu, S. (1994). AIDS risk behavior among drug injectors in New York City: Critical gaps in prevention policy. In D. Feldman (Ed.), *Global AIDS policy* (pp. 215–235). Westport, CT: Bergin and Garvey.

Coyle, S. L. (1993). *The NIDA HIV counseling and education intervention model: Intervention manual*. Rockville, MD: National Institute on Drug Abuse.

Crane, L. R. (1991). Epidemiology of infections in intravenous drug abusers. In D. P. Levine & J. D. Sobel (Eds.), *Infections in intravenous drug abusers*. New York: Oxford University Press.

Des Jarlais, D. C., Hagan, H., Friedman, S. R., Friedmann, P., Goldberg, D., Frischer, M., Green, S., Tunving, K., Ljungberg, B., & Wodak, A. (1995). Maintaining low HIV seroprevalence in populations of IDUs. *Journal of the American Medical Association, 274*, 1226–1231.

Des Jarlais, D. C., Marmor, M., Paone, D., Titus, S., Shi, Q., Perlis, T., Jose, B., & Friedman, S. (1996). HIV incidence among injecting drug users in New York City syringe-exchange programmes. *Lancet, 348*, 987–991.

Diaz, T., Chu, S. Y., Byers, R. H., Hersh, B., Conti, L., Rietmeijer, C., Mokotoff, E., Fann, S., Boyd, D., & Iglesias, L. (1994). The types of drugs used by HIV-infected injection drug users in a multistate surveillance project: Implications for intervention. *American Journal of Public Health, 84*, 1971–1975.

Drug Enforcement Administration. (1993, September). *The National Narcotics Intelligence Consumers Committee (NNICC) Report 1992: The Supply of Illicit Drugs to the United States.* Washington, DC: DEA Intelligence Division.

Edlin, B., Irwin, K., Faruque, S., McCoy, C., Word, C., Serrano, Y., Inciardi, J., Bowser, B., Schilling, R., & Holmberg, S. (1994). Intersecting epidemics: Crack cocaine use and HIV infection among inner-city young adults. *New England Journal of Medicine, 331*, 1422–1427.

Frank, B., & Galea, J. (1996). Current drug use trends in New York City. In *Community epidemiology work group: Epidemiologic trends in drug abuse* (National Institute on Drug Abuse Pub. No. 96-4128, Vol. II, pp. 170–185). Rockville, MD: NIH/NIDA.

Freitas, P. M. (1985). Narcotic withdrawal in the emergency department. *American Journal of Emergency Medicine, 3*, 456–460.

Friedman, S. R., Perlis, T., Atillasoy, A., Goldsmith, D., Neaigus, S., Gu, X. C., Sotheran, J. L., Curtis, R., Jose, B., Telles, P., & Des Jarlais, D. C. (1996). Changes in modes of drug administration and in drugs that are administered: Implications for retrovirus transmission. *Publicacion Oficial de la Sociedad Española Interdisciplinaria de SIDA, 7*, 49–51.

Fullilove, M. T., & Fullilove, R. E. (1989). Intersecting epidemics: Black teen crack use and sexually transmitted disease. *Journal of the American Medical Women's Association, 44*, 146–153.

Fullilove, R. E., Fullilove, M. T., Bowser, B., & Gross, S. (1990). Risk of sexually transmitted disease among black adolescent crack users in Oakland and San Francisco, Calif. *Journal of the American Medical Association, 263*, 851–855.

Garfein, R. S., Vlahov, D., Galai, N., Doherty, M., & Nelson, K. (1996). Viral infections in short-term injection drug users: The prevalence of the hepatitis C, hepatitis B, HIV, and HTLV viruses. *American Journal of Public Health, 86*, 655–661.

Gawin, F. H., & Ellinwood, E. H. (1988). Cocaine and other stimulants. *New England Journal of Medicine, 318*, 1173–1182.

Gorman, M. E., Morgan, P., & Lambert, E. Y. (1995). Qualitative research considerations and other issues in the study of methamphetamine use among men who have sex with other men. In E. Y. Lambert, R. S. Ashery, & R. H. Needle (Eds.), *Qualitative methods in drug abuse and HIV research* (NIDA/NIH Pub. No. 95-4025, pp. 156–181).

Greenblatt, J. (1996). Office of Applied Studies, SAMHSA. Personal communication.

Hagan, H., Des Jarlais, D. C., Friedman, S. R., Purchase, D., & Alter, M. (1995). Reduced risk of hepatitis B and hepatitis C among injection drug users in the Tacoma syringe exchange program. *American Journal of Public Health, 85*, 1531–1537.

Heathcote, J., Cameron, C. H., & Dane, D. S. (1974). Hepatitis-B antigen in saliva and semen. *Lancet 1 (7847)*, 71–73.

Holmberg, S. (1996). The estimated prevalence and incidence of HIV in 96 large US metropolitan areas. *American Journal of Public Health, 86*, 642–654.

Inciardi, J. A. (1993). Kingrats, chicken heads, slow necks, freaks, and blood suckers: A glimpse at the Miami sex-for-crack market. In M. S. Ratner (Ed.), *Crack pipe as pimp: An ethnographic investigation of sex-for-crack exchanges* (pp. 37–68). New York: Lexington Books.

Kane, M. (1995). Global programme for control of hepatitis B infection. *Vaccine, 13*, S47–S49.

Kaplan, C. D., Janse, H. J., & Thuyns, H. (1986). Heroin smoking in the Netherlands. In *Community epidemiology work group: Epidemiologic trends in drug abuse* (pp. 35–42). Rockville, MD: National Institute on Drug Abuse.

Koester, S. (1994). The context of risk: Ethnographic contributions to the study of drug use and HIV. In R. J. Battjes, Z. Sloboda, & W. C. Grace (Eds.), *The context of HIV risk among drug users and their sexual partners* (NIDA/NIH Pub. No. 94-3750, pp. 202–217).

Koester, S., & Hoffer, L. (1994). "Indirect sharing": Additional HIV risks associated with drug injection. *AIDS & Public Health Policy, 9*, 100–105.

Lemon, S. M., & Thomas, D. L. (1997). Vaccines to prevent viral hepatitis. *New England Journal of Medicine, 336,* 196–204.

Leonhardt, K. K., Gentile, F., Gilbert, B. P., & Aiken, M. (1994). A cluster of tuberculosis among crack house contacts in San Mateo County, California. *American Journal of Public Health, 84,* 1834–1836.

Levine, O. S., Vlahov, D., Koehler, J., Cohn, S., Spronk, A., & Nelson, K. (1995). Seroepidemiology of hepatitis B virus in a population of IDUs. *American Journal of Epidemiology, 142,* 331–341.

Levine, O. S., Vlahov, D., & Nelson, K. (1994). Epidemiology of hepatitis B virus infections among IDUs: Seroprevalence, risk factors, and viral interactions. *Epidemiologic Reviews, 16,* 418–436.

McCoy, C. B., Shapshak, S. M., Shah, S. M., McCoy, H. V., Rivers, J. E., Page, B. J., Chitwood, D. D., Weatherby, N. L. Inciardi, J. A., McBride, D. C., Mash, D. C., & Watters, J. D. (1994). HIV-1 prevention: Interdisciplinary studies and reviews on efficacy of bleach and compliance to bleach prevention protocols. In *Proceedings, workshop on needle exchange and bleach distribution programs* (pp. 255–283). Washington, DC: National Academy Press.

Metzger, D. (1997). Drug abuse treatment as AIDS prevention. In *Interventions to prevent HIV risk behaviors* (pp. 93–98). Washington, DC: NIH Consensus Development Conference (Programs & Abstracts). NIH/OMAR.

Murphy, E. L., Bryzman, S., Williams, A. E., Co-Chien, H., Schreiber, G. B., Ownby, H. E., Gilcher, R. O., Kleinman, S. H., Matijas, L., Thomson, R. A., Nemo, G. J., (1996), for the *REDS* Investigators. Demographic determinants of hepatitis C virus seroprevalence among blood donors. *Journal of the American Medical Association, 275,* 995–1000.

Musto, D. F. (1989, Summer). America's first cocaine epidemic. *Wilson Quarterly,* 59–64.

Musto, D. F. (1991, July). Opium, cocaine and marijuana in American history. *Scientific American,* 40–47.

National Institute of Justice. (1996). *1995 drug use forecasting: Annual report on adult and juvenile arrestees.* Washington, DC: U.S. Department of Justice/NIJ.

National Institute on Drug Abuse. (1994). *Metropolitan area drug study: Prevalence of drug use in the DC metropolitan area household and nonhousehold populations, 1991* (Technical Report #8). Rockville, MD: NIH/NIDA.

National Institute on Drug Abuse. (1996). *Community epidemiology work group: Epidemiologic trends in drug abuse* (Vol. I and II., Pub. No. 96-4128). Rockville, MD: NIH/NIDA.

National Institute on Drug Abuse. (1997). *Heroin abuse and addiction* (NIDA Research Report Series, NIH Publication No. 97-4165). Rockville, MD: NIH/NIDA.

National Institutes of Health. (1987). *Interventions to prevent HIV risk behaviors (programs & abstracts).* NIH Consensus Development Conference.

Neaigus, A., Friedman, S. R., Jose, B., Goldstein, M., Curtis, R., Ildefonso, G., & Des Jarlais, D. (1996). High-risk personal networks and syringe sharing as risk factors for HIV infection among new drug injectors. *Journal of Acquired Immune Deficiency Syndromes & Human Retrovirology, 11,* 499–509.

Needle, R. H., & Coyle, S. (1997). Community-based outreach risk-reduction strategy to prevent HIV risk behaviors in out-of-treatment injection drug users. In *Interventions to prevent HIV risk behaviors* (pp. 81–86). NIH Consensus Development Conference (Programs & Abstracts). NIH/OMAR.

Needle, R. H., Coyle, S., Cesari, H., Trotter, R. T., Koester, S., Clatts, M. C., Price, L., McClellan, E., Finlinson, A., Bluthenthal, R., Pierce, T., Johnson, J., Jones, S., & Williams, M. (1997). HIV risk behaviors associated with the injection process: Multiperson use of drug injection equipment and paraphernalia in IDU networks. *Substance Use and Misuse.*

Normand, J., Vlahov, D., & Moses, L. (Eds.). (1995). *Preventing HIV transmission: The role of sterile needles and bleach.* Washington, DC: National Academy Press.

Office of National Drug Control Policy. (1996a). *The national drug control strategy: 1996.* Executive Office of the President.

Office of National Drug Control Policy. (1996b). *Pulse check: National trends in drug abuse.* Executive Office of the President.

Office of National Drug Control Policy. (1997). *The national drug control strategy: 1997.* Executive Office of the President.

Pelletier, A. R., DiFerdinando, G. T., Greenberg, A. J., Sosin, D., Jones, W., Bloch, A., & Woodley, C. (1993). Tuberculosis in a correctional facility. *Archives of Internal Medicine, 153,* 2692–2695.

Porter, J. (1993). Crack users' cracked lips: An additional HIV risk factor. (Letter). *American Journal of Public Health, 83,* 1490.

Ratner, M. S. (Ed.). (1993). *Crack pipe as pimp: An ethnographic investigation of sex-for-crack exchanges.* New York: Lexington.

Rhodes, F., & Malotte, C. K. (1996). HIV risk interventions for active drug users: Experience and prospects. In S. Oskamp & S. C. Thompson (Eds.), *Understanding and preventing HIV risk behavior* (pp. 207–236). Thousand Oaks, CA: Sage.

Rotheram-Borus, M. J. (1997). Interventions to reduce heterosexual transmission of HIV. In *Interventions to prevent HIV risk behaviors* (pp. 63–70). NIH Consensus Development Conference (Programs & Abstracts). NIH/OMAR.

Selwyn, P. A., Sckell, B. M., Alcabes, P., Friedland, G., Klein, R., & Schoenbaum, E. (1992). High risk of active tuberculosis in HIV-infected drug users with cutaneous anergy. *Journal of the American Medical Association, 268,* 504–509.

Shah, S. M., Shapshak, P., Rivers, J. E., Stewart, R., Weatherby, N., Xin, K., Page, J., Chitwood, D., Mash, D., Vlahov, D., & McCoy, C. (1996). Detection of HIV-1 DNA in needle/syringes, paraphernalia, and washes from shooting galleries in Miami: A preliminary laboratory report. *Journal of Acquired Immune Deficiency Syndromes & Human Retrovirology, 11,* 301–306.

Stephens, R. C., Simpson, D. D., Coyle, S. L., McCoy, C. B., & the National AIDS Research Consortium. (1993). Comparative effectiveness of NADR interventions. In B. S. Brown & G. M. Beschner (Eds.), *Handbook on risk of AIDS.* Westport, CT: Greenwood.

Substance Abuse and Mental Health Services Administration (SAMHSA). (1996a). *Preliminary Estimates from the 1995 National Household Survey on Drug Abuse* (Advance Report No. 18). SAMHSA, Office of Applied Studies.

Substance Abuse and Mental Health Services Administration (SAMHSA). (1996b). *Preliminary Estimates from the Drug Abuse Warning Network* (Advance Report No. 14). Washington, DC: SAMHSA, Office of Applied Studies.

Thomas, J. C., Schoenbach, V. J., Weiner, D. H., Parker, E. A., & Earp, J. A. (1996). Rural gonorrhea in the southeastern United States: A neglected epidemic? *American Journal of Epidemiology, 143,* 269–277.

UNAIDS. (1996, July). *The HIV/AIDS situation in mid-1996: Global and regional highlights. Fact Sheet.* New York: United Nations.

Vlahov, D. (1997). The role of needle exchange programs in HIV prevention. In *Interventions to prevent HIV risk behaviors* (pp. 87–92). NIH Consensus Development Conference (Programs & Abstracts). NIH/OMAR.

Wiebel, W. W. (1993). *The Indigenous Leader Model: Intervention Manual.* Rockville, MD: NIH/NIDA.

Wiebel, W. W., Jimenez, A., Johnson, W., Ouellet, L., Jovanovic, B., Lampinen, T., Murray, J., & O'Brien, M. (1996). Risk behavior and HIV seroincidence among out-of-treatment injection drug users: A four-year prospective study. *Journal of Acquired Immune Deficiency Syndromes and Human Retrovirology, 12,* 282–289.

9

Substance Abuse and Disability

Cynthia L. Radnitz
Dennis D. Tirch
Vincent P. Vinciguerra
Alberto I. Moran
Fairleigh Dickinson University
Veterans Affairs Medical Center

Health care professionals who treat individuals with a substance abuse disorder and a disability face a compounded challenge. Not only must they address the general issues of a substance abuse disorder, but also they must address issues that are unique to those with disabilities. This chapter highlights such issues, and examines the implications for treatment created by the interaction of given disabilities and the abuse of addictive substances.

Although there are some commonalities among disabilities, the diverse characteristics of different conditions present unique challenges to the professional. In fact, there is evidence to suggest that substance abuse in persons with acquired disabilities may differ from those with non-acquired disabilities.[1] Thus, the type and severity of the disability will have specific implications for treatment.

PREVALENCE

When investigating the prevalence of substance abuse in individuals with acquired disabilities, such as traumatic brain injury (TBI) and spinal cord injury (SCI), researchers have obtained estimates of abuse at the time of injury, pre-injury, and post-injury. A recent review of studies examining pre-injury drinking patterns among individuals with TBI revealed that at least one-third of patients with moderate to severe injuries had alcohol abuse problems and 36% used illicit drugs pre-injury (Kreutzer, Marwitz, &

Wehman, 1991). Regarding substance abuse at the time of injury, at least 50% of patients with moderate to severe injuries were intoxicated at the time of hospital admission. These findings support the contention that substance abuse plays a major causal role in TBI (Rohe & DePompolo, 1985; Seaton & David, 1990; Sparadeo & Gill, 1989). A comparison of pre-injury to post-injury substance abuse suggests there is a decline in the amount and frequency of consumption for most patients (Kreutzer et al., 1991). However, there remains a substantial percentage of survivors of TBI who are discharged from the hospital and return to using alcohol following rehabilitation (Seaton & David, 1990; Sparadeo & Gill, 1989).

The rate of pre-injury substance abuse is also higher among inpatients with SCI than in the population at large (Heinemann, Goranson, Ginsburg, & Schnoll, 1989; Heinemann, Mamott, & Schnoll, 1990). Heinemann and colleagues (1989) found that prior to injury, 65% of their sample of inpatients with SCI were problem drinkers, and 13% believed they needed treatment for alcohol abuse. On the other hand, Kirubakaran, Kumar, Powell, Tyler, and Armatas (1986) found that pre-injury substance abuse for those with SCI was less prevalent than in the general population. The discrepancy between these studies may be due to sampling from different populations, differences in the comparison samples, differences in latency from pre-injury, or differences in methodology (Radnitz & Tirch, 1995).

High rates of substance abuse intoxication have been noted at the time of spinal cord injury. Heinemann, Donohue, and Schnoll (1988) reported that approximately 62% of a sample of patients with SCI tested positive for alcohol or other drugs at the time of injury. In an investigation of post-injury substance use, O'Donnell, Cooper, Gessner, Shehan, and Ashley, et al., 1981–82) found that 68% of their sample of patients with SCI resumed use of alcohol or other drugs in the late stages of the rehabilitation process. Similarly, Radnitz et al., (1996) found a high prevalence of lifetime substance dependence (37.6%) but not abuse (6.4%) disorders in a sample with SCI. However, few patients met criteria for either current substance abuse (0%) or dependence (3.2%).

A large part of the literature concerning alcohol or other drug use in persons with disabilities pertains to individuals with hearing impairments. One study reported that drinking patterns of individuals with deafness are similar to those of hearing persons (Isaacs, Buckley, & Martin, 1979). Another study found the rate of alcohol problems in persons with hearing impairments to be between 10 and 20% (Boros, 1980–81; Dick, 1989). In 1984 it was estimated that approximately 10% of the 13 million people with hearing impairments in the general population were in need of substance abuse counseling, a figure which approximates that found in the general population (Steitler, 1984). Hence, it appears that substance abuse is no more prevalent in persons with hearing impairment than in the general population.

Despite concerns that the deinstitutionalization of individuals with mental retardation (MR) would provide these individuals with greater access to alcohol and lead to substance abuse problems (Krishef & DiNitto, 1981), recent reviews suggest that this concern is unfounded (Edgerton, 1986; Lottman, 1993). It has been estimated that only 15% to 40% of these individuals drink (Edgerton, 1986; Krishef, 1986) and 5% to 10% are heavy or abusive drinkers (Edgerton, 1986). In fact, the rate of substance abuse problems among persons with MR is probably lower than it is among individuals with other types of disabilities, as well as the general population (Edgerton, 1986; Greer, 1986; Lottman, 1993).

Little has been written concerning epidemiology of alcohol or other drug use disorders among individuals with visual impairment. According to one study, the prevalence of substance abuse in persons who are blind is 8%, a figure that parallels the general population (Peterson & Nelipovich, 1983).

To summarize, among persons with acquired disabilities the prevalence of substance misuse appears to be higher than that in the general population. In contrast, among those whose disabilities were typically not acquired, the prevalence of AOD misuse was at or below that found in the general population.

RISK FACTORS

Individuals with a substance abuse disorder and a disability face risk factors unique to their situation. These factors include the medical, psychological, and social challenges brought on by living with a disability, as well as problematic attitudes that may be imparted by medical staff, family, and peers (Pires, 1989).

Prescription medication misuse has been identified as a risk factor for these individuals (Willweber-Strumpf, Zenz, & Strumpf, 1992). Heinemann, McGraw, Brandt, Roth, and Dell'Oliver (1992) have observed that in a sample of 96 persons with spinal cord injury, 43% of the sample used prescription medication with abuse potential and 24% reported misuse of these drugs on at least one occasion. Hence, the frequent prescription of potentially abused medications to persons with disabilities is an identifiable risk factor in this population. Medication for chronic pain can lead to the development of substance abuse disorders (Vaillant, 1980). Thus, the presence of chronic pain may be a risk factor for developing substance abuse (Finlayson, Maruta, Morse, & Martin, 1986).

The particular character of the disability may also serve as a risk factor for the development of a substance abuse disorder. For instance, traumatic brain injury may increase sensitivity to the effects of alcohol, resulting in greater potential for addiction or dangerous levels of acute intoxication

(Zasler, 1991). Deafness impairs the individual's ability to verbally communicate, which in turn can bring on isolation, and substance abuse to relieve loneliness (Rendon, 1992).

Certain coping styles have been identified as risk factors for substance misuse among persons with disabilities. Examining substance abuse as a coping response, Heinemann, Schmidt, and Semik (1994) assessed drinking patterns in 121 persons with recent spinal cord injury. Pre-injury drinkers were found to use problem-solving coping strategies less frequently than others, to believe that alcohol would help relieve tension, and to think that drinking could facilitate better sleeping patterns and regulate affect. Certain behaviors and attitudes have also been found to correlate with higher substance abuse. Moore and Siegal (1989) assessed 57 orthopedically impaired college students and found that thrill-seeking behavior, sexual activity level, and higher scores on the Perceived Benefits of Drinking Scale correlated with high levels of substance abuse.

In accordance with the theoretical framework advanced by Moore and Polsgrove (1991), four personality characteristics are described as fundamental risk factors in the development of a substance abuse problem: low self-esteem, self-handicapping behavior, low self-control, and sensation-seeking behavior. Such traits regularly receive attention from workers on substance abuse, yet they are ambiguous in their definitions and are lacking in parsimony as logical constructs (Radnitz & Tirch, 1995).

Although research investigating peer pressure as a risk factor for substance abuse in individuals with disabilities is not abundant, there are a few studies that explore this connection. Heinemann, Schnoll, Brant, Maltz, and Keen (1988) found that 61% of individuals with recent spinal cord injuries cited a desire to be sociable as a reason for drinking. Desire for peer acceptance has been found to be a factor influencing the development of substance misuse in those with mental retardation (Moore & Polsgrove, 1991; Selan, 1976; Wenc, 1980–81) and deafness (Isaacs et al., 1979).

ETIOLOGICAL FACTORS

Etiological factors affecting the relationship between disabilities and substance abuse are influenced by whether substance abuse is the cause or the consequence of the disability. For instance, Glass (1980–81), in a study of individuals with visual impairment and alcohol disorders, has suggested the division of substance abusers with disabilities into two subgroups: 1) Type A—wherein substance abuse problems predate a disabling condition, and 2) Type B—in which substance abuse follows the onset of a disabling condition. Although, alcohol is used as a coping mechanism by both the Type A and Type B person with a disability, Type A individuals are conceptualized as having habitually relied upon substance misuse as a way of addressing affective disturbances. Accordingly, Type B individuals are more likely to be open to the development of more adaptive coping methods in psychosocial rehabilitation. Therefore, Type B substance abusers are more likely to recover from an addictive disorder.

Hepner, Kirshbaum, and Landes (1980/81) have discovered four primary etiological pathways underlying the development of an addictive disorder in persons with disabilities. First, individuals with a disability often have greater access to prescription medication due to real ongoing medical needs. Second, the excessive degree of frustration experienced by those with disabilities may lead to the use of alcohol and other substances as a means of coping through "escape." Third, substance abuse may arise as a way for individuals with disabilities to cope with their status as potentially oppressed minorities. While this oppression may not always take an overt form, it may arise from the difficulties of living in a culture that does not universally adapt itself to the needs of those with disabilities. Finally, Hepner et al. (1980/81) suggest that substance misuse might arise as a result of encouragement from health care professionals.

Numerous writers have put forward etiological explanations to account for substance abuse among individuals with specific disabilities. Alcohol and other drugs are involved in 61% of spinal cord injuries (Heinemann, Schnoll, et al., 1988) suggesting that hazardous use of alcohol and other drugs may lead to spinal cord injury (Anderson, 1980–81; Glass, 1980–81; Greer, 1986; Healy, 1993; Motet-Grigoras & Schuckit, 1986; Sweeney & Foote, 1982). Sparadeo and Gill (1989) found that in a sample of 102 patients with head injuries, 56% had a blood alcohol level that contributed to their accidents. Ingraham, Kaplan, and Chan (1992) have noted that substance abuse has been found to causally contribute to traumatic brain injuries, spinal cord injuries, and burns. In the case of lifelong disabling conditions, personality factors and methods of coping may be causal elements in the development of a substance abuse problem. For example, Glass (1980–81) has pointed to "over-identification" with their disability to be an etiological factor among substance misusers who are blind. In a similar vein, Watson, Boros, and Zrimec (1979–80) have suggested that a lack of trust in the larger, hearing culture can lead to alcohol abuse in individuals who are hearing-impaired.

CONSEQUENCES OF SUBSTANCE ABUSE

The adverse health related consequences of substance abuse have been well documented and include diseases of the liver, pancreas, brain, cardiovascular system, respiratory system, endocrine system, and musculoskeletal system. Additionally, persons with disabilities, whose health is already compromised, may be at increased risk for health problems if they abuse alcohol or other drugs. Pneumonia is more likely to develop in persons immobilized after a traumatic injury if they use alcohol (Yarkony, 1993). Persons with spinal cord injuries who drink excessively may stretch their bladders, causing them to lose reflexes and thus preventing control over urinary functioning (O'Donnell et al., 1981–82). Moreover, a chronically distended bladder may trigger dangerously high blood pressure. Zasler (1991) observed that alcohol abuse in persons with traumatic brain injuries can lead to a lowering of the seizure threshold, while heavy alcohol consumption increases the risk of reinjury and has been correlated with increased mortality (Krauss, Morganstein, Fife, Conroy, & Nourjah, 1989)

Substance abuse may lead to increased physical problems in persons living with disabilities due to neglect of self-care. Persons who have sustained traumatic injuries often have catheters placed in their bladders. Individuals who abuse alcohol or other drugs may neglect to catheterize or empty their drainage bags, thus risking urinary tract infections. Also, sitting in a wheelchair often requires frequent lifting to prevent the development of pressure sores. Heavy substance abuse may interfere with this practice, putting the patient at increased risk for pressure sores.

Substance abuse may place persons with disabilities at increased risk for medical problems by interacting with prescription medications. For those individuals with spinal cord injuries who are prescribed benzodiazepines for spasms, alcohol may potentiate the effect of the medication beyond what is clinically indicated (O'Donnell et al., 1981–82). Phenytoin, which is used by individuals with seizure disorders, may have an adverse interaction with alcohol (Zasler, 1991).

After a traumatic injury, substance abuse may adversely impact the rehabilitation process (O'Donnell et al., 1981–82). Frequent intoxication or hangovers may prevent adequate engagement in rehabilitation, resulting in failure to achieve functioning potential. Moreover, nervous system depressants such as alcohol and marijuana may impede movement required during rehabilitation.

Although having a disability may exacerbate the physical consequences of substance abuse, it may buffer the economic consequences (Radnitz, 1994). As a result, there may be fewer incentives for seeking help, as the economic consequences of substance abuse often motivate individuals to present for treatment. Nondisabled persons with addictive disorders often lose their jobs because of intoxication on the job, poor job performance, or excessive absenteeism. Persons with disabilities have a much lower rate of employment than those without disabilities, and they often receive disability compensation (DeVivo, Rutt, Stover, & Fine, 1987). Those receiving disability compensation need not be concerned about the impact of substance abuse on their income.

As with economic consequences, the presence of a disability may also serve to buffer interpersonal consequences. The censure of family and friends experienced by the nondisabled substance abuser may not be experienced by persons with disabilities. Again, the result may be fewer motivational factors for seeking substance abuse treatment. Based on clinical observation, O'Donnell et al. (1981–82) reported that families of individuals with traumatic spinal cord injuries may experience guilt over the injury. Persons with disabilities may be seen as unable to engage in a full range of pleasurable activities, and substance abuse may be perceived as one of the few pleasures of which they can partake.

TRAINING

Specialized training to address substance abuse in those individuals with disabilities has been advocated for administrators and for professionals working in rehabilitation and substance abuse settings. Administrators may need to be educated about methods to prevent substance abuse within their facilities (Heinemann, Schnoll, et al., 1988). Studies have shown that rehabilitation counselors tend to underestimate the prevalence of substance abuse in persons with acquired physical disabilities (Ingraham et al., 1992). Since knowledge of substance abuse is related to comfort in addressing substance abuse issues (Shade-Zeldow et al., 1990, cited in Heinemann, 1993), efforts should be made to educate professionals working in rehabilitation settings. For persons with acquired disabilities, education should focus on identification of substance abuse early in rehabilitation (Heinemann, 1993), especially in distinguishing between those whose substance abuse predated their injury and those who developed the problem after their injury.

Professionals working in rehabilitation settings should also receive education targeting inaccurate beliefs about substance use in persons with disabilities (Greer, 1986). Examples of these counterproductive beliefs include the following: believing that identification of substance abuse would increase stigmatization, or that persons with disabilities are so miserable or so bored that they need to abuse drugs, or that refusing a request for a tranquilizer or painkiller would be cruel or unethical, or that substance abuse problems do not even exist (Pires, 1989). To address these beliefs, Greer (1986) suggests that the rehabilitation team should be made aware of the signs and symptoms of substance abuse.

Although training is indicated for professionals working in substance abuse treatment settings (Boros, 1980–81; Dick, 1989; Rendon, 1992), the importance of tailoring the training to address the issues relevant to particular disabilities should be underscored. For example, to work with clients who are deaf, training in American Sign Language and other relevant skills should be given. Similarly, professionals who work with individuals with SCI should be familiar with pertinent issues like pain management, spasticity, and sexuality. Professionals working with persons with TBI or MR should be familiar with the consequences of cognitive impairment.

ASSESSMENT

Methods of assessing substance abuse in the general population overlap with those that are utilized for individuals with disabilities. However, while commonly used measures may be adequate for assessing substance abuse in the general population, they will not necessarily help the clinician understand how a substance abuse problem and disability interact within a given person. The clinician also must consider whether a change in the mode of administration is needed when assessing those with disabilities. For instance, while assessment of individuals with hearing impairments resembles that conducted in the general population, differences in communication necessitate modifications in procedures (Watson, 1983). Fluency in sign language, paper and pencil measures, lip reading, or an interpreter is essential for effective assessment (Steinberg, 1991). Furthermore, tests that have been standardized, normed, and validated for individuals with hearing impairment are scarce. In the past, clinicians have depended on tests that require minimal verbal instruction (Watson, 1983). More recent research has investigated the use of videotaped, translated, or otherwise modified questionnaires, interviews, and inventories (Steinberg, 1991). Additionally, individuals with hearing impairments and substance abuse face considerable stigmatization and potential isolation (Dick, 1989; Rendon, 1992; Steinberg, 1991). Therefore, if self-report is the only assessment method used, substance abuse problems may be underreported and the use of laboratory tests (e.g., urine toxicology) may be indicated.

For individuals with SCI, adaptations to the mode of assessment may need to be made if they cannot use their hands. In an attempt to adapt the administration of an assessment measure to suit those with SCI, Radnitz et al. (1996) modified their testing battery. Pencil and paper questionnaires were completed verbally when necessary, and motoric components of assessment were adjusted to the capacities of the patient. For example, the Mini-Mental State Exam (Folstein, Folstein, & McHugh, 1975) section requiring the subject to follow serial instructions typically involves the manipulation of paper. Participants were allowed to move a straw in their mouths and blow through it as a substitute for this task. Hence, the cognitive function assessed remained the same, despite the limitations imposed by the individual's disability.

Communication may also be an issue in the assessment of those who are visually impaired. Paper and pencil measures may need to be read to the person or translated into braille. When the mode of communication is altered among patients who suffer sensory impairment, the validity of the instrument is called into question. Although the modification of a measure may retain face validity, the character of responses recorded may be changed. Psychometric evaluation of existing measures adapted for persons with disabilities is needed.

TREATMENT

Although persons with disabilities require special treatment accommodations, there is debate whether programs for the general population can and should make these accommodations, and whether specialized treatment programs should be established. Ideally, a specialized treatment program would have staff dually trained in both substance abuse and the particular disability, would be fully accessible, and would provide an atmosphere where patients need not feel different because of their disability. Nevertheless, considering the proportion of individuals with disabilities who seek treatment for substance abuse problems, it is unlikely that many such programs could be established in a cost-effective manner.

Mainstreaming persons with disabilities into treatment centers designed for the general population presents its own challenges. Overcoming physical barriers requires the availability of ramps, wider doorways, and accessible bathrooms, as well as the provision of specialized vans or ambulances to transport persons in wheelchairs to program activities (Meyers, Branch, & Lenderman, 1988; Pires, 1989). Programmatic barriers are diverse depending on the nature and extent of the disability. For persons with MR or TBI who have cognitive impairment, alterations may need to be made in the content and presentation of program material: for example, shorter sessions, easier reading levels, and frequent repetition of material (Kiley & Brandt, 1993). For those who are blind, the presentation should be auditory or in braille. For those who are deaf, the presentation of material should be made visually or using American Sign Language, and teletypewriting (TTY) devices should be available. Indeed, the presence of a hearing impairment presents particular challenges both for communicating with staff and with patients. For some persons with SCI, MR, TBI, or amputation dressing and other activities of daily living require assistance so that additional time may need to be built into their schedules. Finally, provisions for aftercare may be especially challenging, because aftercare facilities such as AA and NA meetings are often not accessible.

Attitudes held by staff, other patients, and persons with disabilities may also act as barriers to treatment. In some substance abuse treatment facilities, policies have been implemented prohibiting the prescription of some psychotropic medications. This may act as a barrier to persons who need these types of medications for pain or spasticity secondary to the disability. Also, staff may be uneducated as to what the special care needs of persons with disabilities are or they may view the special accommodations necessary for them as a burden and, as a result, come to resent them. The attitudes of other patients may be a barrier to treatment if they function to make the persons with a disability feel excluded. Finally, attitudes may be held by those with disabilities that prevent them from seeking treatment. For example, they may fear being ostracized or self-conscious, as there are unlikely to be many others with their particular disability in a given treatment facility.

CONCLUSIONS

Persons with disabilities are confronted by a number of negative potential consequences when they engage in substance abuse behaviors. Many of these harmful effects are also faced by those without disabilities who develop alcohol or other drug use disorders. However, such problems may be compounded by the characteristics of a disabling condition. Furthermore, there are certain negative sequelae that are specific to given disabilities. Often, those with disabilities are susceptible to unique physical, economic, and social consequences. For example, both family members and health care professionals may express attitudes and engage in behaviors that fail to discourage substance abuse among persons with disability. Guilt, permissiveness, and a lack of understanding of the dangers of substance abuse disorders may combine with socially entrenched misperceptions of the rights and capacities of those with disabilities to encourage the abuse of drugs and alcohol.

A broad distinction can be drawn between substance-abusing individuals with acquired disabilities and persons with lifelong disabilities who suffer from substance abuse disorders. Higher prevalence rates of substance abuse disorders have been found among persons with acquired disabilities than have been found in the general population. Additionally, it has been suggested that substance abuse behaviors may play an etiological role in the acquisition of a disabling condition. Certainly, many individuals who suffer traumatic accidents do so while under the influence of intoxicating substances. Among individuals with non-acquired disabilities, the prevalence of substance misuse problems has been found to be low; however, certain conditions will result in distinct areas of concern for a clinician. The personality implications of a given sensory deficit, for example the lack of trust that those with hearing impairment reportedly feel for the hearing world may create treatment barriers as well as other clinical implications.

In both rehabilitation and substance abuse treatment settings, clinicians working with individuals with disabilities should receive training specific to the issues present in this population. Certain assessment measures may need to be modified to suit persons with disabilities. Potential solutions to such barriers to treatment as accessibility, communication deficits, and personal biases need to be empirically tested and reported on a wider scale. In fact, methodologically sound research on diverse topics in the area of substance abuse and disability is sorely needed to help improve the quality of service delivery to this population.

NOTE

1. In distinguishing acquired from non-acquired disabilities, we use the term "acquired" to refer to those disabling conditions that result from a traumatic injury, primarily spinal cord injury and traumatic brain injury. In doing so, we acknowledge that some persons considered spinal cord injured obtained their spinal lesion as a result of a disease, not a traumatic accident. We also acknowledge that some persons with other disabling conditions such as blindness or deafness, in fact, have acquired disabilities that resulted from traumatic injuries. With these caveats in mind, we nonetheless maintain the distinction of acquired/non-acquired, separating the two according to type of disability even though the distinction is imperfect. We do so because we believe the distinction is helpful for understanding aspects of substance abuse in disability such as prevalence and etiology.

REFERENCES

Anderson, P. (1980–1981). Alcoholism and the spinal cord disabled: A model program. *Alcohol Health and Research World, 5,* 37–41.

Boros, A. (1980–1981). Alcoholism intervention for the deaf. *Alcohol Health and Research World,* 26–30.

DeVivo, M. J., Rutt, R. D., Stover, S. L., & Fine, P. R. (1987). Employment after spinal cord injury. *Archives of Physical Medicine & Rehabilitation, 68,* 494–498.

Dick, J. E. (1989). Serving hearing impaired alcoholics. *Social Work, 34,* 555–556.

Edgerton, R. B. (1986). Alcohol and drug use by mentally retarded adults. *American Journal of Mental Deficiency, 90,* 602–609.

Finlayson, R. E., Maruta, T., Morse, R. M., & Martin, M. A. (1986). Substance dependence and chronic pain: Experience with treatment and follow up results. *Pain, 26,* 175–180.

Folstein, M. F., Folstein, S. F., & McHugh, P. R. (1975). Mini-Mental State: A practical example for grading the cognitive state of patients for the clinician. *Journal of Psychiatric Research, 12,* 189–198.

Glass, E. J. (1980–1981). Problems drinking among the blind and visually impaired. *Alcohol Health and Research World, 5,* 20–25.

Greer, B. G. (1986). Substance abuse among people with disabilities: A problem of too much accessibility. *Journal of Rehabilitation, 52,* 34–38.

Healy, P. C. (1993). Substance abuse in spinal cord injured people. *Psychosocial Process, 6,* 73–76.

Heinemann, A. W. (1993). Prevalence and consequences of alcohol and other drug problems following spinal cord injury. In A. W. Heinemann (Ed.), *Substance abuse & physical disability* (pp. 63–79). Binghamton, NY: Haworth.

Heinemann, A. W., Donohue, R., & Schnoll, S. (1988). Alcohol use by persons with recent spinal cord injury. *Archives of Physical Medicine & Rehabilitation, 69,* 619–624.

Heinemann, A. W., Goranson, N., Ginsburg, K., & Schnoll, S. (1989). Alcohol use and activity patterns following spinal cord injury. *Rehabilitation Psychology, 34,* 191–204.

Heinemann, A. W., Mamott, B. D., & Schnoll, S. (1990). Substance use by persons with recent spinal cord injuries. *Rehabilitation Psychology, 35,* 217–228.

Heinemann, A. W., McGraw, T. E., Brandt, M. J., Roth, E., & Dell'Oliver, C. (1992). Prescription medication misuse among persons with spinal cord injuries. *International Journal of the Addictions, 27,* 301–316.

Heinemann, A. W., Schmidt, M. F., & Semik, P. (1994). Drinking patterns, drinking expectancies, and coping after spinal cord injury. *Rehabilitation Counseling Bulletin, 38,* 35–51.

Heinemann, A. W., Schnoll, S., Brandt, M., Maltz, R., & Keen, M. (1988). Toxicology screening in acute spinal cord injury. *Clinical and Experimental Research, 12,* 815–819.

Hepner, R., Kirshbaum, H., & Landes, D. (1980–1981). Counseling substance abusers with additional disabilities: The center for independent living. *Alcohol Health and Research World, 5,* 11–15.

Ingraham, K., Kaplan, S., & Chan, F. (1992). Rehabilitation counselor's awareness of client alcohol abuse patterns. *Journal of Applied Rehabilitation Counseling, 23,* 18–22.

Isaacs, M., Buckley, G., & Martin, D. (1979). Patterns of drinking among the deaf. *American Journal of Drug and Alcohol Abuse, 6,* 463–476.

Kiley, D., & Brandt, M. (1993). Issues and controversies in chemical dependence services for persons with physical disabilities. In A. W. Heinemann (Ed.), *Substance abuse & physical disability* (pp. 259–269). Binghamton, NY: Haworth.

Kirubakaran, V. R., Kumar, N., Powell, B. J., Tyler, A. J., & Armatas, P. J. (1986). Survey of alcohol and drug misuse in spinal cord injured veterans. *Journal of Studies on Alcohol, 47,* 223–226.

Krauss, J. F., Morgenstein, H., Fife, D., Conroy, C., & Nourjah, P. (1989). Blood alcohol tests, prevalence of involvement, and outcomes following brain injury. *American Journal of Public Health, 79,* 294–299.

Kreutzer, J. S., Marwitz, J. H., & Wehman, P. H. (1991). Substance abuse assessment and treatment in vocational rehabilitation for persons with brain injury. *Journal of Head Trauma Rehabilitation, 6,* 12–23.

Krishef, C. H. (1986). Do the mentally retarded drink? A study of their alcohol usage. *Journal of Alcohol and Drug Education, 31,* 64–70.

Krishef, C. H., & DiNitto, D. M. (1981). Alcohol abuse among mentally retarded individuals. *Mental Retardation, 19,* 151–155.

Lottman, T. J. (1993). Access to generic substance abuse services for persons with mental retardation. *Journal of Alcohol and Drug Education, 39,* 41–55.

Meyers, A. R., Branch, L. G., & Lenderman, R. I. (1988). Alcohol, tobacco, and cannabis use by independently living adults with major disabling conditions. *International Journal of the Addictions, 23,* 671–685.

Moore, D., & Polsgrove, L. (1991). Disabilities, developmental handicaps, and substance misuse: A review. *International Journal of the Addictions, 26,* 65–90.

Moore, D., & Siegal, H. (1989). Double trouble: Alcohol and other drug use among orthopedically impaired college students. *Alcohol Health and Research World, 13,* 118–123.

Motet-Grigoras, C. N., & Schuckit, M. A. (1986). Depression and substance abuse in handicapped young men. *Journal of Clinical Psychology, 47,* 234–237.

O'Donnell, J. J., Cooper, J. E., Gessner, J. E., Shehan, I., & Ashley, J. (1981–1982). Alcohol, drugs, and spinal cord injury. *Alcohol Health and Research World, 4,* 27–30.

Peterson, J., & Nelipovich, M. (1983). Alcoholism and the visually impaired client. *Journal of Visual Impairment and Blindness, 77,* 345–347.

Pires, M. (1989). Substance abuse, the silent saboteur in rehabilitation. *Nursing Clinics in North America, 24,* 291–296.

Radnitz, C. L. (1994). Economic factors and the spinal cord injured substance abuser. *SCI Psychosocial Process, 7,* 123–125.

Radnitz, C. L., Broderick, C. P., Perez-Strumolo, L., Tirch, D., Festa, J., Schlein, I., Walczak, S., Willard, J., Lillian, L. B., & Binks, M. (1996). The prevalence of psychiatric disorders in veterans with spinal cord injury: A controlled comparison. *Journal of Nervous and Mental Disease, 184,* 431–433.

Radnitz, C. L., & Tirch, D. (1995). Substance misuse in individuals with spinal cord injury. *International Journal of the Addictions, 30,* 1117–1140.

Rendon, M. E. (1992). Deaf culture and alcohol and substance abuse. *Journal of Substance Abuse Treatment, 9,* 103–110.

Rohe, D. E., & DePompolo, R. W. (1985). Substance abuse policies in rehabilitation medicine departments. *Archives of Physical Medicine & Rehabilitation, 66,* 701–703.

Seaton, J. D., & David, C. O. (1990). Family role in substance abuse and traumatic brain injury rehabilitation. *Journal of Head Trauma Rehabilitation, 5,* 41–46.

Selan, B. H. (1976). Psychotherapy with the developmentally disabled. *Health and Social Work, 1,* 73–85.

Sparadeo, F. R., & Gill, D. (1989). Effects of prior alcohol use on head injury recovery. *Journal of Head Trauma Rehabilitation, 4,* 75–82.

Steinberg, A. (1991). Issues in providing mental health services to hearing impaired persons. *Hospital and Community Psychiatry, 42,* 380–389.

Steitler, K. A. L. (1984). Substance abuse and the deaf adolescent. In G. B. Anderson & D. Watson (Eds.), *The habilitation and rehabilitation of deaf adolescents.* Wagoner, AR: University of Arkansas Rehabilitation Research and Training Center on Deafness and Hearing-Impairment.

Sweeney, T. T., & Foote, J. E. (1982). Treatment of drug and alcohol abuse in spinal cord injury veterans. *International Journal of the Addictions, 17,* 897–904.

Vaillant, G. E. (1980). Natural history of male psychological health: Antecedents of alcoholism and orality. *American Journal of Psychiatry, 137,* 181–186.

Watson, D. (1983). Substance abuse services for deaf clients: A question of accessibility. *Readings in Deafness, 7,* 13–16.

Watson, E. W., Boros, A., & Zrimec, G. L. (1979–1980). Mobilization of services for deaf alcoholics. *Alcohol Health and Research World, 4,* 33–38.

Wenc, F. (1980–1981). The developmentally disabled substance abuser. *Alcohol Health and Research World, 5,* 42–46.

Willweber-Strumpf, A., Zenz, M., & Strumpf, F. (1992). Medikamentenadhangigkeit bei der Therapie chronischer Schmerzen. *Z. Gesamte Inn. Med.* (Germany), *47,* 312–317.

Yarkony, G. M. (1993). Medical complications in rehabilitation. In A. W. Heinemann (Ed.), *Substance abuse & physical disability* (pp. 93–105). Binghamton, NY: Haworth.

Zasler, N. D. (1991). Neuromedical aspects of alcohol use following traumatic brain injury. *Journal of Head Trauma Rehabilitation, 6,* 78–80.

10

Managed Care and Substance Abuse Treatment

Janice L. Pringle
Linda R. Kostyak
Michael T. Flaherty
St. Francis Medical Center

According to the National Comorbidity Survey, 1991, an estimated 20 million people in the United States have substance abuse disorders. An additional eight million people are estimated to have substance abuse disorders coexistent with other mental disorders (Kessler, McGonagle, Zhao, & Nelson, 1994). When measured in terms of health, productivity, and crime, the estimated economic cost of substance abuse to the nation is a staggering $166 billion per year (Rouse, 1995). On the other hand, an estimated $7 billion is spent annually for treatment of substance use disorders (U.S. Dept. of Health & Human Services, 1989), thus suggesting that people with substance use disorders do not often receive professional help (Kessler et al., 1994). Reasons that account for this discrepancy include the residual effects of historical stigmatization, societal denial of the problem, and treatment systems that fail to adequately address methods for improving access and retention.

In recent years, many employers, policymakers, and consumers have looked to the evolving system of managed health care to control escalating health care costs and improve treatment availability and clinical outcomes for people with substance abuse disorders. However, health care professionals and other consumers have regarded managed care with suspicion and blame cost containment strategies for worsening barriers and limiting access to treatment. Nauert (1997) points out that managed care systems currently regard substance abuse treatment programs as "stepchildren" in that they "generally do not produce high profit margins, they are often under assault by cost-conscious payers, and their clinical leaders may not enjoy the same political clout as their medical and surgical brethren in competing for organizational resources" (p. 49). However, as managed care continues to expand and mature, the role of substance abuse treatment within its framework will demand better definition.

SUBSTANCE ABUSE TREATMENT FUNDING

According to Musto (1992), interest in the abuse of alcohol and drugs can be traced to the latter part of the 19th century, when the disruptive effects of the industrial revolution and unprecedented immigration resulted in a reform movement aimed at protecting the rights of citizens and establishing a moral, if somewhat liberal, order of society. Reformers of the Progressive Era (1890–1910) proposed legislation to regulate a variety of activities and conditions including pollution, water quality, mine safety, food inspection, and most notably, alcohol use. Temperance movement supporters thought alcohol to be responsible for many social evils such as poverty, criminality, political corruption, prostitution, and violence. However, the policy of Prohibition enacted in 1920 as a remedy to alcohol abuse proved ineffective (Reader & Sullivan, 1992).

Concurrent with the movement to end alcohol abuse was an effort to purge the society of narcotic drugs (Musto, 1992). Many legislative measures were enacted to control the trade and manufacture of opium derivatives and direct the treatment of opioid addicts. The Harrison Act of 1914 served to criminalize the use and sale of narcotics, limiting the availability of the only drug treatment at that time, maintenance programs. Despite efforts to provide detoxification and medical treatment to drug users, such as the federally established "narcotic farms" (U.S. Congress, 1929), the addict continued to be regarded as a moral indigent and the source of most social ills. With legislation adopted in 1951 providing mandatory sentencing of offenders, and allowing the death penalty for certain drug-related offenses, attempts to control drug use continued (U.S. Congress, 1956).

As negative public perceptions and punitive legislative actions toward drug use increased, the opposite occurred with alcohol use. The repeal of Prohibition in 1933 opened the door to new therapeutic ideas. Prior to the 1930s, persons with substance use disorders could find little medical help. Those who could afford it would be admitted to private psychiatric hospitals. Those without means would most likely be removed to state mental hospitals that operated on a "custodial-authoritarian model" (Greenblatt, 1978). Early residential treatment programs formed in the late 1800s were open briefly and often remodeled as mental institutions. For example, the Massachusetts State Hospital of Dipsomaniacs and Inebriates opened in 1893 and continued treating alcoholics until 1918, when it became a hospital for shell-shocked World War I veterans (Baumhol & Room, 1987). A revolution in the perception and treatment of alcoholism occurred with the founding of Alcoholics Anonymous in 1935 (Yoder, 1990). The publication of the "Big Book" in 1939 and the national exposure from an article in *The Saturday Evening Post* in 1940, which described a model of institutional care for alcoholism, greatly improved public opinion regarding alcoholism and the treatment of alcoholism.

During the 1940s, Jellinek and others developed a typology of alcoholism that eventually helped to medicalize the condition (Beresford, 1991) and led to the formation of the Yale University Center for Alcohol Studies, the National Committee for Education on Alcoholism (later the National Council on Alcoholism) (Kurtz, 1979), and a respected scientific journal, *The Quarterly Journal of Alcohol Studies* (Hanlon, 1974). In 1945, Connecticut established the first publicly funded alcohol treatment program (Reader & Sullivan, 1992). In 1949, Western Electric Corporation created a program to help alcohol-abusing employees (Hanlon, 1974). By 1958, both the World Health Organization and the American Medical Association defined alcoholism as a disease (Hingson, Matthews, & Scotch, 1979). By 1965, the creation of Medicaid and Medicare programs ensured that the poor and elderly with alcohol or drug use disorders could obtain treatment, although few services existed (Reader & Sullivan, 1992). A small number of outpatient clinics and halfway houses began to emerge throughout this period, but most lacked coordination and consistency.

In 1970, the Hughes Act legislated a federal infrastructure and funding for alcohol abuse treatment and prevention. The effects of this legislation are still felt today. The law furthered the cause of treatment in a number of ways. According to the Institute of Medicine report (1997):

> The act authorized the creation of the National Institute on Alcohol Abuse and Alcoholism (NIAAA) within NIMH, created a National Advisory Council on Alcohol Abuse and Alcoholism to foster policy development, required states to designate alcoholism authorities, established federal formula grants for states to facilitate the creation of comprehensive state plans for the treatment and prevention of alcoholism, mandated treatment and prevention services for federal employees, encouraged hospitals to admit and treat alcoholics, protected the confidentiality of patient records, and funded research. (p. 107)

The NIAAA targeted treatment of the employed alcoholic by training two "occupational alcohol consultants" from each of the 50 states and dispatching them to corporations and labor unions. This work fostered the widespread development of alcoholism intervention programs and eventually, employee assistance programs in both the public and private sectors (Reader & Sullivan, 1992).

Reauthorizations of the Hughes Act (1974, 1976) aided the establishment of independent institutes within the Alcohol, Drug Abuse, and Mental Health Administration (ADAMHA), later renamed the Substance Abuse and Mental Health Services Administration (SAMHSA), and provided incentives to states to adopt the Uniform Act. The Uniform Act "encouraged the development of community-based treatment services and typically specified the creation of emergency detoxification services, short-term inpatient care, residential care in halfway houses, and outpatient services" (p. 107).

By the mid-1970s, a system of federal- and state-funded alcohol abuse treatment programs had been established. Employer awareness prompted approximately 75% of Blue Cross insurance plans to offer coverage for alcohol detoxification (U.S. Department of Labor, 1988). The increasing demand for alcohol use treatment services led to the development of more formalized treatment programs. In many treatment facilities, the "Minnesota model" or the "chemical dependency model" was adopted. The Minnesota model, first designed for alcoholic patients in three Minnesota treatment programs, established the pattern of detoxification followed by 28 days of inpatient monitoring and therapy that was quickly replicated across the United States (Book et al., 1995). To meet the demand of burgeoning programs, states began to form accreditation agencies for both treatment programs and staff. The treatment programs that were developed were faced with a complicated array of funding streams, each with its own eligibility requirements and payment paths (Zarkin et al., 1995).

Many of the events that led to the acceptance and funding of alcohol abuse treatment were parallel for drug abuse. For example, in 1958 the Joint Committee of the American Bar Association and the American Medical Association on Narcotic Drugs released a report that favored increased research on drug abuse rather than increasing punitive measures (Institute of Medicine, 1997). In 1962, the case of *Robinson v. California* deemed the prosecution of individuals based only upon their addiction to be cruel and unusual punishment and recommended treatment not incarceration (Courtwright, Joseph, & Des Jarlais, 1989). Therapeutic communities, beginning with Synanon in 1958 (Brecher, 1972) and Daytop Village in 1963 (Institute of Medicine, 1997) proved that drug abuse was manageable and treatable. In 1965, a newly derived opiate called methadone was tested at Rockefeller University as a stabilizer for heroin addicts, resulting in methadone maintenance as a cost-effective method of treatment (Institute of Medicine, 1997). In 1966, the Narcotic Addict Rehabilitation Act afforded federal funds for the civil commitment and treatment of those addicted to narcotics (Besteman, 1992). By 1968, the number of private and public treatment facilities had grown to 183, primarily in urban areas (Jaffe, 1979). The federal initiative considered of greatest importance, was President Nixon's declaration of the "war on drugs" in 1969. His resolve led to the Comprehensive Drug Abuse

Prevention and Control Act of 1970 and the Special Action Office for Drug Abuse Prevention (SAODAP) that provided a coordinated effort to reduce drug abuse through strict funding guidelines aimed at improving community-based services (Besteman, 1992).

In 1981, with the passage of the Omnibus Budget Reconciliation Act, federal funds were consolidated into the Alcohol, Drug Abuse, and Mental Health Services Block Grant, reducing the totals received by the states by 26% (Lewis, 1988). Although billions of dollars were authorized to fund chemical dependency treatment through the Anti–Drug Abuse Act of 1986 and the 1988 Anti–Drug Abuse Act, two-thirds of the promised monies were not realized by treatment programs, but rather were funneled to law enforcement (Musto, 1992). Unlike alcohol treatment reimbursed by private insurance, drug abuse treatment was funded primarily by public funds. Thus, the consolidation of drug and alcohol programs became inevitable. During the 1980s, treatment for drug and alcohol use disorders became fully integrated within the states under the umbrella of chemical dependency treatment. In essence, by the 1980s drug and alcohol abuse treatments were viewed as viable and legitimate. Numerous public sources were available for funding, including Medicare and Medicaid, federal block grants to states, and a complex array of state and local funding. Commercial insurance companies often covered alcohol abuse services, but resisted any forays into drug abuse services. To counter this problem, states began to issue mandates for insurance coverage of drug abuse treatment. As of 1989, 39 states had such laws (Reader & Sullivan, 1992). As public awareness and available funds grew, so did the demand for services. Hospitals, physicians, free-standing programs, and counselors scrambled to supply the services.

SUBSTANCE ABUSE TREATMENT AND MANAGED CARE

The concept of managed health care is not new. Health maintenance organizations can be tracked a century ago to the industrial revolution. In Tacoma, Washington, in 1906, mill owners and employees "locked in" medical services from Drs. Curan and Yokum by paying them 50 cents per member per month to provide comprehensive treatment (Giles, 1993). During the Great Depression, hospitals once funded by philanthropic support were forced to charge patients fees for services. Hospital use declined while the need for insurance against catastrophic illness rose. Interestingly, prepaid insurance plans began to emerge, but their supporters were met with outrage and law suits from the medical community. In 1932, the American Medical Association (AMA) issued a formal statement opposing prepaid medical coverage, thus leading to the development of Blue Cross, an indemnity or fee-for-service plan that was considered less threatening than capitated services (Mayer & Mayer, 1985). Despite the AMA efforts, other prepaid companies appeared, including the Group Health Association of Washington, D.C., the Group Health Cooperative in Seattle, the Group Health Mutual Insurance Company in Minneapolis, and Kaiser-Permanente in Los Angeles (Giles, 1993). But the prepaid arrangements could not keep pace with the indemnity insurance plans that appealed to employers who were attempting to sell benefits rather than wages to their employees. The indemnity plans were flexible and could be bought for low prices for low-risk groups.

Within the context of the prosperous 1950s and 1960s, cost was not an issue (Reader & Sullivan, 1992). However, by 1971, after a period of inflation in which general medical costs escalated, the Nixon administration prompted the passing of the Health Maintenance Organization Act, which awarded subsidies of more than $200 million to nonprofit groups to develop health maintenance prepaid plans (Iglehart, 1992). The campaign to increase prepaid plans did not reach the projected goals of 1700 HMOs enrolling 40 million members by 1976 (Hadley & Langwell, 1991). The government was even less successful in transforming the Medicare and Medicaid systems into the prepaid arena. Only a handful of HMOs for public clients existed at that time.

As health care insurance expanded, so did the demand for behavioral services. Consumer demand, in addition to reduced social stigma and research touting the effectiveness of behavioral health services, increased the number of employers who included mental health and chemical dependency services in their benefit packages (Institute of Medicine, 1997).

Throughout the late 1970s and mid-1980s, in light of the demand, health care costs continued to increase two to three times the inflation rate. Employers, including the federal government, found themselves paying exorbitant prices for services. The cost of behavioral health care was rising even faster. Some estimates suggested that if left uncontained, health care costs would consume the entire United States Gross National Product by the year 2015 (Giles, 1993). Indemnity health plans were held responsible for this trend. Because these plans reimbursed hospitals and other providers on the basis of reported cost, there were no incentives for providers to trim operating costs. Waste and fraud on the part of the providers was tolerated (Reader & Sullivan, 1992). Meanwhile, individuals could use the behavioral services at will with little cost to themselves. These circumstances were termed the "moral hazard" (Pauly, 1968). The first attempt to contain the "moral hazard" was to implement the diagnostic-related group (DRG) payment schedule in the late 1970s. However, this schedule was applied only to medical services and not mental health services. This partial regulation slowed the rate of increase for medical costs while allowing the rampant escalation of costs for mental health and addictive services (Reader &

Sullivan, 1992). The Institute of Medicine (1997) reports that "as a direct result of these increased costs of employee benefits, companies and insurance plans turned to specialty managed care firms to rein in the costs of care" (p. 94).

By the end of 1995, 161 million Americans were enrolled in a managed health care plan (Institute of Medicine, 1997). The recent increase in health care coverage has also signaled a change in the delivery of substance abuse treatment services. For example, some residential programs reduced their 28-day model to 15 days or less (Shadle & Christianson, 1989). Treatment has become more individually focused and goal-oriented. Outpatient services are favored and intensive outpatient programs have grown rapidly (Wilson, 1993). The integration of substance abuse treatment and ancillary services such as primary medical care has also increased. Primary medical care has been seen as a natural first step in the management of substance abuse disorders as many patients have comorbid conditions such as hepatitis B, tuberculosis, sexually transmitted diseases, AIDS, or other illnesses and conditions directly attributable to the use of drugs and alcohol (Zarkin et al., 1995). An ADAMHA (SAMHSA)-sponsored 3-year demonstration project reported the positive effect of primary medical care on drug treatment outcome (Schlenger et al., 1994). Examples of other ancillary services that are also integrated with substance abuse treatment include mental health services, vocational/educational programming, and services that meet the basic needs of the consumer.

SUBSTANCE ABUSE TREATMENT
AND THE EFFICACY OF MANAGED CARE

The term "managed care" has been used to denote an array of financing plans that are purchased by companies, unions, or the government. The Institute of Medicine (1997) defines managed care as:

> Arrangements for health care delivery and financing that are designed to provide appropriate, effective, and efficient health care through organized relationships with providers. Includes formal programs for ongoing quality assurance and utilization review, financial incentives for covered members to use the plan's providers, and financial incentives for providers to contain costs. . . . Any of a variety of strategies to control behavioral health (i.e., mental health and substance abuse) costs while ensuring quality care and appropriate utilization. Cost-containment and quality assurance methods include the formation of preferred provider networks, gatekeeping (or precertification), case management, relapse prevention, retrospective review, claims payment, and others. (pp. 257–258)

A wide range of managed care organizations exist. The most well-known is the Health Maintenance Organization (HMO), which is designed to provide comprehensive medical and behavioral health services on a prepaid basis (Christianson & Osher, 1994). HMOs can be divided into five types: (1) the *staff model* whereby practitioners are salaried employees of the HMO; (2) the *group model* in which the HMO pays a negotiated, per capita rate to a group of practitioners; (3) the *network model* that allows practitioners to work under contract to the HMO; (4) an *Individual Practice Association (IPA) model* whereby practitioners are compensated by capitation and/or fee-for-service plans; and (5) the *mixed model* that can combine any two or more of the above methods (Institute of Medicine, 1997). A second type of managed care arrangement is called the Preferred Provider Organization (PPO) that is comprised of a network of providers for which members receive financial incentives to visit but they may also choose providers outside of the system at a higher copayment and/or deductible. A third type is called the Point-of-Service (POS) plan that resembles an HMO, but allows for members to obtain provider services outside of the network at a higher fee. A fourth type, the Management Services Organization (MSO), provides practice management and administrative services to an individual or group practice. A fifth type, the Employee Assistance Program (EAP), is used by employees as a first step in seeking help for work-related or personal problems. And finally, the Managed Behavioral Health Care Organization (MBHO), also known as a "carve out," provides the mental health and substance abuse treatment services to members of another managed care organization for which it has been contracted. The notion of a "carve out" is an important one with the management of behavioral health care. It is described by Nauert (1997) as:

> A common practice is to "carve out" mental health and chemical dependence from a larger benefit package and to target cost savings and quality issues specific to behavioral health. Companies then bid out the management of their mental health benefits to a vendor who can oversee case management, claims, administration, and contract negotiations with select providers. (p. 50)

It is felt that the "carve out" will ensure that the services needed in the behavioral sector are not provided at the expense of the more objectively defined general medical services. Mental health care and substance abuse treatment have traditionally received the smallest portion of the health care insurance pie. However, at the end of 1995, 141 million individuals were enrolled in managed behavioral health care: 124 million in specialty programs and 16.9 in Health Maintenance Organizations (HMOs) (Open Minds, 1996).

Approaches to providing health services have changed over the years. Three generations of managed care approaches have been identified. First generation styles focused on extensive utilization review and precertifications by reimbursers who may or may not have the necessary expertise for such decisions. Second generation approaches focused on managing benefits by utilizing networks of providers, capitation, measurement of outcomes, and the sharing of clinical criteria and standards of care (Institute of Medicine, 1997; VanLeit, 1995). Third generation methods are in their infancy, but attempt to develop flexible, comprehensive, and cost-effective mental health care in a continuum of settings, essentially sensitive to the need to provide the most appropriate care (Bartlett, 1994).

To date, a large number of plans still retain the first generation approach. This approach has been criticized by both providers and consumers. The typical first generation approach managed care benefit package allows for 20 sessions of outpatient care and 30 to 60 days of inpatient care per year. These sessions are allotted on the basis of "medical necessity," a vague and often misunderstood concept especially in substance abuse treatment (Pomerantz, 1996). Often, unrealistic limits to care have resulted. Insured substance abuse patients may exhaust their benefits with one inpatient stay, leaving no coverage for relapse or relapse prevention. Approximately 20% of public funding for substance abuse treatment is used by patients who have exhausted their benefits or who are not covered for such services under their plans (Harwood, Thomson, & Nesmith, 1994). It has been noted that these policies continue in light of research that consistently shows treatment success to be positively correlated to the number and length of treatment exposures (Ball & Ross, 1991; Condelli & Hubbard, 1994; Hubbard et al., 1989; McLellan, Arndt, Metzger, Woody, & O'Brien, 1993). One study found that among patients with alcohol and drug abuse disorders, clinicians requested an average of 19.6 inpatient days, but received authorization for an average of only 6.2 days (Wickizer, Lessler, & Travis, 1996).

Typically, the more that a managed care organization is cost-conscious or "bottom line" focused, the less that it spends on mental health services, especially inpatient services. Fee-for-service or indemnity plans may devote 14 to 26% of the total premium to mental health care, while HMOs may dedicate only 3 to 6 % of premium costs (Giles, 1993). Because little formal work has been done by the treatment field to determine best practices, managed care organizations have been unrestricted to develop their own guidelines for authorizing behavioral services. Recently, the American Society of Addiction Medicine (ASAM) and the various state substance abuse programs developed criteria for mandating client placement, continued stay and discharge across a variety of levels of care. In some states, the use of these criteria are mandated for public and commercial managed care organizations. Still, many managed care organizations fight the use of these criteria or refuse to use them at all.

Managed care organizations of all types have also been found to limit substance abuse utilization to acute medical care, omitting the educational, support, and maintenance services that provide care continuity for chronic substance abusers (Larson, Samet, & McCarty, 1997). These services, often called "wraparound" services, have been widely used by state treatment systems and are designed to enhance treatment retention and prevent relapse. The most common services are those that provide housing, child care, transportation, basic needs (food, clothing, utilities), legal assistance, vocational and educational training, employment assistance, family services, medical services, and mental health treatments.

In 1996, the Center for Substance Abuse Treatment (CSAT), a division of SAMHSA, funded a 3-year study of the economic and clinical impact of wraparound services. Acting as the coordinating center for 11 multimodal treatment facilities and seven single county authorities (county agencies that provide case management services), the St. Francis Medical Center is collecting extensive baseline and follow-up data on approximately 3,000 individuals addicted to cocaine or heroin. Results are expected to identify the cost-effectiveness of wraparound services as related to clinical efficacy and pave the way for appropriate policy decisions.

Managed care organizations have also been accused of limiting patient autonomy by unduly influencing health care decisions regarding what providers and what services are most appropriate. With many plans, a primary care physician must authorize the use of all specialty care, including behavioral care and emergency room use. Some managed care plans provide financial incentives to primary care physicians in order to influence the rate at which they may make referrals to specialty care. Because of the general dissatisfaction with this arrangement, President Clinton recommended an HMO "Bill of Rights" to be adopted by Congress to give consumers

- The right to appeal the denial of care
- The right to a "reasonably large" choice of doctors
- The right to have an emergency room visit paid for if a reasonable person would have concluded that the problem was an emergency. (Holmes, 1997)

In addition, patients and providers alike have expressed concerns about the impact of a primary care physician and a third party reviewer on confidentiality issues and the relationship between patient and therapist. The primary care physician or managed care organization may require frequent notifications of the client's progress. Despite a number of federal regulations that protect unauthorized disclosure and restrict even informed disclosure of patient information, the breadth of notification may test legal limits. Managed care organizations may try to coerce the provider into providing unlawful information by threatening reimbursement. Further, claims and utilization review staff of managed care organizations have been known to breach confidentiality with the client's employer or family. As trust is an essential ingredient to the therapeutic relationship, any disruption could be detrimental to the success of the treatment. A number of individuals may choose to self-pay for mental health services rather than risk a breach of confidence through their managed behavioral health care plans.

In a survey of 11 drug treatment programs across the nation, French, Dunlap, Galinis, Rachal, and Zarkin (1996) found that program directors believed that managed care was necessary and inevitable to curb the long waiting lists of patients and inadequate funding. However, in addition to the issues mentioned above, they cited a number of concerns specific to substance abuse treatment. First, they feared the increased burden of rising administrative duties required by MCOs coupled with diminishing administrative staff would further jeopardize patient treatment. Second, they cited the additional reporting required by managed care for public clients as an undue burden to their programs. And finally, they reported that managed care organizations tended to ignore the need for aftercare services, thus increasing the risk of clinical relapse.

Some providers object to the process that managed care organizations use to select providers. Managed care organizations may review a potential provider for his or her history of utilization and contract only with providers who have a track record of inexpensive styles of practice (Christianson & Osher, 1994; Larson et al., 1997). Some managed care organizations have done a poor job of credentialing minority health care professionals or providers. Still others have instituted such cumbersome methods of credentialing that certain providers and professionals are discouraged from applying.

Managed care administrators and purchasers, however, regard complaints and criticisms of managed care practices as reactionary and do not apologize for the limitations placed on providers. Providers have been regarded as entrenched in a liberal yet empirically unsubstantiated pattern of substance abuse treatment (i.e., detoxification followed by a 28-day inpatient stay). Managed care organization administrators and purchasers have felt that this resistance to change, suspecting motivation largely driven by funding issues rather than clinical issues (Holmes, 1997; Reader & Sullivan, 1992).

Whether managed care organizations are judicious or avaricious in their spending habits depends upon one's perspective. However, most managed care organizations recognize the need for sound empirical evidence to support decisions. Thus, a number of evaluations and studies have been undertaken to improve managed care methods and increase client and provider satisfaction.

RESEARCH REGARDING SUBSTANCE ABUSE
TREATMENT AND MANAGED CARE

Concerns about the role of managed care in the treatment of substance
abuse can be captured in three questions:

1. *Access to care*: Will managed care help resolve the dilemma of the
   inaccessibility of care to nearly 40 million people in the United States
   who are projected to need substance abuse treatment? Moreover, will
   those enrolled in managed care organizations qualify but not receive
   appropriate services?
2. *Quality*: Will managed care facilitate and fund appropriate levels of
   treatment that will yield clinical outcomes that reach acceptable
   standards?
3. *Efficiency*: Will managed care be able to reduce or maintain costs so
   that benefits are not cut and access continues to increase to the
   underserved? (adapted from Giles, 1993, p. 29)

Access to Care

Universal access to health care and behavioral health care is a controversial
topic in the United States. There are some camps that view dwindling fiscal
resources as supportive of selective limitation to health care. Other view-
points see access to health care as an entitlement. The final verdict regarding
the role of managed care in providing greater access at less cost (a part of
the health care reform movement) remains to be seen. However, there are
some demonstrated changes in patient access within the structure of health
care in the United States that may be related to managed care.

Currently, managed care organizations have focused on member access
to services. Access standards have been proposed for the National Committee on Quality Assurance's Health Plan Employer Data and Information Set
version 3.0 (Hedis 3.0), the Digital Equipment Corporation, and the American
Managed Behavioral Healthcare Association (AMBHA). Managed care organizations are held to these standards to prevent loss of their accreditation
and contracts. Access is measured in terms of utilization and penetration
rates. Utilization rates refer to waiting time and availability of providers.
Penetration rates are defined as: (1) days and number of visits per 1,000
population, (2) average length of stay, and (3) number of sessions per episode of care (Daniels, Kramer, & Mahesh, 1997; Institute of Medicine, 1997).

A number of studies show that MCOs in general restrict access to some
services, particularly inpatient or residential. A study by Rosenberg (1996)
concludes that HMOs encourage utilization of outpatient services while
hindering utilization of hospital psychiatric expenditures. A comparison of

the days requested by providers (average = 19.6 days) for alcohol or drug use treatment and the resulting days received from the utililization review found that care for psychiatric patients was overall restricted, but care for patients with substance use disorder was even more restricted (average = 6.2 days) (Wickizer et al., 1996). McLellan and colleagues (1996) compared the access of Medicaid recipients before and after the introduction of a managed behavioral carve out. Within the same outpatient programs, managed care clients received shorter treatment stays and fewer professional services than the fee-for-service clients. On the other hand, McFarland, Johnson, and Pople (1994) compared the utilization of 250 seriously mentally ill and with two matched groups enrolled in a Kaiser Permanente HMO. The authors found that seriously mentally ill patients used more services than the other groups, both inpatient and outpatient. Moreover, they maintained their membership in the HMO longer than the others.

The Institute of Medicine (1997) suggests that studies continue to identify the needs of clients, particularly those from special populations whose problem profiles differ from the norm and compare the effects of managed care on access for these special populations. Some studies have suggested that managed care organizations can be selectively restrictive for patients with very severe comorbid psychiatric disorders and specific profiles (i.e., offenders, pregnant and addicted women, older adults, homeless).

Though the recent, albeit sparse research, suggests that access is generally restricted by the presence of managed care, this effect may not be permanent. Managed care organizations may revisit and change their models of access to behavioral health care in light of future research findings, accreditation standards and reported medical offset effects. Although Fraser (1996) cautions against attaching too much weight to offsets, he acknowledges the importance of medical offset effects and defines them as "the realization of enough cost and use reductions in general medical services following psychological intervention to more than pay for the cost of those mental health services" (p. 335).

Quality

Assessing effects of managed care services on quality of service is often determined through the evaluation of clinical outcomes and client satisfaction surveys. Few studies have systematically examined member and provider satisfaction in a managed care setting. However, accreditation standards require managed care organizations to monitor satisfaction and many report their findings in newsletters, annual reports, and information brochures.

Several studies have been conducted on clinical outcomes in a managed care setting. One outcome study conducted by Renz, Chung, Fillman, Mee-

Lee, and Sayama (1995) examined the recidivism rates of managed care vs. nonmanaged care substance abuse patients in a single treatment facility. Contrary to anecdotal reports and the authors' expectations, no significant differences were found. An evaluation of the Southern California Kaiser-Permanente Chemical Dependency Recovery program demonstrated that HMO services were effective in promoting abstinence, especially among patients whose drug of choice was alcohol (Ershoff, Radcliffe, & Gregory, 1996). On the other hand, findings from the RAND medical outcomes study suggested that depressed patients treated within an HMO receive less psychiatric care and may evidence poorer outcomes (Rogers, Wells, & Meredith, 1993). Overall, little quality outcome literature exists. As Renz and associates point out:

> Despite the current ubiquity of managed care, there is little empirical evidence to date that tests the effect of managed care on treatment outcome. In addition, the perceived negative impact of managed care on treatment outcome is based on valuable anecdotal reports but has not been the subject of empirical scrutiny. (p. 287)

Attempts have been made by the providers and the managed care organizations to improve the quality of behavioral health care. One example already mentioned is the development of new client placement criteria such as those established by the American Society of Addiction Medicine (ASAM) in 1987. The Green Spring Alcohol and Drug Detoxification and Rehabilitation Criteria for Utilization Review combines the managed care notions of medical necessity and the provision of least intensive level of care with the ASAM treatment planning model. Predictably, the Green Spring criteria tend to ignore psychosocial aspects of the client. But the effort represents a major step in the integration of managed care with clinical models held by providers (Book et al., 1995).

A similar system for standardizing the administration of HMO services was developed by the Harvard Community Health Plan, a staff model HMO founded in 1969. Approximately 200 clinicians and support staff participated in the creation of the Mental Health Patient Assessment Tool. This instrument is designed to assist clinicians with comprehensive evaluations, administration of benefits, measurement of clinical progress, and support for outcomes research. Input from the staff supported by successful use of the instrument also fostered changes in the delivery system such as the implementation of self-referrals, the development of access standards, the revision of intake triage functions, and the development of additional programs (Abrams, 1993).

The development of future satisfaction and outcome studies will be imperative to determine the quality of managed care organizations. However, at present, judgments regarding the quality of an managed care organization must be based on their accountability to the purchaser, providers, members, and government regulatory agencies. The Institute of Medicine (1997) suggests several methods of maintaining accountability for managed care organizations: (1) accreditation, (2) peer review, (3) state licensure, (4) practitioner credentialing and privileging, (5) public and private sector audits, (6) legal mechanisms through the courts, and (7) the adoption of clinical practice standards and guidelines.

Efficiency

By definition, managed care controls costs. To date, studies uphold this description. Most notable is the study conducted by Callahan, Shepard, Beinecke, Larson, and Cavanaugh (1995) on the Massachusetts Medicaid program. The authors found that managed care reduced expenditures in the first year of operation by 22% by reducing length of hospital stays, number of inpatient admissions, and costs. Similarly, a study by Babigian and associates (1992) found that services for managed care members were less costly than those in traditional plans.

In summary, managed care, though regarded as a necessary evil by some and an unnecessary one by others, has laid claim to the U.S. health care market and appears to be advancing. Clearly, costs to purchasers have been reduced. Whether the resultant decrease in costs will result in improved access, quality, and efficiency remains to be seen.

SUBSTANCE ABUSE TREATMENT
AND THE FUTURE WITH MANAGED CARE

The future role of managed care within substance abuse treatment will be determined in three ways: through integration, innovation, and collaboration.

First, a number of studies suggest that mental health services, including substance abuse treatment services, must be integrated into the full health care delivery system in order to achieve optimal efficiency. For example, one study determined that for every $1 invested by the nation's taxpayers for drug and alcohol treatment, $7 were recouped (Gerstein et al., 1994). The same study determined that treatment produced a decline in criminal activity and hospitalizations. A recent study suggests that, contrary to previous assumptions, the cost of parity between mental health and medical benefits would raise health insurance costs under managed care by only about $1 per enrollee per year (Healthcare Financial Management, 1998). Empirical evidence also indicates that alcohol abuse treatment (and to a less extent, drug abuse treatment) results in medical offset effects or less usage of the medical system (Wickizer, 1994). The Health Insurance Association of America has estimated that the savings in maternity care, physician fees, and hospital charges for each delivery not affected by substance abuse is $48,000 to $150,000 (CSAT, 1995). Moreover, the federal government currently spends over $55 billion to treat the consequences of drug and alcohol abuse (National Center on Addiction and Substance Abuse at Columbia University, 1996). In essence, the nation cannot afford to minimize the importance of substance abuse treatment services.

But managed care organizations, treatment programs, and clinicians must be open to innovation. Treatment outcomes research can continue to advance both clinical and fiscal improvements. Quality of life measurements must be included as important outcome measures (Marwick, 1996). Emphasis must be placed on providing patients with a full range of services with the most appropriate level of care in the most accessible location (Nauert, 1997). This includes:

1. A socioecological model of behavior that emphasizes the importance of context to support functional capacity,
2. Pragmatic treatment that focuses on action-oriented, well-specified interventions and careful monitoring of treatment outcomes,
3. Field-based services that occur in the client's natural environment,
4. Individualized treatment that addresses flexible, collaboratively developed goals,
5. Accountability in which staff members are discouraged from blaming clients for lack of progress and encouraged to focus on the use of creative solutions to problems (VanLeit, 1995).

Innovations may also include automated system designs such as the clinical management information system created by MCC Behavioral Care, Inc. in cooperation with the University of Minnesota (Kane, Bartlett, & Potthoff, 1995). Such systems can help to track information for treatment and organizational revisions.

Most importantly, substance abuse treatment and managed care must form a collaboration. This means that managed care administrators, purchasers, providers, and clients must learn to form a true partnership that will benefit each while maintaining high levels of integrity and flexibility. This level of collaboration may even take the form of provider-based managed care organizations that eliminate the need for an administrative intermediary organization.

Managed care has provided a challenge to substance abuse treatment and vice versa. David Mee-Lee expresses this challenge most eloquently:

If we really focused on patient/client-driven, assessment-based, clinically-driven treatment in the most efficient and effective way, based on accountability and data, that would take care of costs (American Society on Addiction Medicine, Public Workshop, April 18, 1996, Washington, DC as quoted in Institute of Medicine, 1997, p. 20).

ACKNOWLEDGMENT

The authors wish to thank Bethe Anne Ott for her assistance in the preparation of this chapter.

REFERENCES

Abrams, H. S. (1993). Harvard Community Health Plan's mental health redesign project: A managerial and clinical partnership. *Psychiatric Quarterly, 64,* 13–29.

Babigian, H., Mitchell, O., Marshall, P., et al. (1992). A mental health capitation experiment: Evaluating the Monroe-Livingston experience. In R. G. Frank & W. G. Manning (Eds.), *Economics and mental health.* Baltimore: Johns Hopkins University Press.

Ball, J. C., & Ross, A. (1991). *The effectiveness of methadone maintenance treatment: Patients, programs, services, and outcome.* New York: Springer-Verlag.

Bartlett, J. (1994). The emergence of managed care and its impact on psychiatry. *New Directions for Mental Health Services, 63,* 25–35.

Baumhol, J., & Room, R. (1987). Inebriety, doctors, and the state alcoholism treatment institutions before 1940. In M. Galanter (Ed.), *Recent developments in alcoholism, Volume 5* (pp. 135–174). New York: Plenum.

Beresford, T. P. (1991). The nosology of alcoholism research. *Alcohol Health and Research World, 15,* 260–265.

Besteman, K. J. (1992). Federal leadership in building the national drug treatment system. In Institute of Medicine, *Treating drug problems, Volume 2.* Washington, DC: National Academy Press.

Book, J., Harbin, H., Marques, C., Silverman, C., Lizanich-Aro, S., & Lazarus, A. (1995). The ASAM and Green Spring Alcohol and Drug Detoxification and Rehabilitation Criterial for utilization review. *The American Journal on Addictions, 4,* 187–197.

Brecher, E. M. (1972). *Licit and illicit drugs.* Boston: Little, Brown.

Callahan, J. J., Shepard, D. S., Beinecke, R. H., Larson, M. J., & Cavanaugh, D. (1995). Mental health/substance abuse treatment in managed care: The Massachusetts Medicaid experience. *Health Affairs, 14,* 174–184.

Christianson, J. B., & Osher, F. C. (1994). Health Maintenance Organizations, health care reform, and persons with serious mental illness. *Hospital and Community Psychiatry, 45,* 898–905.

Condelli, W. S., & Hubbard, R. L. (1994). Relationship between time spent in treatment and client outcomes from therapeutic communities. *Journal of Substance Abuse Treatment, 11,* 25–33.

Courtwright, D., Joseph, H., & Des Jarlais, D. (1989). *Addicts who survived: An oral history of narcotic use in America, 1923–1965.* Knoxville: University of Tennessee Press.

CSAT (Center for Substance Abuse Treatment). (1995). *Producing results: A report to the nation.* Rockville, MD: Substance Abuse and Mental Health Administration, Center for Substance Abuse Treatment.

Daniels, A., Kramer, T., & Mahesh, N. (1997). Quality assessment and improvement. In K. M. Coughlin (Ed.), *The 1998 outcomes & guidelines sourcebook.* New York: Faulkner & Gray.

Ershoff, D., Radcliffe, A., & Gregory, M. (1996). The Southern California Kaiser-Permanente Chemical Dependency Recovery Program evaluation: Results of a treatment outcome study in an HMO setting. *Journal of Addictive Diseases, 15,* 1–25.

Fraser, J. S. (1996). All that glitters is not always gold: Medical offset effects and managed behavioral health care. *Professional Psychology Research and Practice, 27,* 335–344.

French, M. T., Dunlap, L. J., Galinis, D. N., Rachal, J. V., & Zarkin, G. A. (1996). Health care reforms and managed care for substance abuse services: Findings from eleven case studies. *Journal of Public Health Policy, 17,* 181–203.

Gerstein, D. R., Johnson, R. A., Harwood, H. J., Fountain, D., Suter, N., & Malloy, K. (1994). *Evaluating recovery services: The California drug and alcohol treatment assessment (CALDATA).* Fairfax, VA: Lewin-VHI and National Opinion Research Center at the University of Chicago.

Giles, T. R. (1993). *Managed mental health care: A guide for practitioners, employers, and hospital administrators.* Boston: Allyn & Bacon.

Greenblatt, M. (1978). *Psychopolitics.* New York: Grune & Stratton.

Hadley, J. P., & Langwell, K. (1991). Managed care in the United States: Promises, evidence to date and future directions. *Health Policy, 19,* 91–118.

Hanlon, J. J. (1974). *Public health: Administration and practice.* St. Louis, MO: Mosby.

Harwood, H. J., Thomson, M., & Nesmith, T. (1994). *Healthcare reform and substance abuse treatment: The cost of financing under alternative approaches.* Fairfax, VA: Lewin-VHI.

Healthcare Financial Management. (1998, January). *Expanding mental health benefits* [on-line]. Available: http://www.olivehealthcare.com/mhnews1.html

Hingson, R., Matthews, D., & Scotch, N. A. (1979). The use and abuse of psychoactive substances. In H. E. Freeman, S. Levine, & L. G. Reeder (Eds.), *Handbook of medical sociology* (3rd ed.). Englewood Cliffs, NJ: Prentice-Hall.

Holmes, L. (1997, November 24). The problem(s) with managed care. In *Mental Health Resources* [on-line]. Available: http://mentalhealth.tqn.com/library/weekly/aa112497.htm

Hubbard, R. L., Marsden, M. E., Rachel, J. V., Harwood, H. J., Cavanaugh, E. R., & Ginzburg, H. M. (1989). *Drug abuse treatment: A national study of effectiveness.* Chapel Hill: University of North Carolina Press.

Iglehart, J. K. (1992). Health policy report: The American health care system—Managed care. *The New England Journal of Medicine, 327,* 743–748.

Institute of Medicine. (1997). Edmunds, M., Frank, R., Hogan, M., McCarty, D., Robinson-Beale, R., & Weisner, C. (Eds.). *Managing managed care: Quality improvement in behavioral health.* Washington, DC: National Academy Press.

Jaffe, J. H. (1979). The swinging pendulum: The treatment of drug users in America. In R. I. DuPont, A. Goldstein, & J. O'Donnell (Eds.), *Handbook on drug abuse.* Rockville, MD: National Institute on Drug Abuse.

Kane, R. L., Bartlett, J., & Potthoff, S. (1995). Building an empirically based outcomes information system for managed mental health care. *Psychiatric Services, 46,* 459–461.

Kessler, R. C., McGonagle, K. A., Zhao, S., & Nelson, C. B. (1994). Lifetime and 12-month prevalence of DSM-III-R psychiatric disorders in the U.S. *Archives of General Psychiatry, 51,* 8–19.

Kurtz, E. (1979). *Not-God: A history of Alcoholics Anonymous Center City.* Minneapolis: Hazelden Press.

Larson, M. J., Samet, J. H., & McCarty, D. (1997). Managed care of substance abuse disorders: Implications for generalist physicians. *Alcohol and Other Substance Abuse, 81,* 1053–1069.

Lewis, J. S. (1988). Congressional rites of passage for the rights of alcoholics. *Alcohol Health and Research World, 12,* 240–251.

Marwick, C. (1996). Managed care may feature behavioral medicine. *Journal of the American Medical Association, 275,* 1144–1146.

Mayer, T., & Mayer, G. (1985). HMOs: Origins and development. *The New England Journal of Medicine, 312*, 590–594.

McFarland, B., Johnson, R., & Pople, C. (1994, May). *Severely mentally ill HMO members*. Paper presented at the annual meeting of the American Psychiatric Association, Philadelphia.

McLellan, A. T., Arndt, I. O., Metzger, D. S., Woody, G. E., & O'Brien, C. P. (1993). The effects of psychosocial services in substance abuse treatment. *Journal of the American Medical Association, 269*, 1953–1959.

McLellan, A. T., Meyers, M. A., Hagan, T., et al. (1996, February). Local data supports national trend of decline in substance abuse system. *Connections*, 5–8.

Musto, D. F. (1992). Historical perspectives on alcohol and drug abuse. In J. H. Lowinson, P. Ruiz, & R. B. Millman (Eds.), *Substance abuse: A comprehensive textbook* (2nd ed., pp. 2–14). Baltimore: Williams & Wilkins.

National Center on Addiction and Substance Abuse at Columbia University. (1996). *Substance abuse and federal entitlement programs* [on-line]. Available: http://www.casacolumbia.org/pubs/feb95/sa_int.htm

Nauert, R. C. (1997). Managed behavioral health care: A key component of integrated regional delivery systems. *Journal of Health Care Finance, 23*, 49–61.

Open Minds. (1996). *Managed behavioral health market share in the United States, 1996–1997*. Gettysburg, PA: Open Minds.

Pauly, M. (1968). The economics of moral hazard: Comment. *American Economic Review, 21*, 531–537.

Pomerantz, J. M. (1996). Managed care and mental health [Letter to the editor]. *The New England Journal of Medicine, 335*, 57.

Reader, J. W., & Sullivan, K. A. (1992). Private and public insurance. In J. H. Lowinson, P. Ruiz, & R. B. Millman (Eds.), *Substance abuse: A comprehensive textbook* (2nd ed., pp. 1067–1081). Baltimore: Williams & Wilkins.

Renz, E. A., Chung, R., Fillman, T. O., Mee-Lee, D., & Sayama, M. (1995). The effect of managed care on the treatment outcome of substance use disorders. *General Hospital Psychiatry, 17*, 287–292.

Rogers, W., Wells, K., & Meredith, L. (1993). Outcomes for adult outpatients with depression under prepaid or fee-for-service financing. *Archives of General Psychiatry, 50*, 517–525.

Rosenberg, S. (1996). Health Maintenance Organization penetration and general hospital psychiatric services: Expenditure and utilization trends. *Professional Psychology: Research and Practice, 27*, 345–348.

Rouse, B. A. (Ed.). (1995). *Substance abuse and mental health statistics sourcebook* (DHHS Publication No. SMA 95-3064). U.S. Department of Health and Human Services.

Schlenger, W. E., Roland, E. J., Kroutil, L. A., Dennis, M. L., Magruder, K. M., & Ray, B. A. (1994). *Evaluating services demonstration programs: A multistage approach*. Research Triangle Park, NC: Research Triangle Institute.

Shadle, M., & Christianson, J. B. (1989). The impact of HMO development on mental health and chemical dependency services. *Hospital and Community Psychiatry, 40*, 1145–1151.

United States 70th Congress, Public Law No. 672. (1929, January 19). To establish two United States narcotic farms for the confinement and treatment of persons addicted to the use of habit-forming drugs who have been convicted of offenses against the United States.

United States 82nd Congress, Public Law No. 255. (1956, July 18). To amend the penalty provision applicable to persons convicted of violating certain narcotic laws.

United States Department of Labor, Bureau of Labor Statistics. (1988). *Employee benefits in medium and large firms* (Bulletin 2336). Washington, DC: U.S. Government Printing Office.

United States Department of Health & Human Services. (1989). *National drug and alcoholism treatment unit survey* (DHHS Publication No. ADM 89-1626). Rockville, MD: Author.

VanLeit, B. (1995). Managed mental health care: Reflections in a time of turmoil. *The American Journal of Occupational Therapy, 50*, 428–434.

Wickizer, T. (1994). Medical cost-offset associated with chemical dependency treatment. In *Forecasting the cost of chemical dependency treatment under managed care: The Washington State study* (DHHS Publication No. SMA 95-3045, Technical Assistance Publication [TAP] Series, No. 15, Financing Subseries, Volume II). Washington, DC: Substance Abuse and Mental Health Services Administration (SAMHSA).

Wickizer, T. M., Lessler, D., & Travis, K. M. (1996). Controlling inpatient psychiatric utilization through managed care. *American Journal of Psychiatry, 153*, 339–345.

Wilson, C. V. (1993). Substance abuse and managed care. *New Directions for Mental Health Services, 59*, 99–105.

Yoder, B. (1990). *The recovery resource book.* New York: Simon & Schuster.

Zarkin, G. A., Galinis, D. N., French, M. T., Fountain, D. L., Ingram, P. W., & Guyett, J. A. (1995). Financing strategies for drug abuse treatment programs. *Journal of Substance Abuse Treatment, 12*, 385–399.

11

Criminal Justice Responses to Adolescent Substance Abuse

Richard Dembo
Kimberly Pacheco
University of South Florida

For many reasons, intervening with adolescents experiencing substance abuse problems remains a critical need for the juvenile justice system. First, there has been a growing recognition that youths' participation in crime is closely related to their substance use. Second, youth crime, particularly violent crime, has been increasing among adolescents in recent years; much of this increase can be traced to youth involvement in drug trafficking activities. Third, recent evidence from national surveys indicate an increase in substance use among young people. Of particular concern is an increase in substance use among young adolescents, with its threat of another drug epidemic among these youths in the next 10 years. Fourth, demographic projections indicate a substantial increase in U.S. youth population in the next 10 years, which threatens to place enormous pressure on an already overburdened juvenile justice system.

Responding effectively to adolescent substance abuse presents immense challenges to juvenile justice agencies. In most communities, these agencies have limited personnel and service resources. Most of the resources that are available are directed to "deep-ended" youths—that is, those who are committed to residential programs. This emphasis has increased in recent years in response to the legislative movement across the U.S. to "get tough" on adolescent offenders. In the face of these developments, prevention and community-based intervention efforts have engendered little enthusiasm among punishment oriented legislators, which, unfortunately, has impeded the growth and maturity of these programs.

While there is increasing evidence that treatment of individuals with substance abuse problems can result in significant decreases in delinquency and crime, the field of adolescent substance abuse treatment remains in its infancy (Dembo, Williams, & Schmeidler, 1993). The growing recognition that substance abuse among youths is related to difficulties in a number of areas of experience (such as family relationships, physical abuse and sexual victimization, educational performance, and emotional/psychological functioning) needs to result in innovative, systems-oriented approaches to address these problems.

In a previous paper, Dembo, Williams, and Schmeidler (1993) presented a summary of the needs of troubled youths entering or involved with the juvenile justice system, and reviewed efforts to address their substance abuse problems. Writing this chapter presented an opportunity to survey major changes in the juvenile justice system's efforts to identify adolescents with substance abuse problems, and to respond to them. In particular, Juvenile Assessment Centers (JAC) have been established in various locations in Florida and Kansas. These innovative programs are in the process of making significant changes at the front end of the juvenile justice system. While there has been an increase in "get tough" policies to deal with serious youth offenders, with a corresponding reduction in treatment resources, JAC facilities have assumed the important role of seeking to reduce the flow of youths deeper into the juvenile justice system.

In this chapter, we will focus on the operation of the Hillsborough County JAC, which is serving as a prototype for other JACs. Particular attention will be given to the manner in which law enforcement, state juvenile justice and substance use/mental health agencies, and various service providers work together and share information. As will be seen, JAC facilities represent an exciting, innovative development in juvenile justice.

THE CONTINUING NEED OF JUVENILE OFFENDERS FOR INTERVENTION SERVICES

Research has indicated that many youths entering the juvenile justice system are experiencing multiple personal, educational, and family problems (Dembo et al., 1996). Among the problems most consistently reported by researchers are: physical abuse (Dembo, Dertke, Borders, Washburn, & Schmeidler, 1988), sexual victimization (Dembo et al., 1989; Mouzakitis, 1981), poor emotional/psychological functioning (Dembo, Williams, LaVoie, et al., 1990; Teplin & Swartz, 1989), poor educational functioning (Dembo, Williams, Schmeidler, & Howitt, 1991) and alcohol and other drug use (Dembo, Williams, LaVoie, 1990; U.S. Department of Justice, 1983a, b). Many of these youths' difficulties can be traced to family alcohol or other drug use, mental health, or crime problems, usually beginning at an early age (Dembo, Williams, Wothke, Schmeidler & Brown, 1992; Garbarino & Gilliam, 1980).

In addition, there is increasing awareness that juveniles who are likely to be victims or perpetrators of crime because of substance abuse are also at high risk for being infected by or transmitting the human immunodeficiency virus (HIV). Wish, O'Neil, Crawford, and Baldau (1992) have identified persons having contact with the justice system as an important HIV/AIDS risk-reduction target group. Inciardi and colleagues (Inciardi & Pottieger, 1991; Inciardi, Pottieger, Forney, Chitwood & McBride, 1991) have noted that minorities and inner-city youths in general are particularly at risk for drug-related HIV infection.

Minority and inner-city youth are being socialized in communities and families that are often economically and socially stressed. The psychosocial strain suffered by these youth often increases their risk for future substance use, delinquency, and crime (Nurco, Balter, & Kinlock, 1994); and provides impediments to their development as socially responsible and productive adults (Le Blanc, 1990). Further, these youths and their families are seriously underserved (Arcia, Keyes, Gallagher, & Herrick, 1993; Dembo, Turner, Borden, Schmeidler, & Manning, 1995; Dembo, Williams, Wish, & Schmeidler, 1990; Sirles, 1990; Tolan, Ryan, & Jaffe, 1988). Innovative, holistic strategies (Steiger & Knobel, 1991) are needed to improve the availability, accessibility, service linkage, and delivery of services to high-risk youths and their families.

The barriers to such services are considerable. In most jurisdictions juvenile justice systems and associated programs are sanction-oriented; their structures and procedures often result as much from cumulative political and historical forces and service program fads as from purposeful design. Most U.S. juvenile justice jurisdictions are also crisis-oriented, working with inadequate fiscal, physical, and personnel resources. Guidry (1991) notes that juvenile justice agencies typically have an episodic interest in troubled youth. Interest is focused on the judicially imposed consequences of illegal behavior, with court-imposed intervention coming only after repeated court appearances. At that point, many youths have developed a long list of failures in informal or loosely structured programs, developed serious problems at school, and established a pattern of delinquent behavior, including substance abuse.

JUVENILE ASSESSMENT CENTERS: AN INNOVATIVE APPROACH TO PRELIMINARY SCREENING AND IN-DEPTH ASSESSMENT OF JUVENILE OFFENDERS

At the same time, reaching these youths in early adolescence provides an excellent opportunity to involve them in health and human service intervention services before their problems become more serious. Early intervention can reduce the probability they will continue criminal and high health-risk behavior into adulthood (Klitzner, Fisher, Stewart, & Gilbert, 1991), and help reduce the enormous cost to society of crime, substance abuse, and mental illness (Dembo, Williams, Schmeidler, & Christensen, 1993; Institute for Health Policy, 1993; Klitzner et al., 1991; Rice, Kelman, Miller, & Dunmeyer, 1990).

The establishment of Juvenile Assessment Centers, such as the Hillsborough County JAC in Tampa, Florida, represents a creative response to these needs. JACs recognize the complexity and correlates of substance abuse, and the need to bring together relevant community organizations that provide services to juveniles (Dembo & Brown, 1994). The Tampa JAC has recast the front end of the juvenile justice system in Hillsborough County, increased coordination among various stakeholder agencies, and resulted in improved efficiency in the processing of arrested youths.

Brief History of the Hillsborough County Juvenile Assessment Center

The Tampa JAC officially began operations in early 1993, with major funding supplied by the Anti–Drug Abuse Act of 1988. Numerous groups and individuals were involved in the conceptualization, planning, and implementation of the JAC. Major catalysts in the development of the JAC were the Hillsborough County Anti-Drug Alliance, the Hillsborough County Sheriff's Office, and the Hillsborough County School Board. In particular, Hillsborough County has an Anti-Drug Alliance that advises the County Commissioners on substance abuse issues. The Anti-Drug Alliance includes representatives from a variety of agencies, including law enforcement, substance abuse service providers, and the State Department of Health and Rehabilitative Services. The Alliance provided a forum for the establishment of the Tampa JAC.

During 15 months of self-education, consensus-building, and development of trust and rapport, the JAC planning group decided to initiate operations in a staggered fashion. The Tampa JAC began operations in January 1993 by opening its Truancy Intake Center. Youths who were picked up for truancy by Tampa Police Department officers or Hillsborough County Sheriff Office deputies began to be brought to the truancy center for evaluation and services. Four months later, the JAC delinquency component opened with processing initially being limited to youths arrested on felony or weapons misdemeanor charges. In July 1994, the Tampa JAC began to accept youths arrested on other misdemeanor charges.

The Tampa JAC as a Prototype

Recognizing that there were significant gaps in problem identification, assessment, referral, and access to services by youth at high risk of substance abuse and associated health issues, as well as delinquent behavior, the

Florida legislature began providing funds to support the establishment of JACs throughout the state. In June 1993, during a special session of the Florida legislature, $1.2 million was appropriated to support the development of three additional JACs. The following year, the legislature passed a new Juvenile Justice Bill that, among other things, provided $2 million to help establish eight more JAC programs. Legislative language includes the stated intent to establish JAC facilities in all Florida metropolitan areas. To date, JACs have opened in Orlando, Ft. Lauderdale, St. Petersburg, and Tallahassee. Additional JACs are in various stages of being established in Pensacola, West Palm Beach, Sarasota, Ft. Myers, and Bradenton. Juvenile Assessment Centers based on the Tampa model also are being established throughout the state of Kansas.

In various communities, as key stakeholders assemble to plan the local JAC program, variations on the Tampa JAC model are emerging. In most cases, however, the basic elements and functions of the model include: (1) centralized location of relevant agencies to permit the efficient completion of required legal and social service interventions for at-risk youths and their families; (2) screening, diagnosis and, if indicated, linkage of arrested and other high-risk juveniles with community-based service providers; (3) case management of juveniles assigned to justice system diversion programs; and (4) tracking (usually limited to the purpose of determining referral disposition).

Operation of the Tampa JAC

Arrested youths are brought to the Tampa JAC facility by law enforcement personnel via a "sallyport." Upon entering the JAC, an exchange of official forms occurs between the arresting officer, sheriff's deputies operating JAC's secure wing and State Department of Juvenile Justice (DJJ) staff. Within minutes, the arresting officer is free to return to his or her assigned duties. Once law enforcement and DJJ personnel have completed their admission tasks (see below), the juveniles are further processed by DJJ detention intake and JAC assessor staff.

The Tampa JAC is coordinated by the Agency for Community Treatment Services (ACTS), Inc., a private not-for-profit substance abuse treatment agency. The assessment center is located with the treatment agency's 20-bed adolescent detoxification and stabilization program (the Addiction Receiving Facility) with full-time nursing staff, and medical, psychological, and psychiatric back-up services. The staff who provide these core treatment services as well as those who perform assessment and case management services are available 24 hours a day. This physical consolidation of services contributes greatly to operational efficiency and cost savings (e.g., reduced transportation costs, cross-trained staff serve as multi-position back-ups).

JAC assessors complete preliminary screening of arrested youths, and, if indicated, refer juveniles to specific services, such as Treatment Alternatives to Street Crime (TASC) and Delinquency (Psychological) Assessment Team (DAT) services. All procedures are designed and delivered in conformity with pertinent state law. The outcomes of the referral process are tracked (Dembo & Brown, 1994). JAC assessors also obtain identifying information, such as social security number and the names and locations of significant others, permitting tracking of the youths once they leave the JAC or community-based service programs.

Tampa JAC operations rely heavily on its comprehensive information system, which has three integrated subsystems: (1) preliminary screening data, (2) in-depth assessment data, and (3) referral and referral outcome data (Dembo & Brown, 1994). The information system reflects the components of the JAC's operational activities, which are modelled after the National Institute on Drug Abuse Adolescent Assessment/Referral System (NIDA/AARS) (Rahdert, 1991).

Arrested youths delivered to the JAC for screening submit to on-site breathalyzer and EMIT® urine testing for other drugs (cannabinoids, cocaine, benzodiazepines, amphetamines, opiates, and PCP). All youths processed at the center undergo a preliminary screening process using the NIDA Problem Oriented Screening Instrument for Teenagers (POSIT) to identify potential problems in any of 10 psychosocial functioning areas. The reliability, and discriminant and predictive validity of the POSIT has been established (Dembo, Turner, Borden, et al., 1995; Dembo et al., 1994). Responses to the POSIT are computer scored. The results, based on cut-off scores and red flag items recommended by the AARS manual together with breathalyzer or urine test findings (positive for alcohol or other drug use), are used to determine whether to proceed with more in-depth assessments. Experience indicates that a significant proportion of served youth have recently used an illicit drug (30% of arrested youths processed at the center during February 1996 were EMIT®-positive for marijuana and 4% were for cocaine) or are experiencing potential problems in one or more areas probed by the POSIT.

Again, as recommended by the AARS manual, the in-depth assessment protocol includes the Personal Experience Inventory (PEI; Winters & Henley, 1989) and the National Youth Survey Delinquency Scale (Elliott et al., 1983). Further, information is collected on the youths' sexual victimization (based on the work of Finkelhor, 1979), physical abuse (based on the work of Straus, 1979), and medical histories. Screening and assessment information collected to date indicate that the mental health or substance abuse service needs of arrested juveniles have been significantly unattended or unmet (Dembo, Turner, Borden, et al., 1995).

As noted earlier, JAC operational procedures begin with justice system tasks. On delivery by an arresting officer, juveniles are first fingerprinted and photographed. Florida DJJ detention intake staff complete a Detention Risk Assessment Instrument on the youth (Dembo et al., 1994). A file on the youth is opened or reopened on the JAC information system. Demographic and current arrest information are entered into the computer by assessors, who have received data entry training. On-line computer communications with the Florida Department of Health and Rehabilitative Services in Talla-hassee can print reports of any delinquency and abuse histories. Similarly, JAC staff have computer terminal access to selected county school system specified information on youths' educational history.

On the basis of current charges and arrest history, Florida DJJ delin-quency intake staff determine whether the youth should be placed in secure detention, on home detention, or released to the supervision of a parent, guardian, or responsible relative. Youths released from the JAC to their parents, guardians, or other relatives are scheduled, if needed, for an ap-pointment to receive in-depth assessments by TASC or DAT staff located at the JAC. Youths meeting state-established detention criteria are transported to the local detention center by a van operated by JAC staff 24 hours a day. Detained youths have in-depth assessments completed by counselors from another local service provider that is contracted by detention center admin-istrators to operate a triage-screening unit.

If the assessed youth is already under DJJ supervision, their DJJ coun-selor is notified of the new arrest. If the youth is not currently under DJJ supervision, but is arrested on felony or weapon misdemeanor charges, he or she will be assigned a DJJ counselor. If the youth is arrested on other misdemeanor charges, and is not detention eligible, he or she will be as-signed to case management staff located at the JAC.

JUVENILE ASSESSMENT CENTERS: A FOCAL POINT FOR EARLY INTERVENTION SERVICES

It is important to refer youths who are identified as having a potential substance abuse or mental health problem for additional assessment and, if indicated, placement in needed services. A number of innovative early intervention programs for arrested youths (cf. Klitzner et al., 1991) are being implemented at the Tampa JAC.

Placement in a Nonjudicial Diversion Program

The major purpose of the JAC misdemeanor case management unit is to review the arrest histories and current charges of youths arrested on mis-demeanor offenses to determine their eligibility for involvement in a nonju-dicial diversion program: the Juvenile Alternative Services Program (JASP) or arbitration. Admission of guilt is required for a youth to be accepted in either diversion program. JASP is a 60-day program, which provides immediate sanctions to misdemeanor offenders. It has a number of program components, such as community work service, victim restitution, and counseling services that provide short-term individual, adolescent, group, and family counseling. The arbitration program involves a trained arbitrator (not a judge) hearing the case against a youth, and obtaining relevant information from the youth, the victim, and arresting officer. On the basis of this information, the arbitrator decides on sanctions against the youth. These sanctions can include community service hours, victim restitution, participating in a counseling program, or any combination of these sanctions.

The parents or guardians of misdemeanor youths are called to pick him or her up at JAC the same day they are processed, and to meet with the youth's case manager. The case manager informs the youth's parents or guardians of the legal issues surrounding their child, the results of the youth's preliminary screening, and their recommendation to arbitration or JASP. The case manager is also expected to inform the parents or guardians about their child's specific service needs.

The case managers' recommendations to arbitration or JASP are forwarded to the state attorney's office, where they are usually approved. Youths placed in the arbitration or JASP program are carried on the caseloads of JAC misdemeanor case managers until the youth successfully completes the program to which he or she is assigned. If the youth fails to complete the program, the misdemeanor case manager makes a recommendation to the state attorney's office to reinstate the youth in the program, place the youth in another program, or file a delinquency petition against him or her. If a delinquency petition is filed, the misdemeanor case manager transfers the case to a DJJ case manager.

Linking Youths With Community-Based Substance Abuse and Mental Health Services

DJJ or JAC misdemeanor case managers will make service recommendations that seek to match the service needs of arrested youths processed at the center. JAC assessor staff make direct referrals to the Addiction Receiving Facility if the youth appears to be under the influence of alcohol or other drugs upon entering the center, reports using alcohol or other drugs the day of arrest, or reports a pattern of frequent substance use during the preliminary screening process. Following stabilization and evaluation at the Addiction Receiving Facility, the youth may be referred to an outpatient or residential treatment program.

A unit of TASC and DAT staff are located adjacent to the JAC facility. This unit coordinates with JAC operations, and serves as referral resources for substance abuse or mental health services, respectively. Each morning, TASC/DAT staff review the dossiers on arrested youths processed at JAC the preceding day who are not placed in the juvenile detention center. On the basis of these dossier reports, and the results of the youths' urine tests, staff determine whether a referral should be made to receive TASC or DAT services. The parents or guardians of youths assigned to receive TASC/DAT services will be contacted by telephone or mail and invited to make an appointment for a free in-depth assessment.

The outcomes of youths referred to various services are tracked for 90 days to learn whether the youth has received the recommended service. These data are valuable in providing insights into how the JAC referral process can be improved.

JUVENILE ASSESSMENT CENTERS: PROVIDING IN-HOME INTERVENTION SERVICES TO JUVENILE OFFENDERS

The Youth Support Project (YSP) is a family intervention project that operates out of the Tampa JAC. The YSP is implementing a systems-oriented approach to family preservation called the Family Empowerment Intervention (FEI) (Cervenka, Dembo, & Brown, in press). Funded by the National Institute on Drug Abuse for 5 years, the YSP is now in its third year. This innovative randomized, experimental, prospective longitudinal study, involves four interview data collection waves and recidivism analyses.

A distinctive feature of the FEI is that the families are served by field consultants, who are not trained therapists—although they are trained by, and perform their work under the direction of, a licensed clinician. The FEI is an intensive family systems intervention delivered in the home. The field consultant assigned to the family meets with the family a minimum of three times a week for approximately ten weeks. Each family meeting lasts one hour. All household members are expected to be present for these meetings.

The choice of paraprofessionals is based on a cost-effectiveness argument, and is supported by experimental research indicating that, at least for some treatments, paraprofessionals produce outcomes that are better than those under control conditions, and similar to those involving professional therapists (Christensen & Jacobson, 1994). Further, by requiring less previous therapy training, the FEI will facilitate the opportunities that this treatment can be funded, given the financial limitations now facing agencies that provide services to juvenile offenders.

The focus of the project is on providing intervention services to youths, with less serious offense histories, and their families. Accordingly, youths processed at the Tampa JAC who are arrested on misdemeanor charges and recommended for arbitration or other diversion programs are oversampled for inclusion in the project (80%), as compared to youths with felony arrest histories (20%). Ultimately, 720 Black, Latino, and Anglo, male and female arrested youths processed at the JAC and their families will be involved in the project. Three hundred and sixty youths and their families will be randomly assigned to receive FEI, and 360 youths will be randomly placed in an extended services (ES) group. Extended services group families are able to use an extensive resource file in order to gain referrals to other agencies in the community. This resource system enables project research staff to provide families with information about different community agen-cies and assist families in obtaining appropriate referrals to meet their needs. Families involved in the YSP receive services for up to 4 years.

ADOLESCENT DRUG COURT

Background

The drug court movement began in the 1980s with the explosion of cocaine, crack, and PCP use. Increased law enforcement activity focused more closely on drug-related crimes and put greater emphasis on the apprehension of street dealers. As a result, many state and local criminal courts began to be inundated with felony drug cases (U.S. Dept. of Justice, NIJ, 1993a, b).

The strain that was placed on the court system led to a search for more effective ways to handle the increased number of drug arrests. One solution to this problem was the development of the concept of drug courts. The drug court concept departed from the traditional approach where the court frequently sanctioned the offenders "out" to treatment as a condition of their probation. In contrast, the drug court brought drug treatment to the criminal justice population (U.S. Dept. of Justice, NIJ, 1995). The first diver-sionary treatment adult drug court in the U. S. was designed and imple-mented in Dade County, Florida in 1989 (U.S. Department of Justice, 1993b). Since that time, many other jurisdictions have followed suit: for example, Ft. Lauderdale, Chicago, and Portland, Oregon (U.S. Department of Justice, BJA, 1993a). The rationale behind the court-based drug treatment approach was guided by the notion that providing defendants an opportunity for self-improvement and drug treatment would reduce the demand for illicit drugs and, hence, involvement in crime and reinvolvement in the court system (U.S. Department of Justice, NIJ, 1993b, c).

Core Elements of a Drug Treatment Court

One of the most important elements necessary for the effective operation of a drug court is the collaborative effort among a variety of criminal justice agencies, courts, and treatment providers. All the key agencies involved in drug courts need to be on the same team, making the same demands on the defendant. They all need to have one goal to fulfill, which is to keep the defendant out of the court system and off drugs (U.S. Department of Justice, 1993b, U.S. Department of Justice, NIJ, 1995; U.S. Department of Justice, NIJ, 1993c).

Just as important as the collaborative interrelationships among criminal justice agencies is the working relationship between the courts and the treatment providers. The treatment program must be tailored to serve the purpose of criminal processing while facilitating successful treatment for drug-involved defendants (U.S. Department of Justice, 1993b, U.S. Department of Justice, NIJ, 1995).

A treatment drug court cannot succeed without the central role and leadership of the judiciary. Drug courts are led by a drug court judge who not only oversees the case processing aspect of criminal cases, but who is also actively involved in reviewing the defendants' status in their treatment program. The judge serves as the overall facilitator of treatment by resolving criminal justice issues while helping overcome problems that stand in the way of treatment progress.

Tampa's Adolescent Drug Court

On March 28, 1995, the Tampa JAC began voluntary drug testing of all juvenile arrestees. As indicated earlier, on-site testing results have indicated high rates of the recent use of marijuana, and, secondarily, cocaine among these youths. The Tampa Adolescent Drug Court was established to intervene with these youths. It is an early intervention program designed to reach drug-involved youth at a critical stage, and is modeled after the Miami Drug Court (U.S. Department of Justice, 1993c). Tampa's juvenile drug court is the first of its kind, although Pensacola, Florida is in the process of establishing its own juvenile drug court.

The Tampa JAC plays a critical role in the life of the Adolescent Drug Court by screening all youths who are processed at the center as well as making referrals of eligible youths to the program. To be eligible for the program, a youth must be charged with a felony or misdemeanor possession of an illegal drug, an alcohol-related offense, or a nonviolent crime determined to have been motivated by drug dependency. The youth must be physically and mentally stable to receive treatment and must have a low recidivism rate, as indicated by a first- or second-time felony or multiple misdemeanor arrest on a drug charge. The youth must also have a responsible adult that agrees to attend counseling with him or her. In sum, youths are screened for the program on the basis of their POSIT results, urinalysis results, current charges, and past criminal history (Adelson & Labart, 1995).

Each youth admitted to the program is required to submit to random drug tests, make regular court appearances, and be willing to complete any other sanctions the court or treatment program imposes (Labart, 1995a). Each participant is assigned a case manager shortly after intake and prior to the first court appearance. The case manager will act as a liaison for the youth in the court, as well as develop treatment plans, service contracts and monitor the youth's progress in the program.

The Adolescent Drug Court is designed as a 9-month program and is divided into four phases. Phase I of the program is the stabilization and detoxification stage. Each youth is admitted to the ACTS Addiction Receiving Facility for 3 to 5 days for a comprehensive evaluation. This evaluation is primarily psychosocial in nature and collects information regarding medical history, criminal history, substance use/abuse, family functioning, educational performance, history of abuse/neglect, mental health status, and peer involvement. After Phase I each client is referred to ACTS Youth Outpatient Treatment Program to begin Phase II.

Phase II is an intensive day treatment program designed to last between 2 and 13 weeks. Clients who do not benefit from an outpatient program can be referred to a residential program by the court. Treatment is focused on sobriety through a 12-step model, self-esteem growth, and building family communications. In this phase, clients attend group counseling, individual counseling, and family counseling sessions, as well as participate in support groups such as Al-Anon or NA. Random urine tests are given twice a week at the discretion of the counselor. If a client relapses, a referral can be made to Phase I of the program.

Phase III of the program focuses on continued sobriety with an emphasis on decision-making skills, peer relationships, and educational/vocational issues. This phase is designed to last for approximately 12 weeks. The client continues attending group, individual, and family counseling sessions, along with support groups. Random urine tests are given once a week at the discretion of the counselors.

Phase IV, the final program stage, lasts for the duration of the program. During this phase, emphasis is placed on the client's continued involvement in support groups and counseling sessions that will sustain drug-free living. The client continues attending group counseling sessions and support groups, and submits urine specimens for testing three to four times a month (Labart, 1995b).

The juvenile's progress is monitored by a Drug Court judge throughout the four treatment phases. If a client does not participate successfully in treatment, the judge may sanction him or her back to juvenile court to be processed on their current charges. The judge will successfully discharge a client from treatment once the client (1) submits clean urines for at least six months; (2) successfully completes outpatient or residential treatment; (3) continues with his or her education plans or is continuously employed; and (4) completes any sanctions imposed by the courts, such as restitution payment, a letter of apology, community service hours, and payment of fines and client fees. Once a client successfully completes the Adolescent Drug Court program, his or her current charges will be dismissed (Labart, 1995a).

CONCLUSIONS

A national commitment to help troubled youths is needed to reduce their substance abuse and delinquency. Youths involved in the juvenile justice system, especially those with substance abuse or mental health problems, consume a large and growing amount of state resources as they grow older. Early intervention is needed for these youths to reduce the likelihood they will move further into the juvenile, and, ultimately adult, justice systems. Studies have documented the enormous cost to our society of crime and drug abuse (Institute for Health Policy, 1993; Rice et al., 1990).

Juvenile Assessment Centers are ideal places to complete required legal activities as well as initiate innovative, early intervention efforts to address delinquent behavior and related psychosocial problems of troubled youth. Juvenile Assessment Centers are recasting the front end of the juvenile justice systems in the communities in which they operate. They represent an exciting development in the 1990s to address, in a more comprehensive way, the complex issues presented by youth crime.

ACKNOWLEDGMENT

The preparation of this manuscript was supported by Grant #1-R01-DA08707-03, funded by the National Institute on Drug Abuse, and by a grant from the Florida Department of Juvenile Justice.

REFERENCES

Adelson, V., & Labart, E. (1995). [Tampa's Adolescent Drug Court Procedure Manual]. Unpublished raw data.

Arcia, E., Keyes, L., Gallagher, J. J., & Herrick, H. (1993). National portrait of sociodemographic factors associated with underutilization of services: Relevance to early intervention. *Journal of Early Intervention, 17,* 283–297.

Cervenka, K. A., Dembo, R., & Brown, C. H. (in press). A family empowerment intervention for families of juvenile offenders. *Aggression and Violent Behavior: A Review Journal.*

Christensen, A., & Jacobson, N. S. (1994). Who (or what) can do psychotherapy: The status and challenge of nonprofessional therapies. *Psychological Science, 5,* 8–14.

Dembo, R., & Brown, R. (1994). The Hillsborough County Juvenile Assessment Center. *Journal of Child and Adolescent Substance Abuse, 3,* 25–43.

Dembo, R., Dertke, M., Borders, S., Washburn, M., & Schmeidler, J. (1988). The relationship between physical and sexual abuse and tobacco, alcohol and illicit drug use among youths in a juvenile detention center. *International Journal of the Addictions, 23*, 351–378.

Dembo, R., Turner, G., Borden, P., Schmeidler, J., & Manning, D. (1995). Screening high risk youths for potential problems: Field application in the use of the Problem Oriented Screening Instrument for Teenagers (POSIT). *Journal of Child and Adolescent Substance Abuse, 3*, 69–93.

Dembo, R., Turner, G. S., Chin Sue, C., Schmeidler, J., Borden, P., & Manning, D. (1994). An assessment of the Florida Department of Health and Rehabilitative Services Detention Risk Assessment Instrument on youths screened and processed at the Hillsborough County Juvenile Assessment Center. *Journal of Child and Adolescent Substance Abuse, 4*, 45–77.

Dembo, R., Turner, G. S., Chin Sue, C., Schmeidler, J., Borden, P., & Manning, D. (1995). Predictors of recidivism to a juvenile assessment center. *International Journal of the Addictions, 30*, 1425–1452.

Dembo, R., Turner, G., Schmeidler, J., Chin Sue, C., Borden, P., & Manning, D. (1996). Development and evaluation of a classification of high risk youths entering a juvenile assessment center. *International Journal of the Addictions, 31*, 303–322.

Dembo, R., Williams, L., LaVoie, L., Berry, E., Getreu, A., Wish, E. D., Schmeidler, J., & Washburn, M. (1989). Physical abuse, sexual victimization and illicit drug use: Replication of a structural analysis among a new sample of high risk youths. *Violence and Victims, 4*, 121–138.

Dembo, R., Williams, L., LaVoie, L., Getreu, A., Berry, E., Genung, L., Schmeidler, J., Wish, E. D., & Kern, J. (1990). A longitudinal study of the relationships among alcohol use, marijuana/hashish use, cocaine use and emotional/psychological functioning problems in a cohort of high risk youths. *International Journal of the Addictions, 25*, 1341–1382.

Dembo, R., Williams, L., & Schmeidler, J. (1993). Addressing the problems of substance abuse in juvenile corrections. In James A. Inciardi (Ed.), *Drug treatment in criminal justice settings.* Newbury Park, CA: Sage.

Dembo, R., Williams, L., Schmeidler, J., & Christensen, C. (1993). Recidivism in a cohort of juvenile detainees: A 3-1/2 year follow-up. *International Journal of the Addictions, 26*, 1197–1221.

Dembo, R., Williams, L., Schmeidler, J., & Howitt, D. (1991). *Troubled lifestyles: High risk youth in Florida.* Washington, DC: U.S. Department of Education.

Dembo, R., Williams, L., Wish, E. D., & Schmeidler, J. (1990). *Urine testing of detained juveniles to identify high-risk youth.* Washington, DC: U.S. Department of Justice.

Dembo, R., Williams, L., Wothke, W., Schmeidler, J., & Brown, C. H. (1992). The role of family factors, physical abuse and sexual victimization experiences in high risk youths' alcohol and other drug use and delinquency: A longitudinal model. *Violence and Victims, 7*, 245–266.

Elliott, D. S., Ageton, S. S., Huizinga, D., Knowles, B. A., & Canter, R. J. (1983). *The prevalence and incidence of delinquent behavior: 1976–1980.* Boulder, CO: Behavioral Research Institute.

Finkelhor, D. (1979). *Sexually victimized children.* New York: The Free Press.

Garbarino, J., & Gilliam, G. (1980). *Understanding abusive families.* Lexington, MA: Lexington.

Guidry, J. (1991, June 18). Cloak of evil not worn by adults alone. *Tampa Tribune* (Florida).

Inciardi, J. A., & Pottieger, A. E. (1991). Kids, crack, and crime. *Journal of Drug Issues, 21*, 257–270.

Inciardi, J. A., Pottieger, A. E., Forney, M. A., Chitwood, D. D., & McBride, D. C. (1991). Prostitution, IV drug use, and sex-for-crack exchanges among serious delinquents: Risks For HIV infection. *Criminology, 29*, 221–235.

Institute for Health Policy. (1993). *Substance abuse: The nation's number one health problem.* Waltham, MA: Author.

Klitzner, M., Fisher, D., Stewart, K., & Gilbert, S. (1991). *Report to the Robert Wood Johnson Foundation on strategies for early intervention with children and youth to avoid abuse of addictive substances.* Bethesda, MD: Pacific Institute for Research and Evaluation.

Labart, E. (1995a). [13th Judicial Circuit Juvenile Drug Court Procedure Manual]. Unpublished raw data.

Labart, E. (1995b). [ACTS, Inc., Outpatient Treatment Manual for Juvenile Drug Court]. Unpublished raw data.

Le Blanc, M. (1990). *Family dynamics, adolescent delinquency and adult criminality*. Paper presented at the Society for Life History Research Conference.

Mouzakitis, C. M. (1981). Inquiry into the problem of child abuse and juvenile delinquency. In R. J. Hunner & Y. E. Walker (Eds.), *Exploring the relationship between child abuse delinquency.* Montclair, NJ: Allenheld, Osmum.

Nurco, D. N., Balter, M. B., & Kinlock, T. (1994). Vulnerability to narcotic addiction. *Journal of Drug Issues, 24*, 293–314.

Rahdert, E. R. (Ed.). (1991). *The adolescent assessment/referral system*. Rockville, MD: National Institute on Drug Abuse.

Rice, D. P., Kelman, S., Miller, L. S., & Dunmeyer, S. (1990). *The economic costs of alcohol and drug abuse and mental illness*. San Francisco: University of California, San Francisco, Institute for Health and Aging.

Sirles, E. A. (1990). Dropout from intake, diagnostics, and treatment. *Community Mental Health Journal, 26*, 345–360.

Steiger, J. C., & Knobel, D. (1991). *Profiles of juvenile offenders in Washington state Division of Juvenile Rehabilitation Facilities: Results from a 1990 survey of youth in residence*. Olympia, WA: Washington Department of Social and Health Services.

Straus, M. A. (1979). Measuring intrafamily conflict and violence: The conflict tactics (CT) scales. *Journal of Marriage and the Family, 41*, 75–88.

Teplin, L. A., & Swartz, J. (1989). Screening for severe mental disorder in jails. The development of the Referral Decision Scale. *Law and Human Behavior, 13*, 1–18.

Tolan, P., Ryan, K., & Jaffe, C. (1988). Adolescents' mental health service use and provider, process, and recipient characteristics. *Journal of Clinical Child Psychology, 17*, 229–236.

U.S. Department of Justice. (1983a). *Prisoners and alcohol* (ACJ-86223). Washington, DC: Bureau of Justice Statistics Bulletin.

U.S. Department of Justice. (1983b). *Prisoners and drugs* (NCJ87575). Washington, DC: Bureau of Justice Statistics Bulletin.

U.S. Department of Justice. (1993a). *Special drug courts* (NCJ-144531). Washington, DC: Bureau of Justice Assistance.

U.S. Department of Justice. (1993b). *Justice and treatment innovation: The drug court movement* (NCJ-149260). Washington, DC: National Institute of Justice.

U.S. Department of Justice. (1993c). *Miami's "drug court," a different approach* (NCJ-142412). Washington, DC: National Institute of Justice.

U.S. Department of Justice. (1995). *The drug court movement*. Office of Justice Programs. Washington, DC: National Institute of Justice.

Winters, K. C., & Henley, G. A. (1989). *Personal Experience Inventory manual*. Los Angeles: Western Psychological Services.

Wish, E. D., O'Neil, J., Crawford, J. A., & Baldau, V. (1992). Lost opportunity to combat aids: Drug users in the criminal justice system. In T. Mieczkowski (Ed.), *Drugs, crime, and social policy*. Boston: Allyn & Bacon.

12

Criminal Justice Responses to Adult Substance Abuse

Timothy W. Kinlock
University of Baltimore and
Friends Research Institute

Thomas E. Hanlon
David N. Nurco
University of Maryland School of Medicine and
Friends Research Institute

This chapter summarizes research findings on the effectiveness of criminal justice responses to adult substance abuse. The focus is on heroin and cocaine primarily, because, in contrast to the use of other substances, increased use of heroin and cocaine typically results in an increase in criminal activity among offenders (Nurco, Hanlon, & Kinlock, 1991). Initially, pertinent issues and a brief historical overview of criminal justice–based interventions will be addressed. Subsequently, the focus will be on the effectiveness of various interventions, such as compulsory supervision and mandatory treatment; police crackdowns; parole and probation; incarceration; and more recently developed sanctions, such as intensive supervision parole/probation (ISP); shock incarceration; and in-prison treatment. Emphasis will be placed on methodological considerations, particularly the use of outcome measures, in order to illustrate the extent of the knowledge regarding assessment of these approaches. In the conclusion, unanswered questions and suggestions for future research and policy will be addressed.

BACKGROUND AND PERTINENT ISSUES

Since the early 1980s, increased national concern over substance abuse, especially heroin and cocaine, have had a profound impact on such criminal justice interventions as mandatory treatment, police crackdowns, parole, probation, and incarceration. The 1980s also ushered in a period of strong conservative views that stressed the notion that the sources of deviant and criminal behavior reside within individuals and not in society. One consequence of this thinking was a de-emphasis on treatment and rehabilitation and the increased reliance on criminal justice sanctions as a means of reducing substance abuse and its related crime.

Research has indicated that some of these approaches, mainly mandatory treatment, can be effective in reducing narcotic addiction and crime. However, an emphasis on the arrest and incarceration of substance abusers has also caused problems by overburdening the criminal justice system and taxing the limited availability of personnel and other resources necessary for providing meaningful treatment. As a result, dramatic increases in the proportions of substance abusers under criminal justice supervision, severe prison overcrowding, and a lack of programs designed to meet the needs of substance-abusing offenders have become pressing concerns. These concerns have been exacerbated by high rates of recidivism, relapse to substance abuse, and HIV infection among drug-involved prisoners. In response to this situation, new criminal justice interventions aimed at drug-abusing inmates have been recently developed (Inciardi, 1993; MacKenzie & Uchida, 1994).

Evaluations of the effectiveness of criminal justice approaches have heretofore contained some important limitations. First, they have focused on only one phase of correctional system involvement, that of separately evaluating either in-prison treatment or supervision of clients in the community. Despite emphasis on continuity of care, substance abuse treatment research has rarely examined the relative effectiveness of approaches that combine both institutional interventions and aftercare in the community. Second, except for studies that have assessed mandatory treatment (which have typically used self-report data), community-based research, including that on ISP and shock incarceration, has used arrest, conviction, and reincarceration data as principal indicators of deviant activity. Such measures are gross underestimates of the extent of such activity, including illicit drug use. Self-report studies, in which confidentiality of data and immunity from prosecution have been assured, have consistently found that less than 1% of crime reported by substance abusers results in arrest (Ball, 1991; Inciardi, 1986; Inciardi & Pottieger, 1986, 1991, 1994). These and other methodological problems have consistently hampered a meaningful assessment of criminal justice interventions.

While self-reports of substance use and crime are generally reliable and valid when obtained for research purposes from substance abusers who are entering treatment programs in the community or who are already incarcerated (Chaiken & Chaiken, 1982; Hser, Anglin, & Chou, 1992; Inciardi, 1986; Wish & Gropper, 1990), they are less likely to be valid for individuals who are being evaluated for initial disposition following arrest. New arrestees tend to underreport recent substance abuse, even in a voluntary, confidential research interview (Wish & Gropper, 1990). Moreover, probationers and parolees are more likely to deny involvement in substance abuse and crime if they know that urinalysis monitoring is not required and if they perceive that the researchers are associated with the criminal justice system. Because of these circumstances, urine testing is increasingly being used to determine recent substance abuse among such individuals.

HISTORICAL PERSPECTIVE

Criminal justice responses to substance abuse in the United States have focused primarily on narcotic drugs such as heroin. The development of approaches aimed at nonnarcotic drug abuse is a more recent phenomenon. Among nonnarcotic drugs, cocaine currently commands the most attention by both law enforcement personnel and criminal justice researchers because of high rates of abuse and the association of the abuse of this particular drug with increased criminal activity.

Since the passage of the Harrison Act in 1914, which banned the over-the-counter sale of narcotics and cocaine in the United States, the history of responses to substance abuse in our nation has been cyclic. Criminal justice sanctions, including deterrence, arrest, and incarceration, have dominated during periods when the social and political climate was conservative: from the 1920s through the 1950s and again from 1980 to the present. In contrast, treatment and rehabilitation were emphasized during more liberal periods such as the 1960s and 1970s.

During the past 30 years, the changing social and political climate of the United States, combined with other factors, has contributed to dramatic changes in criminal justice policies with regard to substance abuse. Throughout the 1960s, when rehabilitation was dominant within the criminal justice system, offenders were generally given indeterminate sentences and were provided treatment based on their individual needs (Cullen & Gilbert, 1982). This policy was largely based on the medical model. Professionals, typically psychologists and psychiatrists on parole boards, were responsible for determining the nature of the offender's problem, the nature of treatment based on that problem, and when the problem was sufficiently alleviated so the inmate could be released from supervision or custody.

Several events in the late 1960s and early 1970s led to a change in the abovementioned approach. Many more liberal-minded Americans were of the opinion that events such as the Vietnam War, the civil rights movement, women's rights and opportunity, and the increased prevalence of prison riots brought into question the humaneness of correctional policies. Such events were construed as evidence that the criminal justice system was not fair to offenders because it forced them to undergo interventions that were not of their choice and because others, namely parole boards, decided how long they should be incarcerated. Moreover, there was concern that the system was unfair to minorities, as most prisoners participating in riots over adverse circumstances and unfair treatment were African American. Thus, as a means of reducing discrimination, a determinate system of sentencing based on the severity of the offender's crime was preferred in addition to the abolition of parole boards and treatment be given only with consent. For entirely different reasons, many Americans with conservative views were also upset about the rehabilitation policy and the indeterminate nature of sentences within the criminal justice system. They felt that the criminal justice system was "soft" on crime because many offenders did not serve their full sentences. They contended that indeterminate sentencing resulting from parole actions contributed to the rise in the crime rate during the late 1960s and early 1970s (Lilly, Cullen, & Ball, 1995).

As a consequence of the general ambiance of dissatisfaction arising from both perspectives, the emphasis shifted from that of rehabilitation to a policy of "just desserts" (retribution), incapacitation, and deterrence. Determinate sentences and adherence to uniformly accepted sentencing guidelines became more common, and parole boards were given less discretional power and influence. In addition, several literature reviews published at that time (Lipton, Martinson, & Wilks, 1975; Martinson, 1974; Sechrest, White, & Brown, 1979) were interpreted as evidence that "nothing works," giving policymakers further justification for de-emphasizing rehabilitation.

In the 1980s, the emphasis shifted toward increased punishment. Crime was considered an individual matter as reflected in the popularity of Wilson and Herrnstein's (1985) theory of the causes of crime. According to this theory, crime and drug use were considered the result of biological and psychological abnormalities in certain individuals as opposed to social or economic inequalities. When the causes of drug use and crime are viewed as resulting from individual deficiencies, the response is typically more punitive. Evidence of this type of response is reflected in increased arrests and incarcerations accounted for, in part, by the "war on drugs" and "zero tolerance" policies emphasized during the 1980s (Inciardi, 1993; Lilly et al., 1995). Against this backdrop, public concern over crack cocaine led to even tougher sentences against drug dealers and users (Inciardi, 1993; Wexler, 1994).

As might be expected, this latest shift in policy contributed to increases in the prevalence of both lifetime (ever used) and regular substance abuse among criminal justice–involved populations as more substance abusers were being sent to prison. While studies have consistently revealed high rates of use among incarcerated individuals, there is strong evidence that this problem has been increasing. Barton (1980, 1982) conducted two surveys of 10,400 and 5,300 inmates during 1974 and 1978, respectively. In the 1974 survey, 61% of the subjects admitted lifetime use of illicit drugs; approximately 25% reported daily or near-daily use. These rates increased to 68 and 40%, respectively, in the 1978 survey. Harlow (1991) reported even higher lifetime and regular use rates among a sample of 395,554 inmates interviewed in 1989. Seventy-eight per cent of these respondents reported having lifetime use of illicit drugs, while 58% reported regular drug use. Moreover, data from Drug Use Forecasting (DUF), a nationwide urinalysis testing system, indicated that during 1994, 66% of over 27,000 arrestees from 24 U.S. cities tested positive for recent drug use (National Institute of Justice [NIJ], 1995a), compared to 61% in 1991. In 1994, 22 cities had positive rates over 50%; six had positive rates over 70%.

Drug use rates among arrestees and prisoners are approximately two to nine times higher than for the general population (Johnston, O'Malley, & Bachman, 1995a, 1995b; National Institute on Drug Abuse [NIDA], 1992). There is an even greater disparity between the two populations with regard to heroin and cocaine use, which are more likely than other drugs to be associated with increased criminal activity, AIDS, and other adverse health consequences. For example, among Harlow's inmate sample noted above, 70% reported heroin use and 24% cocaine use in the month preceding the offense. In contrast, among household residents interviewed at about the same time (NIDA, 1992) only .1% used heroin and 2% used cocaine in the month preceding interview.

In recent years, there has been a gradual increase in combining sanctions with treatment, partially because of the increasing number of substance abusers in the criminal justice system. The past 10 years has witnessed the development of a number of new approaches to the management of substance-abusing individuals, such as in-prison treatment, intensive supervision/probation (ISP), home detention, shock incarceration, boot camp prisons, and interventions encompassing both prison and parole periods. These new programs, together with the more traditional practices of arrest, incarceration, and deterrence, along with mandatory treatment, presently comprise the major criminal justice–based interventions for substance abuse in the United States.

RESEARCH FINDINGS ON CRIMINAL JUSTICE INTERVENTIONS

Compulsory Supervision/Mandatory Treatment

Among the most encouraging findings concerning criminal justice interventions are those associated with compulsory supervision and mandatory treatment of drug abusers. These interventions use legal pressure combined with a monitoring, or surveillance, component. One of the most ambitious evaluations of treatment outcomes in the United States was the Drug Abuse Reporting Program (DARP), which involved over 4,000 clients (Simpson & Sells, 1982). This research found that methadone maintenance, therapeutic communities, and outpatient drug-free treatment programs were superior to detoxification only and intake only (i.e., no treatment) in reducing illicit drug use and criminal activity at 3- to 6-year follow-up. Moreover, as found in subsequent studies (Collins & Allison, 1983; Hubbard, Collins, Rachal, & Cavanaugh, 1988; Hubbard, Rachal, Craddock, & Cavanaugh, 1984), marked improvement among court-referred clients tended to occur during the first three months of treatment, especially with methadone maintenance, suggesting a compliance factor associated with court-mandatory entry and program surveillance. After this initial change, improvement tended to continue over time as individuals developed the necessary motivation to stay in treatment.

Three of the studies cited above (Collins & Allison, 1983; Hubbard et al., 1984, 1988) concerned research conducted by the Research Triangle Institute (RTI) with the Treatment Alternatives to Street Crimes (TASC) programs. These studies consistently found that clients who were legally induced to enter treatment remained in treatment longer than those who were not. Furthermore, clients under correctional supervision improved as much as clients with no criminal justice involvement in terms of substance abuse, criminal behavior, and employment during the first 6 months of treatment. These findings suggest that some individuals who are coerced into treatment are changed by the experience or are least deterred from abusing drugs and committing crime while in treatment.

Consistent with the above findings, research on the California Civil Addict Program (Anglin & McGlothlin, 1984; McGlothlin, Anglin, & Wilson, 1978) found that court-ordered, drug-free outpatient treatment combined with correctional supervision (including urine monitoring and weekly visits to a parole officer) was associated with significant reductions in narcotic use and crime. A subsequent larger-scale evaluation involved a determination of the program's long-term effectiveness in reducing readdiction (Anglin, 1988). In this longitudinal study, which involved nearly 1,000 subjects, Anglin compared two groups of people with narcotic addiction with similar baseline characteristics over a 20-year follow-up period. One group of subjects had attended the Civil Addict Program while the other group had been released from the program on technical grounds after minimal exposure to supervision. While nearly all subjects became readdicted to narcotics during the follow-up period, the number and length of readdiction periods, as well as the frequency of self-reported crime and arrests, were significantly lower for the treatment group.

Finally, in a more recent analysis, Anglin and Powers (1991) studied 202 people with narcotic addiction who had episodes of each of four different types of interventions: methadone maintenance alone, legal supervision alone, both interventions combined, and neither intervention. Results indicated that legal supervision was better than no intervention with regard to reducing substance abuse and crime, while methadone maintenance was better than legal supervision. Legal supervision combined with methadone maintenance was more effective than methadone maintenance alone in terms of reducing narcotic use. There were no differences with regard to ethnic group or gender in the effectiveness of the interventions.

Police Crackdowns

Police crackdowns are sudden increases in legal sanctions, threats of apprehension, or police officer presence for specific offenses or for all offenses in a specific location (Sherman, 1990). Crackdowns concentrate police resources on specific problems, including drug distribution, by providing for significant increases in police visibility and sanctions (Worden, Bynum, & Frank, 1994). Despite their recent popularity, the effectiveness of police crackdowns remains a source of debate, largely because of methodological problems in evaluations. While the findings of some of the few systematic, objective examinations of crackdown effects have been favorable, the lack of controlled conditions has made it difficult to attribute the findings to the intervention in question (Kinlock, 1994; Worden et al., 1994). Further, national databases, including the Uniform Crime Reports (UCR), typically do not obtain drug-related information essential to evaluating crackdown effectiveness. Similar to available evidence on the drug-relatedness of violent crime (Goldstein, Brownstein, & Ryan, 1992), such databases are limited because they do not provide information on whether the arrestee was a drug user, whether drugs were being used at the time of arrest, and the types of drugs that were involved (Kleiman & Smith, 1990). As noted earlier, official crime data also provide substantial underestimates of the amount of criminal activity committed by individuals prior to their arrest.

Other research on the effectiveness of police crackdowns in curbing heroin and cocaine use has illustrated the difficulty in reducing the demand for, and availability of, drugs. In a review of 18 police crackdown cases, including six on illicit drug distribution and use, Sherman (1990) suggested that curbing illicit drug trafficking may be more difficult than curbing other types of crime. He attributed this to the vibrant market nature of the drug trade, especially the high demand for drugs such as heroin and crack cocaine. Even with large numbers of arrests of both dealers and users, drug markets continue to attract new participants to take the place of those arrested. Subsequent ethnographic observations by Goldstein (1992) are consistent with those of Sherman concerning this phenomenon.

Parole/Probation

Despite above findings linking legal supervision to reduced drug abuse and crime, there has not been improvement in the management of the majority of offenders serving sentences on parole and probation. As Petersilia (1995) noted, current federal efforts have focused almost exclusively on incarceration, largely ignoring the needs and behavior of the 3½ million adults on parole and probation. Similar to jail and prison inmates, adults on parole and probation have steadily increased in number since 1980, and a disproportionately high number of these individuals have been substance abusers. However, significant decreases in community corrections' budgets have contributed to major reductions in both the availability of drug treatment services and the quality and quantity of correctional supervision (Petersilia, 1995). These policies, together with the decline of our inner cities, fewer legitimate employment opportunities, and reduced funding for social service, health care, and child care (Lilly et al., 1995) have contributed to high rates of relapse to substance abuse and crime among parolees and probationers (Petersilia, 1995).

Incarceration

Despite their recent popularity, policies increasing the likelihood of incarceration of substance abusers have been associated with several adverse consequences. A discouraging finding of follow-up studies of incarcerated individuals with narcotic addiction has been that most of their jail or prison sentences have been followed by relapse to narcotic addiction. Maddux and Desmond (1981) reported that of 584 incarceration periods of one week or longer for 248 narcotic addicts studied over a 15-year period, 66% were followed by readdiction within one month and 94% by readdiction within one year. More recently, Nurco (1990) indicated that of 318 jail or prison sentences of at least one month for 355 people with narcotic addiction examined over a 13-year period, 78% were followed by readdiction within one month and 88% within one year. As noted previously, narcotic addiction is associated with increased crime rates. Concerning a broader spectrum of substance abuse, Chaiken and Chaiken (1982) found that among former prisoners, those with the highest rates of serious crime were most likely to abuse substances and violate parole.

The increased availability of illicit drugs, particularly cocaine and heroin, and the resulting "war on drugs" have also contributed to prison overcrowding and overburdening resources elsewhere in the criminal justice system. In 1984, there were over 463,000 state and federal prisoners nationwide, which, at that time, was 20% over capacity. On December 31, 1994, the number of persons being held in federal and state prisons reached a record high of 1,053,738—a 319% increase over the total number for 1980 (NIJ, 1995b). Also, the percentages of prisoners serving a drug sentence increased from 8% in 1980 to 26% in 1993. Further, despite the size of the substance-abusing prisoner population, treatment resources have been minimal. The U.S. General Accounting Office (1991) estimated that only 20% of over 500,000 state inmates with substance abuse problems received treatment. In addition, although substance abuse treatment was available for prisoners in most states, only a single treatment modality was typically offered.

Newer Approaches

Because of significant increases in prison crowding and in the number of drug abusers in the criminal justice system, some new "alternatives to incarceration"—such as ISP, home detention, electronic monitoring, and shock incarceration—have emerged in recent years. These interventions are viewed by some as alternatives to incarceration, as the rationale underlying them involves the observation that the offenders would otherwise have been sent to prison.

ISP Programs

Of the alternative approaches to incarceration, the most commonly used and frequently evaluated has been intensive supervision parole/probation (ISP). Although there is no standard ISP program nationwide, this approach generally involves smaller caseloads and more frequent contacts and drug testing than are involved in traditional probation and parole. The rationale underlying ISP is that smaller caseloads and closer surveillance of offenders will result in reduced drug use and crime. Research findings indicating that the effectiveness of substance abuse treatments was enhanced by mandatory supervision from the criminal justice system was a major consideration in the development of the ISP approach (Turner, Petersilia, & Deschenes, 1994).

Perhaps the most ambitious, rigorous assessment of ISP involved 569 probationers at five sites participating in the Bureau of Justice Assistance's "Intensive Supervision Program for Drug Offenders" (Turner, Petersilia, & Deschenes, 1992; Turner et al., 1994). Probationers at each site were randomly assigned to either ISP or to a control condition involving routine probation/parole supervision. Outcome measures at 12-month follow-up included urinalysis testing results for drug use, arrests, and technical violations. Results indicated that ISP clients had undergone significantly more urine tests, drug counseling, and parole/probation contacts than control clients. While precise details on, and statistical comparisons of, the proportions of drug-positive ISP and control probationers were not reported, ISP clients in four of the five sites had significantly more technical violations for drug use than did non-ISP offenders. Furthermore, although there were no differences between the two groups in arrests or drug-related arrests, ISP offenders were more likely than controls to have been incarcerated while on parole, mainly for technical violations for drug use. At 1-year follow up, 39% of the ISP offenders had been jailed (compared to 28% of controls); 13% of the ISP group had been committed to prison (compared to 10% of those on routine supervision). ISP offenders also spent more time incarcerated during the follow-up period (73 days) than did controls (56 days).

In a review of the above and other less precise evaluations of ISP programs, Deschenes, Turner, and Petersilia (1995) noted that such approaches have not substantially reduced drug use among offenders or prison crowding. Also, they observed that because of variations across jurisdictions in sanctions and program implementation, questions remained regarding the effectiveness of ISP as either a prison diversion or supervision enhancement program. In an attempt to address such questions, both types of programs were implemented in Minnesota and subsequently evaluated in a randomized field experiment involving 300 offenders. Outcome measures at 1-year follow-up included urinalysis results, arrests, and technical violations. Results showed no differences between experimental and control subjects in either positive tests for drug use or arrests (Deschenes et al., 1995).

In spite of the above findings, the effectiveness of ISP programs cannot be precisely determined because of several methodological limitations. As mentioned previously, the use of arrest, conviction, and reincarceration data makes it difficult to determine the effectiveness of these programs on the type, amount, and severity of criminal activity actually committed by offenders. Further, urinalysis results obtained from evaluations of ISP programs were limited for several reasons. First, analyses for percentage of positive tests were not conducted separately by type of drug(s). As noted earlier, frequent use of heroin and cocaine are more likely than other drug use patterns to be related to increased criminal activity and adverse health consequences. Thus, by grouping all drugs together into a single category, it was difficult to estimate the differential risks ISP and control groups experienced with respect to criminal behavior and drug-related illnesses. Also, the analyses focused on the percent of offenders testing positive at least once during the follow-up period. Because use of this procedure combines infrequent with regular drug users, one cannot obtain estimates of the number of offenders who were addicted to, or dependent upon, a particular drug or combination of drugs.

Shock Incarceration

Shock incarceration, or "boot camp" programs use military structure and discipline, physical training, and strict rules to facilitate the development of prosocial behavior (MacKenzie, 1994). Beginning in Georgia in 1983, such programs have expanded to 29 states and the Federal Bureau of Prisons (MacKenzie & Souryal, 1994). Although their use was not originally intended as a substance abuse intervention strategy, it became increasingly clear that many offenders who were entering shock programs had histories of extensive drug involvement. As a consequence, drug treatment and education and urine monitoring were incorporated into shock incarceration programs. Results of a 1992 national survey of shock programs indicated that all jurisdictions reported having some type of drug treatment or education component, as well as urine monitoring (MacKenzie, 1994). As was noted with ISP, this survey found that there was no standard shock incarceration program nationwide; the type (modality) and duration of drug treatment/education varied considerably across programs.

There have been few evaluations of the effectiveness of shock incarceration in reducing substance abuse. Two studies, one conducted by the New York Department of Correctional Services (1992) and the other by Shaw and MacKenzie (1990), indicated that offenders with a legal history of drug involvement were associated with fewer rearrests. A subsequent investigation by Shaw and MacKenzie (1991), however, found no differences between drug-abusing and non-drug-abusing offenders. These investigators also found that substance abusers (defined as individuals with prior drug arrests or persons who were recommended for substance abuse counseling by parole or probation agents) were more likely than other offenders to have a positive urinalysis result during a one-year community supervision period.

In summarizing the above findings, MacKenzie (1994) concluded that large differences among programs in terms of goals, activities, and aftercare make it difficult to precisely evaluate their effectiveness. Furthermore, she noted that shock programs' short duration (on average, 4 months) was generally insufficient to produce any long-term benefits. From these observations, MacKenzie concluded that shock incarceration programs should extend the time available for treatment. She also concluded that more information is needed about the links between treatment programs and supervision, how the transition in treatment can be successfully coordinated from the prison phase to the community, and what types of programs are effective, both in general and for different types of offenders.

While MacKenzie's recommendations are commendable, other improvements are needed with regard to the selection of outcome measures. As in the evaluations of ISP, arrest and incarceration rates have been the primary dependent variables and urinalysis results have not been differentiated with regard to type and extent of drug use.

In-Prison Treatment Programs

In a 1990 report by the National Criminal Justice Association, state and local policymakers were called upon to explore treatment options to help address urgent problems concerning the increasing numbers of drug-involved offenders entering an already overburdened criminal justice system and the failure of the criminal justice system to break the cycle of addiction and crime. The recommendations made have been subsequently endorsed by corrections officials, treatment personnel, researchers, and policymakers (National Task Force on Correctional Substance Abuse Strategies, 1991). Within the past few years, concerns raised by the report have contributed to a significant shift in emphasis of corrections in the United States away from security and control and toward a model stressing treatment and rehabilitation (Wexler, 1994), resulting in new prison-based substance abuse treatment alternatives.

Among the most promising in-prison interventions are therapeutic communities, case management approaches, and innovative programs combining in-prison treatment with aftercare in the community. In addition to addressing drug-related issues, these approaches provide life-skills training and counseling to help clients confront various serious problems that they will likely encounter upon release to the community, such as finding legitimate jobs, educational opportunities, and suitable living arrangements. Researchers have emphasized that therapeutic communities are particularly relevant to successful rehabilitation efforts because of the isolation of their participants from the rest of the prison population (Chaiken, 1989; Inciardi, 1993). Such isolation is considered necessary in order to minimize the influence of drugs, violence, and other norms and values regarding drug use and crime typically found in prison environments. The primary goal of such therapeutic communities is to change negative patterns of thinking and feeling that predispose one to drug use.

Wexler and Lipton (1993) found that while a variety of in-prison substance abuse treatment programs have been successful in reducing relapse and officially recorded recidivism rates, the most promising results came from therapeutic communities. In their studies, inmates receiving treatment had lower relapse, rearrest, and recidivism rates following release than comparison groups. Dropouts had higher relapse and rearrest rates than those who completed treatment. In addition, Falkin, Wexler, and Lipton (1990) reported that in-prison programs are most effective when they have a competent staff, support from correctional authorities, adequate resources, therapy aimed at alleviating problems beyond substance abuse, and the provision of continuity of care after inmates are paroled. These authors, along with Weinman and Lockwood (1993), have emphasized that interventions based on social learning theories designed to meet individual needs are most likely to be successful.

Similar to investigations of most other criminal justice-based interventions, the above studies have focused on official crime data as indicators of criminal activity. Consequently, their findings on the extent of such activity among program participants should be reviewed with caution. Furthermore, despite an emphasis on continuity of care, the studies did not examine the relative effectiveness of institutional intervention and aftercare in the community.

Other Programs

Comprehensive evaluations of the effectiveness of other alternative sanctions to reduce substance abuse, such as home detention and electronic monitoring, are especially lacking. Further, these approaches may be used as part of, or in combination with, other interventions such as shock incarceration and ISP (MacKenzie, 1994; Turner et al., 1994). These circumstances make it difficult to disentangle the effects of one type of surveillance from another. Not until systematic study, including random assignment to combined approaches, is undertaken on a sizable number of subjects will the specific advantages of these new techniques be discernible.

UNANSWERED QUESTIONS AND FUTURE DIRECTIONS

Several important methodological issues concerning the evaluation of surveillance-oriented programs involve the lack of standardization of disciplinary procedures within the criminal justice system. First, investigators of ISP, shock incarceration, and intensive urine monitoring programs have observed extensive variations, both within and across jurisdictions and among parole and probation agents, in their responses to drug use infractions (MacKenzie, 1994; Nurco, Hanlon, Bateman, Toledano, & Kinlock, 1993; Turner et al., 1992). Sites and officers have tended to vary considerably, in both the type and severity of sanctions to evidence of drug use among offenders under surveillance. Second, surveillance-oriented programs typically increase the amount of deviance brought to the attention of probation and parole agents (Jernigan & Kronick, 1992). As a consequence, the number of technical violations increases, as noted in the above evaluation of ISP conducted by Turner et al. (1992). Further, depending on the nature of sanctions employed, such circumstances may significantly increase the number of offenders who are incarcerated on the basis of technical violations of probation and parole (Turner et al., 1992).

Little attention has been paid to factors that influence the adjustment of parolees in their return to the community (Martin & Inciardi, 1993; McMurray, 1993). There are several reasons why interventions begun within the institution need to be extended to this transitional period. First, inmates with histories of heroin and cocaine abuse typically have urgent needs for housing and legitimate employment upon release, as well as the need to avoid association with drug abusers (Martin & Inciardi, 1993). Also, as noted earlier (Maddux & Desmond, 1981; Nurco, 1990), most people with narcotic addiction relapse within one month of release from incarceration. Such readdiction episodes are often accompanied by increased criminal activity (Hanlon, Nurco, Kinlock, & Duszynski, 1990). Further, overburdened caseloads and inadequate resources make it more difficult for corrections officials to ensure that employment and stable residences have been secured for prospective parolees.

Because of these circumstances, new research and intervention efforts are being focused on this transitional period encompassing both prison and community-based aftercare. One such effort involves the development of a case management approach that applies an Assertive Community Treatment (ACT) model for parolees with a history of substance abuse who are released from the Delaware prison system. In this program, which targets offenders whose substance-abusing behavior has placed them at risk for HIV infection, intervention is provided in five stages, with the fifth stage occurring approximately 6 months after release. Beginning with evaluation and assessment, ACT clients receive, in succession, the following services: intensive drug treatment, including individual and group counseling, AIDS education, family therapy, life skills planning with an emphasis on educational and vocational training, relapse prevention, and finally, case management designed to support the client's transition into community life.

Preliminary analysis of 6-month follow-up data suggest at least limited support for the effectiveness of the ACT program (Martin & Inciardi, 1993). In these analyses, data on relapse to drug use, relapse to injection drugs, unprotected sex, and rearrest were available on 258 drug-involved offenders—114 randomly assigned to ACT and 144 who were randomly assigned to standard parole supervision. Outcome data were obtained from a variety of assessments and from HIV and urine tests. Results indicated modest reductions in the probability of relapse to both illicit and injection drugs among ACT clients when contrasted with standard parole clients. However, ACT clients were more likely to be rearrested than standard parole clients during the follow-up period. More detailed, long-term analyses, including the use of confidential self-reports of criminal activity, as well as official arrest records, urine testing, and HIV testing, are forthcoming.

Martin and Inciardi noted that their findings should be viewed with caution, as results may change with the completion of the 6-month follow-up data collection (456 subjects completed the baseline interview) and the examination of longer-term effects at 18-month follow-up. Moreover, they noted that outpatient case management may not be the best alternative for many prison releases with extensive histories of substance abuse because many of these offenders are victims of child physical and sexual abuse and have cognitive problems, psychological dysfunction, unrealistic thinking, and severe defects in educational and employment skills. Thus, substance abuse may be more appropriately viewed as a response to a series of social and psychological disturbances. Such disturbances and their root causes may need to be addressed by intensive long-term treatment, including residential treatment.

Another new intervention approach, DOPERS-based modular treatment (DMT), currently being evaluated by the present authors, focuses on changing drug-abusing offenders' irrational beliefs and thinking errors that contribute to substance abuse and criminal lifestyles (Nurco, 1993). Three distinct DMT modules are intended for different types of substance abusers: 1) those whose substance abuse stems from their criminal lifestyles; 2) those with chronic lifelong problems with a drug of choice; and 3) those whose substance use is situational. This study, conducted in Baltimore, consists of two phases: 1) pre-release (the last 6 months of incarceration); and 2) aftercare (the first 6 months of parole).

The study compares treatment outcomes with respect to drug use (both self-report and regular urine testing results); criminal activity; and psychological, social, and interpersonal functioning over an 18-month period for four groups of prisoners with a history of substance abuse. There are equal proportions of males and females in each group. In each six-month phase of the study, subjects are randomly assigned to either experimental (DMT) plus standard correctional programming (SPS), or SPS alone. Thus, DMT is offered to one group during both pre-release and parole phases; to one group during pre-release only; and to one group during parole only. A fourth group of subjects is not offered DMT during either period.

This project, which began data collection in July 1995, is to our knowledge the first study to examine the relative effectiveness of specialized treatment for different types of drug-involved offenders across prison and parole systems using the same treatment staff over the entire treatment course. This work is also apparently the first to compare the relative effectiveness of specialized treatment offered at pre-release, specialized treatment offered at aftercare, and standard correctional programming. With regard to outcome assessment, in contrast to most evaluations of criminal justice interventions, measures of recidivism include self-reports of crime obtained under confidential conditions, as well as rearrest and reincarceration.

With regard to the assessment of police crackdowns, several writers have emphasized the need to employ experimental designs with tighter controls and random assignment of locations to crackdown interventions (Kinlock, 1994; Sherman, 1990; Worden et al., 1994). Such experiments could involve geographic locations or "hot spots" in which open drug trafficking (Sherman, 1990; Weisburd & Green, 1994) and drug-related violence (Harries, 1990) are prevalent. Drug hot spots can be identified by ethnographic methods (Goldstein, 1989), computer mapping technology (Herbert, 1993), and citizen and police reports (Weisburd & Green, 1994). As Sherman (1990) suggested, controlled experiments could be set up in drug hot spots that use intermittent, unpredictable, repetitive, and brief crackdowns on constantly shifting targets. Using data on specific drug-related problems, described below, these designs, covering smaller areas, allow for more intensive, concentrated observation.

As Eck (1989) emphasized, problems created by drugs are primarily local neighborhood problems. Eck noted that establishing a central collating section of local government to collect data on drug-related problems would be a significant advantage over having the data scattered across many agencies in inconsistent formats and not tied to local subdivisions. Along with police information, such data sources could include: drug-related school disciplinary actions, drug-related housing agency renovations, car accidents caused by drugs, drug-related emergency medical calls, drug-related hospital admissions, medical examiner reports, and drug test results. Such data could be supplemented with confidential self-reports of neighborhood residents, including drug abusers, and incorporated into the abovementioned designs.

Also, there is evidence that researchers and police can collaborate to develop and use innovative methods to collect data on drug-related problems. Such procedures have been useful in determining the drug-relatedness of over 2,000 violent crimes occurring in New York State during the 1980s and the primary cause (psychopharmacological, economic-compulsive, systemic, or multiple) and specific substances involved (Goldstein, Brownstein, Ryan, & Bellucci, 1989; Goldstein et al., 1992). In such a classification, psychopharmacological violence results from the short- or long-term effects of the ingestion of a drug; economic-compulsive violence stems from the need to obtain money to purchase drugs; and systemic violence emanates from attempts to settle disputes between participants in the drug distribution system. In these studies, data concerned both the relationships between and the drug involvement of victims and perpetrators; potentially drug-related features of events; and characteristics of crime scenes (e.g., drug market, shooting gallery). In the evaluation of future police crackdowns targeting both the distribution and use of crack, powder cocaine, and heroin, similar data collection procedures would appear particularly useful for assessing the extent of violence associated with these drugs.

Concerning ISP and shock incarceration, evaluation research needs to ensure consistency of response to technical violations across both sites and parole/probation officers. Further, outcome measures should include confidential self-reported crime, as well as arrests and incarcerations. To facilitate valid self-reports under such circumstances, researchers should provide subjects with the assurance offered by a federal certificate of confidentiality (Inciardi, 1986), which protects against the release of sensitive information provided by subjects to any law enforcement authority, court, or grand jury.

In conclusion, researchers and policymakers need to emphasize that given the diversity among substance abusers, no single approach is likely to be effective for all individuals. As a corollary of this, future research needs to determine the types of interventions that are most effective for different types of substance abusing offenders. Such a view contrasts sharply with the history of public responses to substance abuse in the United States, which have swung back and forth between an overemphasis on criminal justice sanctions and one on treatment and rehabilitation. As a consequence, substance abuse policy has been dictated more by the nature of the social and political climate than by substance abuse research findings. Further, researchers and policymakers need to impress upon others that not all substance abusers are alike. Regardless of the prevailing policy at any given time, there has been general consensus, although erroneous, that substance abusers basically comprise a homogeneous group of individuals. Finally, both researchers and policymakers should be adamant in recommending that, as opposed to past practices, law enforcement and treatment sectors work in concert, rather than in competition, with one another.

REFERENCES

Anglin, M. D. (1988). The efficacy of civil commitment in treating narcotic addiction. In C. G. Leukefeld & F. M. Tims (Eds.), *Compulsory treatment of drug abuse: Research and clinical practice* (NIDA Research Monograph 86) (pp. 8–34). Rockville, MD: National Institute on Drug Abuse.

Anglin, M. D., & McGlothlin, W. H. (1984). Outcome of narcotic addict treatment in California. In F. M. Tims & J. P. Ludford (Eds.), *Drug abuse treatment evaluation: Strategies, progress, and prospects* (NIDA Research Monograph 51) (pp. 57–80). Rockville, MD: National Institute on Drug Abuse.

Anglin, M. D., & Powers, K. I. (1991). Individual and joint effects of methadone maintenance and legal supervision on the behavior of narcotic addicts. *Journal of Applied Behavioral Science, 27*, 515–531.

Ball, J. C. (1991). The similarity of crime rates among male heroin addicts in New York City, Philadelphia and Baltimore. *Journal of Drug Issues, 21*, 412–427.

Barton, W. (1980). Drug histories and criminality: Survey of inmates of state correctional facilities, January 1974. *International Journal of the Addictions, 15*, 233–258.

Barton, W. (1982). Drug histories and criminality of inmates of local jails in the United States (1978): Implications for treatment and rehabilitation of the drug abuser in a jail setting. *International Journal of the Addictions, 17*, 417–444.

Chaiken, M. R. (1989, October). *Prison programs for drug-involved offenders* [National Institute of Justice Research in Action]. Washington, DC: U.S. Department of Justice.

Chaiken, J. M., & Chaiken, M. R. (1982). *Varieties of criminal behavior.* Santa Monica, CA: Rand Corporation.

Collins, J. J., & Allison, M. (1983). Legal coercion and retention in drug abuse treatment. *Hospital and Community Psychiatry, 34,* 1145–1149.

Cullen, F. T., & Gilbert, K. E. (1982). *Reaffirming rehabilitation.* Cincinnati: Anderson.

Deschenes, E. P., Turner, S., & Petersilia, J. (1995). A dual experiment in intensive community supervision: Minnesota's prison diversion and enhanced supervised release programs. *The Prison Journal, 75,* 330–356.

Eck, J. (1989). *Police and drug control: A home field advantage.* Washington, DC: Police Executive Research Forum.

Falkin, G. P., Wexler, H. K., & Lipton, D. S. (1990, May). *Drug treatment in state prisons. Report to the National Academy of Sciences.* New York: Narcotic and Drug Research, Inc.

Goldstein, P. J. (1989). Drugs and violent crime. In N. A. Weiner & M. E. Wolfgang (Eds.), *Pathways to criminal violence* (pp. 16–48). Newbury Park, CA: Sage.

Goldstein, P. J. (1992, March 25). *The relationship between drugs and violence.* Paper presented at the University of Maryland, College Park.

Goldstein, P. J., Brownstein, H. H., & Ryan, P. (1992). Drug-related homicide in New York: 1984 and 1988. *Crime and Delinquency, 38,* 459–476.

Goldstein, P. J., Brownstein, H. H., Ryan, P., & Bellucci, P. A. (1989). Crack and homicide in New York City, 1988: A conceptually based event analysis. *Contemporary Drug Problems, 16,* 651–687.

Hanlon, T. E., Nurco, D. N., Kinlock, T. W., & Duszynski, K. R. (1990). Trends in criminal activity and drug use over an addiction career. *American Journal of Drug and Alcohol Abuse, 16,* 223–238.

Harlow, C. W. (1991). *Drugs and jail inmates, 1989* [Bureau of Justice Statistics Special Report]. Washington, DC: U.S. Department of Justice.

Harries, K. (1990). *Serious violence: Patterns of homicide and assault in America.* Springfield, IL: Thomas.

Herbert, E. (1993, April). NIJ's drug market analysis program. *National Institute of Justice Journal.*

Hser, Y., Anglin, M. D., & Chou, C. (1992). Reliability of retrospective self-report by narcotics addicts. *Psychological Assessment, 4,* 207–213.

Hubbard, R. L., Collins, J. J., Rachal, J. V., & Cavanaugh, E. R. (1988). The criminal justice client in drug abuse treatment. In C. G. Leukefeld & F. M. Tims (Eds.), *Compulsory treatment of drug abuse: Research and clinical practice* (pp. 42–68). (NIDA Research Monograph 86). Rockville, MD: National Institute on Drug Abuse.

Hubbard, R. L., Rachal, J. V., Craddock, S. G., & Cavanaugh, E. R. (1984). Treatment outcome prospective study (TOPS): Client characteristics and behaviors before, during, and after treatment. In F. M. Tims & J. P. Ludford (Eds.), *Compulsory treatment of drug abuse: Research and clinical practice* (pp. 57–80). (NIDA Research Monograph 86). Rockville, MD: National Institute on Drug Abuse.

Inciardi, J. A. (1986). *The war on drugs: Heroin, cocaine, and public policy.* Palo Alto, CA: Mayfield.

Inciardi, J. A. (1993). Drug-involved offenders: Crime-prison-treatment. *The Prison Journal, 73,* 253–256.

Inciardi, J. A., & Pottieger, A. E. (1986). Drug use and crime among two cohorts of women narcotics users: An empirical assessment. *Journal of Drug Issues, 16,* 91–106.

Inciardi, J. A., & Pottieger, A. E. (1991). Kids, crack, and crime. *Journal of Drug Issues, 21,* 257–270.

Inciardi, J. A., & Pottieger, A. E. (1994). Crack-cocaine use and street crime. *Journal of Drug Issues, 24,* 293–314.

Jernigan, D. E., & Kronick, R. F. (1992). Intensive parole: The more you watch, the more you catch. *Journal of Offender Rehabilitation, 17,* 65–76.

Johnston, L. D., O'Malley, P. M., & Bachman, J. G. (1995a). *National survey results on drug use from the monitoring the future study, 1975–1994. Vol. I: Secondary school students*. Rockville, MD: National Institute on Drug Abuse.

Johnston, L. D., O'Malley, P. M., & Bachman, J. G. (1995b). *National survey results on drug use from the monitoring the future study, 1975–1994. Vol. II: College students and young adults*. Rockville, MD: National Institute on Drug Abuse.

Kinlock, T. W. (1994). Problem-oriented data collection: Toward improved evaluation of police drug crackdowns. *American Journal of Police, 13*, 59–94.

Kleiman, M. A. R., & Smith, K. (1990). State and local drug enforcement: In search of a strategy. In M. Tonry & J. Q. Wilson (Eds.), *Drugs and crime: Vol 13. Crime and justice: A review of research* (pp. 159–202). Chicago: University of Chicago Press.

Lilly, J. R., Cullen, F. T., & Ball, R. A. (1995). *Criminological theory: Context and consequences* (2nd ed.). Thousand Oaks, CA: Sage.

Lipton, D., Martinson, R., & Wilks, J. (1975). *The effectiveness of correctional treatment*. New York: Praeger.

MacKenzie, D. L. (1994). Shock incarceration as an alternative for drug offenders. In D. L. MacKenzie & C. D. Uchida (Eds.), *Drugs and crime: Evaluating public policy initiatives* (pp. 215–230). Thousand Oaks, CA: Sage.

MacKenzie, D. L., & Souryal, C. (1994). *Multisite evaluation of shock incarceration*. Washington, DC: National Institute of Justice.

MacKenzie, D. L., & Uchida, C. D. (Eds.). (1994). *Drugs and crime: Evaluating public policy initiatives*. Thousand Oaks, CA: Sage.

Maddux, J. F., & Desmond, D. P. (1981). *Careers of opioid users* [Praeger Studies on Issues and Research in Substance Abuse]. New York: Praeger.

Martin, S., & Inciardi, J. A. (1993). A case management treatment program for drug-involved prison releasees. *The Prison Journal, 73*, 319–331.

Martinson, R. (1974). What works?—Questions and answers about prison reform. *The Public Interest, 35*.

McGlothlin, W. H., Anglin, M. D., & Wilson, B. D. (1978). Narcotic addiction and crime. *Criminology, 16*, 106–128.

McMurray, H. L. (1993). High risk parolees in transition from institution to community life. *Journal of Offender Rehabilitation, 19*, 145–161.

National Criminal Justice Association. (1990). *Treatment options for drug-dependent offenders: A review of the literature for state and local decision makers*. Washington, DC: U.S. Department of Justice, Bureau of Justice Assistance.

National Institute on Drug Abuse. (1992). *National household survey on drug abuse: Main findings*. Rockville, MD: Author.

National Institute of Justice. (1995a). *Drugs and crime, 1994: 1994 drug use forecasting annual report on adult and juvenile arrestees*. Washington, DC: U.S. Department of Justice.

National Institute of Justice. (1995b). *Prisoners in 1994*. Washington, DC: Bureau of Justice Statistics, U.S. Department of Justice.

National Task Force on Correctional Substance Abuse Strategies. (1991, June). *Intervening with substance abusing offenders: A framework for action*. Washington, DC: U.S. Department of Justice, National Institute of Corrections.

New York Department of Correctional Services. (1992). *The fourth annual report to the legislature on shock incarceration and shock parole supervision*. Albany: Department of Correctional Services and Division of Parole.

Nurco, D. N. (1990). *Social support and drug-free living among parolees*. Research proposal submitted to the National Institute on Drug Abuse, April 3, 1990.

Nurco, D. N. (1993). *Drug abuse treatment of criminal justice-involved populations*. Research proposal submitted to the National Institute on Drug Abuse, October 1, 1993.

Nurco, D. N., Hanlon, T. E., & Kinlock, T. W. (1991). Recent research on the relationship between illicit drug use and crime. *Behavioral Sciences and the Law, 9*, 221–242.

Nurco, D. N., Hanlon, T. E., Bateman, R. W., Toledano, E., & Kinlock, T. W. (1993). Policy implications derived from an experimental intervention involving drug-abusing offenders. *The Prison Journal, 73*, 332–342.

Petersilia, J. (1995). A crime control rationale for reinvesting in community corrections. *The Prison Journal, 75*, 479–496.

Sechrest, L., White, S., & Brown, E. (Eds.). (1979). *The rehabilitation of criminal offenders: Problems and prospects.* Washington, DC: National Academy of Sciences.

Shaw, J. W., & MacKenzie, D. L. (1990, November). *Boot camps: An initial assessment of the program and parole performance of drug-involved offenders.* Paper presented at the Annual Meeting of the American Society of Criminology, Baltimore, MD.

Shaw, J. W., & MacKenzie, D. L. (1991). Shock incarceration and its impact on the lives of problem drinkers. *The American Journal of Criminal Justice, 16*, 63–96.

Sherman, L. W. (1990). Police crackdowns: Initial and residual deterrence. In M. Tonry & N. Morris (Eds.), *Crime and justice: A review of research* (Vol. 12, pp. 1–48). Chicago: University of Chicago Press.

Simpson, D. D., & Sells, S. B. (1982). *Evaluation of drug abuse treatment effectiveness: Summary of the DARP follow-up research* (NIDA Treatment Research Report). Rockville, MD: National Institute on Drug Abuse.

Turner, S., Petersilia, J., & Deschenes, E. (1992). Evaluating intensive probation/parole (ISP) for drug offenders. *Crime and Delinquency, 29*, 34–61.

Turner, S., Petersilia, J., & Deschenes, E. P. (1994). The implementation and effectiveness of drug testing in community supervision: Results of an experimental evaluation. In D. L. MacKenzie & C. D. Uchida (Eds.), *Drugs and crime: Evaluating public policy initiatives* (pp. 231–252). Thousand Oaks, CA: Sage.

U.S. General Accounting Office. (1991, September). *Drug treatment: Despite new strategy, few federal inmates receive treatment* [Report to the Committee on Government Operations, House of Representatives]. Washington, DC: Author.

Weinman, B. A., & Lockwood, D. (1993). Inmate drug treatment programming in the Federal Bureau of Prisons. In J. A. Inciardi (Ed.), *Drug treatment and criminal justice* (pp. 194–208). Newbury Park, CA: Sage.

Weisburd, D., & Green, L. (1994). Defining the street-level drug market. In D. L. MacKenzie & C. D. Uchida (Eds.), *Drugs and crime: Evaluating public policy initiatives* (pp. 61–76). Beverly Hills, CA: Sage.

Wexler, H. K. (1994). Progress in prison substance abuse treatment: A five year report. *Journal of Drug Issues, 24*, 349–360.

Wexler, H. K., & Lipton, D. S. (1993). Reform to recovery: Advances in prison drug treatment. In J. A. Inciardi (Ed.), *Drug treatment and criminal justice* (pp. 209–227). Newbury Park, CA: Sage.

Wilson, J. Q., & Herrnstein, R. J. (1985). *Crime and human nature.* New York: Simon & Schuster.

Wish, E. D., & Gropper, B. A. (1990). Drug testing in the criminal justice system. In M. Tonry & J. Q. Wilson (Eds.), *Drugs and crime* [Crime and Justice: A Review of Research, Vol. 13] (pp. 321–391). Chicago: University of Chicago Press.

Worden, R. E., Bynum, T. S., & Frank, J. (1994). Police crackdowns on drug abuse and trafficking. In D. L. MacKenzie & C. D. Uchida (Eds.), *Drugs and crime: Evaluating public policy initiatives* (pp. 95–113). Thousand Oaks, CA: Sage.

13

Regulation of Sale and Distribution

Joseph F. Spillane
Center for Studies in Criminology and Law
University of Florida

The societal impact of substance abuse has been well documented. A recent report published by the Robert Wood Johnson Foundation (1993) cited estimates that placed the cost of illegal drug abuse in the United States at $67 billion. In recent years, reducing the problems associated with drugs has emerged as one of the most visible public policy questions. The primary legal response during this era of heightened concern has been the effort to limit the sale and distribution of problematic drugs. Reducing substance abuse by controlling drug distribution is itself an old idea; throughout the 20th century, governments have sought to limit access to drug supplies.

The basic premise behind the regulation of distribution and sale is that reductions in drug availability will be accompanied by corresponding decreases in demand. Achieving a reduction in demand for a drug will then reduce the problems and costs associated with its consumption. This method of control does not seek to reduce the desire to consume, but to reduce the ability to satisfy that desire.

Any thorough discussion regarding the limitation of drug distribution must also acknowledge, however, the multiple objectives that legal controls serve. Drug sellers often face the charge of not merely supplying existing demand, but of actively cultivating new usage, and thereby assuming a moral responsibility. Viewing drug sellers in this light, whether as agents of moral decline or as factors in the etiology of substance abuse, has prompted tough legal penalties aimed at distribution. Other objectives can include: preserving neighborhood safety; reducing violence; controlling organized criminal enterprises; satisfying foreign policy objectives; maintaining professional standards among physicians and pharmacists; and generating revenue through taxation. Given the multiple objectives of drug regulation, it is not surprising that legal controls have thrived in periods of both therapeutic optimism and pessimism regarding to the treatment of substance abuse.

This review begins with an examination of the current state of historical research on the development of drug regulation, from the relatively open markets of the 19th century to the tightly controlled illicit markets of the late 20th century. This chapter continues with an overview of research on contemporary drug control, including a detailed review of several areas of significant new study. Finally, this chapter concludes by exploring the literature on current policy debates, including the ongoing academic controversy over drug legalization.

CONTROLLING DISTRIBUTION: THE HISTORICAL DIMENSION

Until the last quarter of the 19th century, drugs were available to consumers with few or no legal restrictions. Neither American and European law made much distinction between various methods by which drug products could be sold to the public, nor did the law attempt to define which drugs might be considered more or less dangerous. Because of the relative ease with which consumers could purchase drugs such as morphine and cocaine, numerous scholars have concluded that the 19th century was a kind of "dope-fiend's paradise" (Brecher, 1972), although some recent historical research suggests that this portrait is almost surely overdrawn (Baumohl, 1992). Paradise or not, it is certainly true that, addicted or not, consumers could purchase most drug supplies directly from druggists or other retailers, by mail order, or through proprietary and patent medicine preparations.

Dissatisfaction with unregulated drug distribution was widespread by the close of the 19th century, and advocates of reform called for legal control of drug supplies. Most arguments in favor of regulation tended to begin with an assumption that drug sales could be identified as either legitimate or illegitimate, and conclude with a call to certify these distinctions through legal rules. One product of this legitimate/illegitimate approach to dealing with drug distribution was a dual quality to future drug control. Subsequently, one area of drug control tended to focus on legitimate sales—defining what those were, and regulating "legitimate" sellers. The second area of drug control focused on illegitimate sales, especially the street vendors who supplied the burgeoning black market in opiates and cocaine.

The first area, the regulation of legitimate supply, largely focused on the medical and pharmaceutical professions, as well as the legal drug industry.

Recent historical work suggests that formal regulation of these sources of supply built upon existing informal self-regulation (Spillane, 1994). At the turn of the century, the most important dimension to maintaining a legitimate drug trade appears to have been the avoidance of indiscriminate drug sales, especially to those already addicted. Leading American physician H. C. Wood, Jr., summarized the logic of self-regulation in 1916:

> The education of the general public as to the danger of narcoticism both the individual and to the community rests chiefly upon the pharmaceutical and medical professions. But we ourselves need to be taught our own shortcomings. Physicians must be brought to an appreciation of the fact that the too ready recourse to the hypodermic needle has led many a victim to life-long slavery. Did you as pharmacists realize the devil that lurks in the cough syrups, and other narcotic patent medicines, which you so thoughtlessly hand across the counter, you would forever banish this class of preparations from your shelves. Would you destroy the happiness, ruin the body and mind of your fellow-men for a few paltry pieces of silver he gives you? (Wood, 1916)

Appreciating past experience with professional self-regulation seems especially useful in light of recent studies that highlight similar issues that the "medicalization" of drug control might pose for contemporary society (Levine, 1993).

Formal regulation of the legal drug supply focused on the translation of these professional standards into legal rules. In the United States, state-level controls often relied on the agency of state boards of medicine or pharmacy, which controlled professional licensing. The federal government became involved with regulating the nation's drug supply with the passage of the 1906 Pure Food and Drugs Act. While the act did not create a class of prohibited drugs, or even a category of prescription drugs, it did set standards for purity and labeling; these standards were used to remove a number of drug products thought to be abused, such as those containing opiates or cocaine. The dual quality to the Pure Food and Drugs Act is reflected in the historical literature, some of which emphasizes the importance of protecting unwitting consumers from dosing themselves with potentially addicting drugs (Young, 1961, 1990), and some of which emphasizes the desire of organized physicians and the pharmaceutical industry to assert their exclusive control over the nation's drug supply (Estes, 1988; Starr, 1982; Temin, 1980).

Traditional regulators of medicine and pharmacy have continued to play an important role in substance abuse control. In 1938, passage of the Food, Drug and Cosmetic Act in the wake of the Elixir Sulfanilamide disaster created a large class of drugs that would henceforth be available only on a physician's prescription. For the first time, the Food and Drug Administration (FDA) began to try to limit the distribution of certain non-narcotic drugs of abuse. Among the first were the barbiturates—the introduction of Phenobarbital and many barbiturate derivatives having resulted in widespread reports of their misuse and toxicity. Throughout the 1940s and 1950s, FDA inspectors initiated numerous prosecutions of pharmacists who failed to comply with federal rules regarding the distribution of both amphetamines and barbiturates (Jackson, 1976; Swann, 1994; Temin, 1980).

In 1951, the Durham–Humphrey Amendment continued the process begun 13 years earlier by creating two classes of drugs—prescription and nonprescription—into which all drug products had to be classified. Prescription drugs included those defined as habit-forming, and those that were toxic or dangerous (Swann, 1994). To strengthen enforcement efforts directed against amphetamines, barbiturates, hallucinogens, and other non-narcotic drugs of abuse, the FDA created a Bureau of Drug Abuse Control (BDAC). During the 1960s and 1970s, new drug problems continued to emerge out of the legal pharmaceutical industry and medical practice. These included methamphetamine (Methedrine) in the late 1960s (Inciardi, 1992), and methaqualone (Quaalude) in the early 1970s (Goode, 1993). In 1968 the functions of BDAC were merged into what would become the Drug Enforcement Administration (DEA), dealing with drugs from both licit and illicit sources.

The second area of drug control, the control of illicit distribution, focused on drug use and sale that had relatively weak connection to "legitimate" purposes. Briefly summarized, historical research suggests that there are four salient features to the control of illicit distribution.

First, control efforts focused most intensely on those drugs that lacked any medical or professional base of distribution, and which were largely employed for "nonmedical" reasons. Opium smokers, for example, used the drug for pleasure, and distribution and sale took place in the opium den rather than the doctor's office or the drugstore. Second, control of illicit distribution relied more heavily on the traditional apparatus of the criminal justice system. To limit opium smoking, local law enforcement employed widespread arrests of sellers, and the forcible closure of opium dens and other distribution points.

Third, illicit drug sellers supplying nonmedical markets were thought to play a much more active role in increasing the incidence of drug abuse. Where 19th-century views of addiction tended to emphasize the enslaving properties of drugs, concerns over the illicit drug markets of the early 20th century emphasized the role of the seller, and the ways in which the drug dealer captured customers. Leonard Scott of the U.S. Public Health Service captured the tone when he called the drug addict the "bond-servant of the drug peddler." While Scott urged a nonpunitive approach to addicts, he also urged "a relentless war on the fiendishly cruel and rapacious drug vendor . . . though it cost you millions in money it will not only be doing an act of justice but it will repay you richly when the final reckoning comes" (Scott,

1923). Such an approach to drug control emphasized the moral necessity of punishing drug sellers.

Fourth, legal controls on underground drug markets tended to focus on specific drugs of abuse, rather than on the drug supply more generally. Early anticocaine measures, for example, tended to prohibit or limit only those forms of cocaine that seemed popular among nonmedical consumers. In 1913, the New York State legislature passed the Delahanty measure, which banned sales of flake or crystal cocaine (the form most often used for cocaine sniffing). It did not restrict the sale of large crystal cocaine, used in the preparation of cocaine solutions—the form of cocaine employed in medical and dental practice.

The involvement of the federal government in the control of the illicit drug traffic began in earnest following passage of the Harrison Narcotics Act of 1914. The Harrison Act took the form of a revenue measure, which required distributors of narcotics (defined as opiates and cocaine) to register. In its original form, there was little to the legislation beyond the licensing of professionals; policing the illicit traffic appeared to remain with the states. Yet the Treasury Department, which had been assigned to enforce the Harrison Act, quickly adopted the position that the purpose of the law should be a federal prohibition on nonmedical narcotic use. Since registered professionals were henceforth the only legal sources of supply, all unregistered persons in possession of opiates or cocaine violated the law.

The stepped-up enforcement activities of the Narcotics Division (which became the Federal Bureau of Narcotics in 1930) were accompanied by an expanded control over the import and export of narcotics. In 1922, the Narcotic Drugs Import and Export Act (Jones–Miller Act) imposed a range of reporting requirements, restricted imports, and mandated fines and imprisonment for violations.

Efforts to eliminate illicit markets gradually emerged as the dominant arena of substance abuse control in the United States. The two chief preoccupations of Harry J. Anslinger, the first commissioner of the Federal Bureau of Narcotics (FBN), profoundly influenced the shape of 20th-century drug law enforcement. First, Anslinger made international controls a priority; the fastest route to eliminating the problem of substance abuse, Anslinger argued, would be to prevent narcotics from entering the country. Anslinger and the FBN pursued a variety of bilateral and multilateral agreements. With the Narcotics Limitation Convention of 1931, Anslinger secured a leadership position for the United States in international drug control it has yet to relinquish.

Second, Anslinger kept the FBN's focus squarely on nonmedical drug problems. While he largely avoided the problems posed by amphetamines and barbiturates, Anslinger eagerly pursued the control of marijuana. By the mid-1930s, the use of marijuana had been widely publicized; despite a lengthy history of medical use, however, marijuana's therapeutic connections were tenuous at best. Distribution took place almost entirely outside of licit channels, giving the FBN an opportunity to pursue a high-profile campaign. The resulting Marijuana Tax Act of 1937 set the tone for subsequent drug legislation, with near-total prohibition and tough penalties. Penalties for violations involving the sale and distribution of narcotics generally were dramatically increased with the passage of the Boggs Act of 1951 and the Narcotics Control Act of 1956. Both enhanced federal authority over drug law enforcement, and introduced severe mandatory minimum sentences for violators.

Historical studies of drug control have produced an important body of work that places current policy in context. Much of the research on the United States has focused on the development of legislation at the federal level (Musto, 1987; Young, 1961), or on the activities of the Federal Bureau of Narcotics both domestically (Kinder, 1992; McWilliams, 1989, 1992) and internationally (Kinder & Walker, 1986; Nadelmann, 1993). Other historical scholarship has highlighted international drug control more generally (McAllister, 1992; Taylor, 1969; Walker, 1981, 1991). The work of David Courtwright (1982) illustrates the ways in which drug control efforts influenced patterns of use. In addition to work on the United States, important historical work has detailed development in Great Britain (Berridge & Edwards, 1981; Kohn, 1992; Parssinen, 1983) and the Netherlands (de Kort & Korf, 1992).

CONTEMPORARY CONTROL
OF SALE AND DISTRIBUTION

The control of drug distribution remains one of the primary components of substance abuse policy, as it has been throughout the 20th century. In recent years, however, the legal control of drug sellers has assumed an unprecedented importance in the United States. These developments are visible on a rhetorical level, as the language of drug control has become increasingly attentive to drug sellers. The National Drug Control Strategy for 1989 illustrates the point:

> The first challenge facing our criminal justice system is to help reclaim neighborhoods that have been rendered unsafe by drugs. For it is in neighborhoods that drugs pose an immediate threat to local residents and the quality of their lives. Drug dealers harass, intimidate, and assault pedestrians. They entice and coerce children to join their ranks. Crack houses accelerate the deterioration of already rundown residential blocks. Parks and public spaces become havens for illicit activity. In such neighborhoods, drugs are sold freely and openly and buyers fear no criminal sanction. Residents are left alone with the task of protecting their lives and property, while trying to keep their children away from a life of drug use. (U.S. Office of National Drug Control Policy, 1989)

During the 1980s, the articulation of policy goals often shifted toward sellers rather dramatically, and coincided with calls for more vigorous drug law enforcement, together with more certain and severe penalties.

The current importance of distribution control extends far beyond rhetorical significance; by almost any measure, such efforts now take place on an unprecedented scale. One estimate of drug control expenditures at all levels of government placed the figure at $28 billion in 1990, much of which was devoted to the control of distribution and sale (Reuter, 1992). As a measure of activity, drug arrests also indicate the enormous scope of control efforts, with over 1 million arrests annually for drug law violations in the United States. On the state level, these higher numbers have also translated to higher prison populations, placing a strain on correctional systems and state budgets. In California, prison commitments of drug offenders increased from approximately 1,500 in 1980 to 22,600 in 1990 (Zimring & Hawkins, 1994).

Finally, the scope of control efforts may be matched by the growing importance of the drug distribution networks themselves. Illicit economies have always been important, but a number contemporary observers have raised new concerns over the centrality of drug distribution in some communities (Bourgois, 1989; Model, 1993). The growth of crack cocaine and the declining licit economies in areas of concentrated poverty have encouraged the development of large-scale criminal enterprises, further deteriorating the quality of life (Currie, 1993; Johnson, Williams, Dei, & Sanabria, 1990; Simon, 1993). Drug selling has increasingly become a symbol of urban social pathology, or linked to studies of the "underclass" phenomenon (Auletta, 1982; Duster, 1987; Wilson, 1987), although some have questioned how these connections are made (Kornblum, 1993).

Contemporary efforts to control drug sale and distribution may be divided into four basic approaches: international control, interdiction, disrupting traffickers, and retail-level enforcement. International control efforts are primarily directed at disrupting international drug trafficking organizations, as well as seizing or destroying illicit drugs at various stages of production. The logic of stopping drug distribution at the source often combines with a moralistic viewpoint that mirrors the traditional images of the street-level dealer—drug cartels and even national governments are accused not merely of supplying demand, but of insidiously cultivating drug consumption in foreign markets (Kinder, 1992). As with drug control more generally, the reduction of substance abuse is but one goal of international action; a number of studies have demonstrated that conflicts with other interests, such as foreign policy, can compromise the potential for success (Moore, 1990).

Interdiction involves the disrupting shipments of illicit drugs in transit. The apparent simplicity of "sealing the borders" against the flow of heroin and cocaine led to an enormous investment of resources during the 1980s and 1990s. One result of that investment has been a dramatic increase in drug seizures—nearly 100 tons of cocaine were seized by the U.S. Coast Guard and Customs in 1992 alone. But despite enormously increased seizures of drugs, research detailing the relative lack of impact on consumption in the United States suggests interdiction may not be so successful (Kleiman, 1992; Reuter, 1988).

Disrupting drug trafficking organizations refers to the set of drug control policies that aim to disrupt distribution at the higher levels of the trade, an approach described as "getting Mr. Big" by Kleiman and Smith (1990). In addition to targeting high-level individuals, this area of control focuses on the capacity of criminal enterprises to "do business." Limiting the ability of drug distributors to carry out necessary financial transactions is just one of the areas which some recent research describes as promising (Moore, 1990).

Retail-level drug control focuses on the lower levels of distribution, where sellers are both more numerous and more visible to law enforcement. Kleiman (1992) has observed that an approach that focuses on retailers has the potential to disrupt illicit drug markets, although a sense of justice might suggest that higher-level distributors are more blameworthy. Although crackdowns on drug sellers enjoy support of policymakers and the public, the arrests they generate may overwhelm the capacities of criminal justice systems.

Each of these four levels of enforcement have been the subject of a tremendous quantity of scholarly research, and it is hardly possible to summarize all of the important recent work. There are several particularly important areas, however, that promise to illuminate a great deal about the organization and control of drug distribution. Three of these areas will be discussed here, including the economics of drug distribution, the consequences of control, and the social context of drug selling.

The economics of drug selling represents an area of research that has been the focus of considerable attention recently. Much of this work focuses on evaluating the basic economic premise of drug control—if drug supplies are reduced, costs will rise, which will diminish overall drug use (Reuter & Kleiman, 1986). Other studies emphasize the structure of drug distribution, including the organization of drug networks, roles of sellers, and price levels (Moore, 1990). Korf (1990) has developed a similar analysis for the legal cannabis markets in Amsterdam, while other work focuses on legal markets for alcohol and tobacco (Kozlowski, Coambs, Ferrence, & Adlaf, 1989). Recent work by Ruggerio and South (1995) on Europe has developed a "market approach" that suggests that illicit economies of drug distribution exist in the context of local economies more generally; this produces somewhat distinctive patterns of drug selling from region to region, from highly individualized to tightly organized. In sum, this area of research promises to highlight the interactions between markets and laws, and thereby evaluate the efficacy of drug control measures.

Studies that describe the consequences of control begin with the premise that efforts to control sale and distribution generate reactions and effects that not only influence drug sellers, but patterns of substance abuse as well. To the extent that legal controls serve to reduce supply and thereby lower demand, such influences may be intentional. Often, however, these effects are not intended. For example, research has demonstrated that control of a particular drug may drive out less potent forms, and encourage the distribution of more potent forms. Relevant examples have included shifts from beer and wine to hard liquor under alcohol Prohibition (Levine & Reinarman, 1993); the shift from powder cocaine to crack in the 1980s (Nadelmann, 1991); or the increased potency of marijuana (Kleiman, 1989). A number of recent studies focus broadly on the consequences of control for consumption, and while their conclusions vary, they share a concern over the impact of legal environments on substance abuse (Kaplan, 1983, 1988; Kleiman, 1989; Michaels, 1987; Nadelmann, 1989; Trebach, 1987; Zimring & Hawkins, 1992).

Finally, exploring the social context of drug selling is yet another means of evaluating the control of sale and distribution. Specifically, this area of research focuses on the lives and social organization of drug sellers. Preble and Casey (1969) led the way with their study of heroin addicts in New York City, which articulated sellers' roles, assessed the impact of distribution structures on heroin addicts, and examined the perceptions of sellers and addicts. Recent ethnographic work has built upon these earlier studies (Adler, 1985; Mieczkowski, 1994; Williams, 1989, 1992). Other research has applied the economic approaches discussed above to the study of drug sellers (Johnson et al., 1985; Reuter, MacCoun, & Murphy, 1990). Recent work on distribution has also included anabolic steroids (Goldstein, 1990), and Ecstasy (Rosenbaum, Morgan, & Beck, 1989). These studies define more clearly the role of the distributor to the problem of substance abuse.

CURRENT DEBATES

The tremendous quantity of current research on drug distribution and sale has generated much useful information, but there remains little consensus regarding the policy implications. The critical debates over the future of drug control have concentrated on three basic issues: which methods of control produce the best results; the appropriate allocation of resources between supply reduction and demand reduction; and drug legalization.

The first of the debates concerns the relative effectiveness of various methods of drug distribution control. As drug budgets have expanded, assessing cost-effectiveness has become an increasingly salient issue. A number of recent studies maintain that, although the control of distribution should be maintained, some approaches are more effective than others (Kleiman & Smith, 1990; Moore, 1990).

The second of the debates deals with the allocation of resources to deal with substance abuse. The question that has generated the most controversy is whether or not a disproportionate amount of drug control dollars are being spent on controlling distribution and sale, rather than on treatment or prevention. While numerous evaluations deal either with drug law enforcement or with the efficacy of treatment (Anglin & Hser, 1990) and prevention (Botvin, 1990), few studies have been able to compare supply and demand programs. An exception is the recent analysis by Rydell and Everingham (1994), which concluded that expanding treatment while cutting back on supply control would make cocaine control more cost-efficient. Positive evaluations of drug treatment, together with a concern over the costs associated with aggressive distribution control, have resulted in a number of recent studies advocating a less punitive drug policy (Currie, 1993; Kleiman, 1992). These kinds of approaches are echoed in the emerging "harm reduction" literature. Harm reduction advocates argue for a nonmoralistic approach to controlling distribution, aimed at minimizing the harm from both substance abuse and its control.

Finally, there is the ongoing debate concerning the legalization of drugs. In discussing legalization proposals, it should be noted at the outset that few such proposals involve the removal of legal controls over drug distribution. Rather, calls for legalization often constitute a return to a regulated, legal market. Some legalization proposals advocate a "medicalization" of drug distribution, not unlike the pre–Harrison Act distribution of cocaine and heroin in the United States. Other proposals urge that currently prohibited drugs become part of a well-regulated, nonmedical market, not unlike the current markets for alcohol and tobacco.

There are many published arguments in favor of legalization, of which a representative few are listed here. Some legalization proposals treat legalization from a libertarian perspective, arguing that interference with drug markets is itself immoral (Friedman & Friedman, 1984; Szasz, 1985, 1992). The larger number of legalization proposals, however, take a cost–benefit approach to drug policy (Nadelmann 1988, 1989; Ostrowski, 1990; Wisotsky, 1990). Cost–benefit arguments for legalization stress the benefits of this policy shift to some extent, but rely heavily on pointing out the costs associated with current efforts to eliminate or control distribution. These are costs associated with substance abuse, but largely products of the legal environment. They include: violence, drug adulteration, the development of organized crime enterprises, and corruption.

The scholarly literature critiquing the claims of legalization is somewhat smaller (Inciardi & McBride, 1991; Wilson, 1990), but raises some significant issues. There are several elements to the scholarly critique of legalization. The first is that legalization proposals tend to be short on the details (Inciardi & McBride, 1991), a criticism that has been addressed somewhat in recent years (Karel, 1991), but that nevertheless remains a failing that—as Zimring and Hawkins (1992) point out—is common to both sides of the legalization debate. The second critique is that drug use will increase under legalization, thereby increasing the costs of substance abuse and negating the benefits of reduced enforcement. This argument relies in part on a much more aggressive portrait of drug distribution; if drug sellers actively develop markets, rather than passively responding to demand, then legalization might allow sellers to greatly increase the number of new drug users. The final critique suggests that the central premise of legalization—that it would put an end to illicit markets—may not be entirely valid (Courtwright, 1992). This perspective is partly historical, for it cites as evidence previous experiences with regulated drug supplies that produced black markets.

Given the varied impulses that motivate the control of drug distribution and sale, it should not be surprising to find widespread disagreement over policy direction. For nearly a century, national governments have sought to deal with the basic problems of substance abuse by restricting consumer access, with limited success. Recent research on the control of distribution and sale, however, has dealt with more than just the success and failures of law enforcement. The studies reviewed above illuminate the relationship of drug distribution to patterns of drug use, a step that promises to identify more effective and realistic policies for reducing the costs of substance abuse.

REFERENCES

Adler, P. A. (1985). *Wheeling and dealing: An ethnography of upper-level drug dealing and smuggling communities.* New York: Columbia University Press.

Anglin, M. D., & Hser, Y. (1990). Treatment of drug abuse. In *Drugs and crime.* Chicago: University of Chicago Press.

Auletta, K. (1982). *The underclass.* New York: Random House.

Baumohl, J. (1992). The "dope-fiend's paradise" revisited: Notes from research in progress on drug law enforcement in San Francisco, 1875–1915. *The Surveyor, 24,* 3–12.

Berridge, V., & Edwards, G. (1981). *Opium and the people: Opiate use in nineteenth century England.* New Haven, CT: Yale University Press.

Botvin, G. J. (1990). Substance abuse prevention: Theory, practice, and effectiveness. In M. Tonry & J. Q. Wilson (Eds.), *Drugs and crime* (pp. 461–519). Chicago: University of Chicago Press.

Bourgois, P. (1989). In search of Horatio Alger: Culture and ideology in the crack economy. *Contemporary Drug Problems, 16,* 619–649.

Brecher, E. M. (1972). *Licit and illicit drugs: The Consumers Union report on narcotics, stimulants, depressants, inhalants, hallucinogens, and marijuana—including caffeine, nicotine, and alcohol.* Boston: Little, Brown.

Courtwright, D. T. (1982). *Dark paradise: Opiate addiction in America before 1940.* Cambridge, MA: Harvard University Press.

Courtwright, D. T. (1992). Drug legalization, the drug war, and drug treatment in historical perspective. In W. O. Walker III (Ed.), *Drug control policy: Essays in historical and comparative perspective* (pp. 42–63). University Park: Pennsylvania State University Press.

Currie, E. (1993). *Reckoning: Drugs, the cities, and the American future*. New York: Hill & Wang.

de Kort, M., & Korf, D. (1992). The development of drug trade and drug control in the Netherlands: A historical perspective. *Crime, Law and Social Change, 17*, 123–144.

Duster, T. (1987). Crime, youth unemployment, and the black underclass. *Crime and Delinquency, 33*, 300.

Estes, J. W. (1988). The pharmacology of nineteenth-century patent medicines. *Pharmacy in History, 30*, 3–18.

Friedman, M., & Friedman, R. (1984). *Tyranny of the status quo*. New York: Harcourt Brace Jovanovich.

Goldstein, P. J. (1990). Anabolic steroids: An ethnographic approach. In *Anabolic steroid use*. Rockville, MD: National Institute on Drug Abuse.

Goode, E. (1993). *Drugs in American society* (4th ed.). New York: McGraw-Hill.

Inciardi, J. A. (1992). *The war on drugs II*. Mountain View, CA: Mayfield.

Inciardi, J. A., & McBride, D. C. (1991). The case against legalization. In J. A. Inciardi (Ed.), *The drug legalization debate* (pp. 45–79). Newbury Park, CA: Sage.

Jackson, C. O. (1976). Before the drug culture: Barbiturate/amphetamine abuse in American society. *Clio Medica, 11*.

Johnson, B. D., Goldstein, P., Preblc, E., Schmeidler, J., Lipton, D. S., Spunt, B., & Miller, T. (1985). *Taking care of business: The economics of crime by heroin abusers*. Lexington, MA: Heath.

Johnson, B. D., Williams, T., Dei, K. A., & Sanabria, H. (1990). Drug abuse in the inner city: Impact on hard-drug users and the community. In M. Tonry & J. Q. Wilson (Eds.), *Drugs and crime* (pp. 9–67). Chicago: University of Chicago Press.

Kaplan, J. (1983). *The hardest drug: Heroin and public policy*. Chicago: University of Chicago Press.

Kaplan, J. (1988). Taking drugs seriously. *The Public Interest, 92*, 32–50.

Karel, R. B. (1991). A model legalization proposal. In J. A. Inciardi (Ed.), *The drug legalization debate* (pp. 80–102). Newbury Park, CA: Sage.

Kinder, D. C. (1992). Shutting out evil: Nativism and narcotics control in the United States. In W. O. Walker III (Ed.), *Drug control policy: Essays in historical and comparative perspective* (pp. 117–142). University Park: Pennsylvania State University Press.

Kinder, D. C., & Walker, W. O. (1986). Stable force in a storm: Harry J. Anslinger and United States foreign policy, 1930–1962. *Journal of American History, 72*, 908–927.

Kleiman, M. (1989). *Marijuana: Costs of abuse, costs of control*. New York: Greenwood.

Kleiman, M. (1992). *Against excess: Drug policy for results*. New York: Basic Books.

Kleiman, M. A., & Smith, K. D. (1990). State and local drug enforcement: In search of a strategy. In *Drugs and crime*. Chicago: University of Chicago Press.

Kohn, M. (1992). *Dope girls: The birth of the British drug underground*. London: Lawrence & Wishart.

Korf, D. J. (1990). Cannabis retail markets in Amsterdam. *The International Journal on Drug Policy, 2*, 23–27.

Kornblum, W. (1993). Drug legalization and the minority poor. In R. Bayer & G. M. Oppenheimer (Eds.), *Confronting drug policy: Illicit drugs in a free society* (pp. 115–135). Cambridge, England: Cambridge University Press.

Kozlowski, L., Coambs, R., Ferrence, R., & Adlaf, E. (1989). Preventing smoking and other drug use: Let the buyers beware and the interventions be apt. *Canadian Journal of Public Health, 80*, 452–456.

Levine, H. G., & Reinarman, C. (1993). From prohibition to regulation: Lessons from alcohol policy for drug policy. In R. Bayer & G. M. Oppenheimer (Eds.), *Confronting drug policy: Illicit drugs in a free society* (pp. 160–193). Cambridge, England: Cambridge University Press.

Levine, R. J. (1993). Medicalization of psychoactive substance use and the doctor-patient relationship. In R. Bayer & G. M. Oppenheimer (Eds.), *Confronting drug policy: Illicit drugs in a free society* (pp. 319–336). Cambridge, England: Cambridge University Press.

McAllister, W. B. (1992). Conflicts of interest in the international drug control system. In W. O. Walker III (Ed.), *Drug control policy: Essays in historical and comparative perspective* (pp. 143–166). University Park: Pennsylvania State University Press.

McWilliams, J. C. (1989). *The protectors: Harry J. Anslinger and the Federal Bureau of Narcotics, 1930–1962*. Newark: University of Delaware Press.

McWilliams, J. C. (1992). Through the past darkly: The politics and policies of America's drug war. In W. O. Walker III (Ed.), *Drug control policy: Essays in historical and comparative perspective* (pp. 5–41). University Park: Pennsylvania State University Press.

Michaels, R. J. (1987). The market for heroin before and after legalization. In *Dealing with drugs: Consequences of government control*. Lexington, MA: Heath.

Mieczkowski, T. (1994). The experiences of women who sell crack: Some descriptive data from the Detroit crack ethnography project. *The Journal of Drug Issues, 24*, 227, 233–248.

Model, S. (1993). The ethnic niche and the structure of opportunity: Immigrants and minorities in New York City. In M. B. Katz (Ed.), *The "underclass" debate: Views from history* (pp. 161–193). Princeton, NJ: Princeton University Press.

Moore, M. H. (1990). Supply reduction and drug law enforcement. In M. Tonry & J. Q. Wilson (Eds.), *Drugs and crime* (pp. 109–157). Chicago: University of Chicago Press.

Musto, D. F. (1987). *The American disease: Origins of narcotic control* (Expanded ed.). New York: Oxford University Press.

Nadelmann, E. A. (1988). The case for legalization. *The Public Interest, 92*, 3–31.

Nadelmann, E. A. (1989). Drug prohibition in the United States: Costs, consequences, and alternatives. *Science, 245*, 939–947.

Nadelmann, E. A. (1991). The case for legalization. In J. A. Inciardi (Ed.), *The drug legalization debate* (pp. 17–44). Newbury Park, CA: Sage.

Nadelmann, E. A. (1993). *Cops across borders: The internationalization of U.S. criminal law enforcement*. University Park: Pennsylvania State University Press.

Ostrowski, J. (1990). The moral and practical case for drug legalization. *Hofstra Law Review, 18*, 607–702.

Parssinen, T. (1983). *Secret passions, secret remedies: Narcotic drugs in British society, 1820–1930*. Philadelphia: Institute for the Study of Human Issues.

Preble, E., & Casey, J. J. (1969). Taking care of business—The heroin addict's life on the street. *The International Journal of the Addictions, 4*, 1–24.

Reuter, P. (1988). Can the borders be sealed? *Public Interest, 92*, 51–65.

Reuter, P. (1992). Hawks ascendant: The punitive trend of American drug policy. *Daedalus, 121*.

Reuter, P., & Kleiman, M. (1986). Risks and prices: An economic analysis of drug enforcement. In M. Tonry & N. Morris (Eds.), *Crime and justice: A review of research* (pp. 289–340). Chicago: University of Chicago Press.

Reuter, P., MacCoun, R., & Murphy, P. (1990). *Money from crime: An economic study of drug dealing in Washington, D.C.* Santa Monica, CA: Rand Corporation.

Robert Wood Johnson Foundation. (1993). *Substance abuse: The nation's number one health problem*. Princeton, NJ: Author.

Rosenbaum, M., Morgan, P., & Beck, J. E. (1989). Ethnographic notes on Ecstasy use among professionals. *The International Journal on Drug Policy, 1*, 16–19.

Ruggerio, V., & South, N. (1995). *Eurodrugs: Drug use, markets and trafficking in Europe*. London: UCL Press.

Rydell, C. P., & Everingham, S. S. (1994). *Controlling cocaine: Supply versus demand programs*. Santa Monica, CA: Rand Corporation.

Scott, L. C. (1923). The case of the drug addict. *Quarterly Bulletin of the Louisiana State Board of Health, 24*, 14–18.

Simon, J. (1993). *Poor discipline: Parole and the social control of the underclass, 1890–1990*. Chicago: University of Chicago Press.

Spillane, J. F. (1994). *Modern drug, modern menace: The legal use and distribution of cocaine in the United States, 1880–1920*. Unpublished doctoral dissertation, Carnegie Mellon University, Pittsburgh, PA.

Starr, P. (1982). *The social transformation of American medicine*. New York: Basic Books.

Swann, J. P. (1994). FDA and the practice of pharmacy: Prescription drug regulation before the Durham-Humphrey Amendment of 1951. *Pharmacy in History, 36*, 55–70.

Szasz, T. (1985). *Ceremonial chemistry: The ritual persecution of drugs, addicts, and pushers.* Holmes Beach, Florida: Learning Publications.

Szasz, T. (1992). *Our right to drugs: The case for a free market*. New York: Praeger.

Taylor, A. H. (1969). *American diplomacy and the narcotics traffic, 1900–1939: A study in international humanitarian reform*. Durham, NC: Duke University Press.

Temin, P. (1980). *Taking your medicine: Drug regulation in the United States*. Cambridge, MA: Harvard University Press.

Trebach, A. S. (1987). *The great drug war*. New York: Macmillan.

U.S. Office of National Drug Control Policy. (1989). *National drug control strategy*. Washington, DC: U.S. Government Printing Office.

Walker, W. O. (1981). *Drug control in the Americas*. Albuquerque: University of New Mexico Press.

Walker, W. O. (1991). *Opium and foreign policy: The Anglo-American search for order in Asia, 1912–1954*. Chapel Hill: University of North Carolina Press.

Williams, T. (1989). *The cocaine kids*. New York: Addison-Wesley.

Williams, T. (1992). *Crackhouse: Notes from the end of the line*. New York: Addison-Wesley.

Wilson, J. Q. (1990). Against the legalization of drugs. *Commentary, 89*, 21–28.

Wilson, W. J. (1987). *The truly disadvantaged: The inner city, the underclass, and public policy*. Chicago: University of Chicago Press.

Wisotsky, S. (1990). *Beyond the war on drugs: Overcoming a failed drug policy*. Buffalo, NY: Prometheus.

Wood, H. C. (1916). Some of the results of the Harrison Anti-Narcotic Law. *Journal of the American Pharmaceutical Association, 5*.

Young, J. H. (1961). *The toadstool millionaires: A social history of patent medicines in America before federal regulation*. Princeton, NJ: Princeton University Press.

Young, J. H. (1990). *Pure food: Securing the federal food and drugs act of 1906*. Princeton, NJ: Princeton University Press.

Zimring, F. E., & Hawkins, G. (1992). *The search for rational drug control*. New York: Cambridge University Press.

Zimring, F. E., & Hawkins, G. (1994). The growth of imprisonment in California. *British Journal of Criminology, 34*, 83–96.

Media Influence

Joseph C. Fisher
InterData
Sanibel, Florida

MEDIA AND BEHAVIOR

For media representations of smoking and drinking and advertisements for alcohol and tobacco products to affect consumer behavior to the point that adverse social, economic, and health consequences occur, two mechanisms are necessary: (1) a means whereby messages carried in the media are observed, processed, and converted into behavior by the viewer; and (2) a mechanism to explain how the incremental consumption attributable, at least in part, to media exposure results in adverse outcomes in aggregate and on an individual basis. In short, there must be theories to explain how media influence behavior, and next how the behavior attributable to media effects eventuates in adverse societal outcomes.

Although there are many theories evoked to explain media effects, the one that informs research in the substance abuse field most often is social learning theory. Codified by Bandura (1977), social learning theory is predicated on an operant conditioning model, suggesting that behavior is shaped by the consequences that follow it. So if the behavior is rewarded or is followed by no negative consequences it is more likely to be acquired, increased, or continued, whereas if negative consequences attend the behavior it becomes less likely in the future.

The unique aspect of social learning theory is not its operant conditioning core, but instead the belief that complex behaviors such as smoking and drinking are learned in a social context. Reinforcement contingencies can

235

occur as a result of personal use of a substance (differential reinforcement), as well as though interaction with others engaged in the behavior (differential association). In addition to providing models of use, significant others hold definitions of the behavior as approved or forbidden that provide a normative context within which personal behavior develops. On an individual basis, then, the acquisition and maintenance of behavior depends on the cumulative history of rewards and punishments experienced when using a substance and contact with models engaged in the behavior and the normative context for permissible use they create.

Especially important when considering media effects is the belief that behavior can be learned, in a sense at a distance, by watching filmed models and the consequences that befall them. This tenet is based in large part on two classic experiments on aggression among preschoolers conducted by Bandura and his colleagues. The first of these (Bandura, Ross, & Ross, 1963) found that subjects were twice as likely as controls to exhibit aggressive behavior if they had been exposed to an aggressive model. In a follow-on study (Bandura, 1965), preschoolers were again exposed to filmed models of aggressive behavior, but in this instance rewards, punishment, or no consequences followed the behavior. Imitations of the behavior were similar for those who saw models who were rewarded or escaped consequence.

The results of these experiments indicate that behavior can be acquired through the observation and imitation of filmed models, even animated ones. Additionally, the consequences accruing to the model as a function of their behavior provides significant learning material for the viewer, behavioral imitation being more likely if the consequences are not negative. Social learning theory in general and these two conclusions in particular have directed much of the research involving media effects on alcohol and tobacco use.

Media content and advertising are intrinsically social constructions so differences in public perception of alcohol and tobacco use mean their treatment in these forms of communication will vary considerably. Images of smoking and drinking appear in the media with starkly different rates, underscoring the prevailing view of each in society. Depictions of smokers and drinkers differ, as do their motives for using the substance and the context in which use takes place. Themes used in advertising to persuade consumers to use alcohol and tobacco products are not the same, the former, capitalizing on public acceptance, contain images of group use for sociability, celebration, and reward, while the latter, seeming to accept outcast status, portrays the smoker as solitary, independent, and free. The messages are clear. To drink is to be one with one's peers; to smoke is an act of independence, if not defiance, by a free thinker.

For smoking, then, any media or advertising effect that serves to initiate, increase, or prolong consumption damages the collective health, but for alcohol the effect is socially consequential only if the rates of alcohol-related adverse outcomes are affected. The mechanism to explain how they might be is the single distribution theory of alcohol prevalence. Briefly, the theory suggests that the distribution of consumption in society is lognormal and that the rate of alcohol-related problems is a function of how many people are in the positively skewed tail of the distribution that exceeds a critical threshold beyond which the problems readily occur. Thus, to the degree media and advertising raise the average level of consumption of absolute alcohol and push more people into the extreme end of the distribution, they will contribute to alcohol-related problems.

It is important that we examine this theory closely because it determines, to a great extent, how research about media effects on alcohol use should be evaluated. First and foremost, it suggests that alcoholics and normal drinkers do not differ or, more correctly, only differ in the annual quantity of alcohol consumed. Media representations can be expected, therefore, to affect consumers uniformly regardless of their current drinking. Additionally, for adverse outcomes to occur it is necessary to demonstrate that the average per capita consumption of raw or absolute alcohol increases, it is not sufficient to show that category consumption (beer, wine, liquor) increases or much less that the consumption or share of a particular brand responds to media messages. In sum, the total consumption of all alcoholic beverages as a system must be considered and shown to increase.

FORMS OF COMMUNICATION

Before beginning our investigation of media effects, it is important to draw a distinction between various forms of mass media representations of alcohol and tobacco. First, we will distinguish between nonconsumptive and consumptive forms of communication. By nonconsumptive, we mean the appearance or use of the substance in a creative presentation the intent of which is unrelated to the consumption of the substance. When shown under these circumstances, alcohol and tobacco tend to be of secondary importance, incidental to the main theme and not central to the scene or the behavior of the characters in it. Nonconsumptive representations occur in all types of mass media including literature, music, films, and broadcast programming.

Consumptive forms of communication differ in that the intent of the message is to affect consumer behavior as it regards the substance. The most obvious form of consumptive communication is advertising, the purpose of which is to influence consumer product choices. More generally, consumptive communication can be segmented by message content (positive or negative) and message intent (promotes use or prevents use).

What is commonly known in commercial circles as "image advertising" involves positive statements about the product form of a substance, the intent of which is to persuade consumers to use more of it. Invariably, the positive aspects of use of the substance generally or the positive attributes of a product form specifically are emphasized. So the aging or blending of a scotch might be stressed in a print ad, or the derived benefits of alcohol use (e.g., as a reward for a job well done) could find its way into a product slogan such as "For all you do, this Bud's for you."

The goal of image advertising is to build brand equity, which can be defined as the willingness of consumers to pay more for a product than a commodity alternative. Typically, it takes an extended period of time and significant advertising investment to build brand equity, and yet the investment usually pays dividends over the long term in the price differential consumers are willing to pay for a product.

The principle issues surrounding advertising for abused substances are associated with the positive aspects of the portrayal of the substance and the clear goal of stimulating consumption. Thus, alcohol and tobacco advertising are criticized because none of the deleterious health effects of product use are presented. Especially egregious in this view is "lifestyle" advertising, which supposedly implies the product and substance are integral to behaviors that are precisely those that are diminished with use (e.g., athletic prowess or sexual performance). Advertising is assumed to be misleading and deceptive as a consequence.

With respect to consumption, the major debate surrounds whether advertising builds primary demand or only affects product choices (as staunchly maintained by the advertising community). If the former, advertising might be expected to induce people to take up the behavior who might otherwise not; might stimulate sufficient incremental consumption to increase the rates of adverse social, economic, and health consequences; and finally could reinforce the behavior, making cessation that much more difficult. If advertising only affects brand choices, a relatively constant amount of demand would be shifted among a set of product choices, or at worst between product categories (e.g., wine to beer) with little if any noticeable impact on aggregate demand, and hence the negative outcomes associated with use.

At times advertising can carry a negative message while attempting to promote use. Typically, this occurs when competitors in a category denigrate each other's products or services for their own benefit. Although competitive advertising can focus on product attributes such as automotive acceleration or the tar or nicotine content of a cigarette, the most often used basis of comparison is price. In essence, then, the hallmarks of competitive advertising are a direct comparison with a named product substitute on the basis of some shared characteristic, usually price.

Competitive advertising is a self-defeating strategy and is assiduously avoided by most companies. It tends to be used when products or services in a category are, for all practical purposes, commodities. Because almost all competitive advertising reduces to price arguments, it is thought to "cheapen" the product. More importantly, consumers are taught to shop on the basis of price, thereby negating the brand equity built with such considerable effort and expense by image advertising.

Given how sensitive consumption of alcohol and tobacco is to price, we might expect competitive advertising to be an effective way to build primary demand. It is perhaps a relief then to find competitive advertising is virtually nonexistent in the alcohol and tobacco categories at the present time. Competitive advertising is included here for completeness and to raise the specter of what it might portend if it were used by alcohol and tobacco manufacturers, but due to its absence from the categories will not be discussed further.

Counteradvertising attempts to limit use by stressing the negative aspects of use or abuse of the substance. To use the example of drunk driving again, the campaign sponsored by Mothers Against Drunk Driving (MADD) is precisely what is meant here by counteradvertising. Images of empty swings and pictures of children killed by drunk drivers dominate the message. Negative consequences are stressed, while the remedy—reduced consumption and abuse—is implied.

Generally, counteradvertising takes two forms. As illustrated above, the first of these are stand-alone advertisements designed to correct the information imbalance created by the preponderance of positive messages carried by image advertisements in the media. These can be sponsored by advocacy groups like MADD or may be part of a government-initiated prevention program that includes a mass media component. Undoubtedly the most well known and thoroughly researched counteradvertising involved antismoking ads broadcast during the late 1960s as part of the Fairness Doctrine ruling by the Federal Communications Commission.

Warning labels are the second form of counteradvertising. Whether carried on product packages or advertisements for the product, the goal of warning labels is to offset manufacturer selling messages by cataloguing the pejorative health consequences of routine use of a substance. The assumption is, advertising creates a climate of misinformation that needs to be corrected and, further, that can be corrected by giving consumers a list of known health risks in warning labels.

NONCONSUMPTIVE COMMUNICATION

Behavioral effects are assumed to be a function of exposure to smoking and drinking images in the media, their frequency, cumulative number, salience, and meaning. As a consequence, the investigation of effects usually begins with a content analysis of the media environment. In simplest terms, this involves counting how many references to alcohol or tobacco are encountered in a media sample and sometimes documenting how the incidence changes over time. The content of the messages is also considered, what it demonstrates or implies about usage, how it could be interpreted by those exposed, and what this might portend for behavioral effects.

All manner of nonconsumptive communications have been content analyzed. These studies can take a prospective as broad as alcohol use in all of Western literature (Montagne, 1988) or as narrow as drinking in the plot and character development of a single novel (Noelke, 1986). Alcohol use as a creative facilitator by literary figures has been studied (Digby & Digby, 1988), as has the appearance of drinking references in magazine articles and editorials (Breed & De Foe, 1978). And because of an abundance of references, country and western music is a favorite genre for those studying alcohol references in popular music (Beckley & Chalfant, 1979; Connors & Alpher, 1989).

Several broad patterns about alcohol portrayals in mass media are apparent from these studies. First, alcohol and drinking references have become more frequent regardless of media type. Second, the nature of the references has changed. Contemporary images of drinking tend to reflect current beliefs about drinking and the etiology of alcoholism. Use of alcohol is seen more often as an everyday and commonplace occurrence. Alcoholism is viewed less as a result of a character flaw or moral deficiency than as a disease or psychological illness. Therapeutic options described have evolved in accordance with this psychological view of causation.

Some of the best content analytic studies have been conducted by Room and Herd (Herd, 1983; Herd, 1986; Herd & Room, 1982; Room, 1987, 1988). In historical analyses of films, the investigators documented a complex and reciprocal relationship between cultural context and alcohol portrayals. Alcohol is seen as a powerful symbolic image, the use of which reflects prevailing social and historical practice. Alcohol use in films also tends to press the outer limits of societal use and in so doing helps extend the definition of acceptable behavior. Thus, although alcohol depictions in films are culturally fixed by prevailing usage norms, they are also instrumental in expanding the boundaries of then current use.

Undoubtedly, the most public and influential medium is television, and its importance as a source of behavioral models has not escaped investigators. Something like a cottage industry has developed around the study of drinking and smoking cues in television programming. Typically, studies of this sort enumerate a sample of programming that is either expected to depict high rates of alcohol and tobacco use, such as fictional prime time shows or soap operas, or is representative of a part of the day (e.g., "prime time"). The sample is thought to be a proxy for the television environment to which the public is exposed and the normative content in which it operates.

Analysis of the televised material is both quantitative and qualitative. Individual scenes are coded for the presence or absence of alcohol, tobacco, or other substances, and whether they are consumed by a major character or simply appear on-screen. The prevalence of cues is usually reported as a percent of programs or scenes that include the substance or behavior and the rate of appearances per hour. On the qualitative side, an attempt is often made to interpret the context and consequences of usage, in the simplest guise whether it is positive, neutral, or negative. Consistent with social learning theory precepts, positive and neutral contexts and consequences are assumed to promote use, while negative use situations and outcomes presumably act against behavioral acquisition by the viewer.

As suggested earlier, published reports of this sort are legion, and we will consider only a few of the more revealing ones here. The first of these are historical studies originally conducted by Breed and De Foe (1978) and continued by Breed, Wallack, and Cruz (Cruz & Wallack, 1986; Wallack, Breed, & Cruz, 1987). The subject matter of the studies was fictional prime time, consisting of situation comedies and dramas and excluding nonfiction programming such as news, sports, and special broadcasts. Both alcohol and tobacco depictions were considered and special attention was paid to major smoking policy events, notably the publication of the first Surgeon General's Report on smoking and health in 1964 and the implementation of the ban of broadcast advertising for cigarettes in 1971.

Prior to the Surgeon General's Report, between 1950 and 1963, tobacco appeared on fictional prime time programming 2.32 times per hour while alcohol was portrayed 2.78 times per hour. After the Surgeon General's Report until the cigarette advertising ban, 1964 to 1970, smoking depictions dropped in half to 1.22 per hour, while drinking incidences grew by half to 4.12. The trend continued after 1971, with smoking portrayals declining by two thirds to 0.44 depictions per hour, whereas alcohol appearances increased to 4.79 times per hour. By 1981–1982, the rate of alcohol depictions grew to 8.72 per hour, three times the original rate, while tobacco incidences were 0.28 per hour, roughly one tenth the rate prior to the Surgeon General's Report. In the final period studied, 1984, alcohol appeared 10.65 and tobacco 0.87 times per hour. Over time, alcohol portrayals on prime time fictional programs increased by a factor of four, from 2.78 to 10.65 per hour, and tobacco appearances declined by 60%, from 2.32 to 0.87 times per hour.

Another interesting pattern in these findings is the relative rates of appearance for alcohol and tobacco over time. Before the Surgeon General's Report was issued, television viewers were about as likely to see a portrayal of tobacco and smoking as they were alcohol and drinking, 2.32 per hour for the former versus 2.78 for the latter. From 1971 onward, a person viewing prime time situation comedies and dramas was 10 times more likely to see alcohol portrayed than tobacco.

This relationship is further demonstrated in Table 14.1, which summarizes the results of studies that examined the prevalence of illicit drugs in television programming as well as alcohol and tobacco. The data gathered by Breed and colleagues was based on a common programming sample definition and counting methodology; therefore, trends over time are identifiable. By comparison, the results summarized in Table 14.1 vary with respect to sample and methodology and the estimates of prevalence for the various substances range widely across the studies. As an example, De Foe, Breed, and Breed (1983), studying only fictional prime time, obtained rates of appearance per hour for alcohol between 4.79 and 8.60. MacDonald and Estep (1985), using a more representative sample of prime time programming, found rates per hour for alcohol ranging from 2.24 to 3.54. Our purpose here is to examine the relative rates in which alcohol, tobacco, and illicit drugs appear in television programming that can be determined within each study.

From Table 14.1 it can be seen that alcohol depictions are much more prevalent than either tobacco or illicit drug appearances. For instance, alcohol appeared five times more often than tobacco in 1973, the earliest study of programming (McEwen & Hanneman, 1974). Similar ratios were reported by Fernandez-Collado and Greenberg (1978) for prime time programs most watched by children; Greenberg, Fernandez-Collado, Graef, Kor-

TABLE 14.1
Prevalence of Abused Substances on Television

		Rate per Hour			
	Year Studied	Alcohol	Tobacco	Illicit Drugs	Programming
MacDonald &	1984	3.54	1.33	0.18	All prime time
Estep, 1985	1983	2.54	0.65	0.30	
	1982	2.24	0.47	0.24	
De Foe et al., 1983	1981	8.60	0.24	—	Fictional prime time
	1979	7.94	0.26	0.03	
	1978	7.62	0.22	—	
	1977	5.52	0.33	—	
	1976	4.79	0.48	0.10	
Greenberg et al.,	1977	2.66	0.48	0.83	Fictional prime
1979	1976	2.19	0.70	0.22	time & Saturday morning
Fernandez-Collado et al., 1978	1976	1.46	0.36	—	Prime time with largest children's audience
McEwen & Hanneman, 1974	1973	1.31	0.26	0.31	All prime time & public television

zenny, and Atkin (1979) for fictional programming on prime time and Saturday morning; and more recently MacDonald and Estep (1985) for all prime time programming. The appearance differential widens when only fictional prime time programming is considered (De Foe et al., 1983) with reported ratios of 10:1 and 16:1 for alcohol and tobacco, respectively.

Rates for depictions of illicit drugs vary from no instances to nearly one per hour. In two cases, McEwen and Hanneman (1974) and Greenberg et al. (1979), tobacco and illicit drugs appeared with roughly equal frequency. MacDonald and Estep (1985) detected two to seven times more tobacco portrayals than ones for illicit drugs. Perhaps most surprising given the preponderance of alcohol images observed, De Foe et al. (1983) found virtually no illicit drug references in prime time situation comedies and dramas. Nonetheless, in the majority of studies the frequency of tobacco appearances more closely parallels that for illicit drugs than for alcohol. In a sense, then, since the broadcast ban on cigarette advertising, tobacco has been treated as if it were an illicit drug in television programming.

Another charge leveled at television drinking portrayals is that they do not accurately reflect the consumption patterns of viewers. Wallack et al. (1987) found that alcohol represented roughly two thirds of all beverage consumption on television, yet actual worldwide consumption was only 16%. In contrast, water and soft drinks, each of which accounted for a third of true beverage consumption in 1984, appeared on television only 3% and 6% of the time, respectively, that year. In light of these findings, the investigators concluded alcohol and drinking images are ubiquitous on television and are presented in an unbalanced fashion, giving the impression that alcohol use is a normal, everyday occurrence all of which "may contribute to the normalization of drinking in American life" (p. 37).

Recent years have seen a continuation of the tradition of counting alcohol and tobacco images on television. Diener (1993) examined soap opera broadcasts in 1986 and 1991 and found typical rates for alcohol, 3–5 per hour, but virtually no depictions of tobacco. Hazan and Glantz (1995) found the rate of tobacco appearances in fictional prime time programs to be 0.70 per hour. And for those who would decry the "wetness" of American programming, Waxer (1992) found that depictions of alcohol consumption on British television were three times more frequent than on similar programs in the United States and Canada.

At this juncture, several conclusions can be drawn regarding the prevalence of alcohol, tobacco and illicit drugs on television:

1. The medium has grown progressively "wetter" over time, with alcohol depictions increasing fourfold in fictional prime time from 1950 to 1984.
2. Tobacco representations have all but disappeared over the same period, with depictions declining by 60–90% depending on the time studied.

3. Despite an increase in the frequency of tobacco portrayals in recent studies, tobacco is still seen less than once per hour in prime time.

4. Tobacco, once seen as often as alcohol on television, appeared about as often as illicit drugs after the Surgeon General's Report and the broadcast ban of cigarette advertising television.

Perhaps the best final statement on this topic was provided by Gerbner, Gross, Morgan, and Signorielli (1981) after their analysis of the Cultural Indicators Database, consisting of 10 years' worth of television programming and 3 years of commercials: "The impression of some people that television characters smoke a great deal is unwarranted and may be derived from old movies. In contrast to the relatively limited amount of smoking, alcohol is hard to escape on television" (pp. 903–904).

Depictions of substance use are likely to involve positive social contexts. Typical are the following: "good-guy" smokers outnumber "bad-guy" smokers and smokers tend to be "high-status role models" as opposed to medium or low status (Hazan & Glantz, 1995); drinking occurs in "normal" contexts such as bars, restaurants, or living rooms (Diener, 1993); drinking motives are pleasant and social with over 80% occurring for hospitality, enjoyment, and celebration reasons (Futch, Lesman, & Geller, 1984); further, solitary drinkers are depicted only 4% of the time (Hansen, 1986); smokers are regularly seen characters almost none of whom want to quit (Cruz & Wallack, 1986); drinking outcomes disproportionately favor consumption being either neutral, 85%, or positive, 9%, whereas depictions of illicit drugs are invariably negative (MacDonald & Estep, 1985); and similarly, 70% of scenes showing alcohol use in soap operas reinforce drinking or show it free of consequences (Lowery, 1980).

The cumulative weight of these images is thought to "glamorize" the substances in question and portray a normative context approving of consumption. The expected impact is described by Greenberg (1981): "It is anticipated that regular viewers of such series [top-rated fictional prime time programs] would be more likely to believe that: 1) everyone does it, 2) it's fun to do it, 3) nothing bad happens to you if you do it, and 4) it's readily available" (p. 203). Thus, television programming, on the strength of generalizations of social learning theory, is concluded to be a significant environmental factor contributing to the start-up, stimulation, and perpetuation of smoking and drinking.

From time to time there have been dissenting opinions expressed about what might otherwise seem to be an inexorable chain of logic. For example, MacDonald (1983) interviewed inveterate soap opera watchers—the majority of whom, unlike content analytic coders, felt that the consequences of alcohol use by characters in the series were predominantly negative. Heilbronn (1988) argued that alcohol is a flexible social symbol that can be used as a creative tool to set context, define characters, and foreshadow consequences. The type of drink a character chooses can be an encapsulated packet of information conveying character, background, personality, and social position. From this perspective, alcohol use on television is seen as a means to glamorize the setting rather than the scene glamorizing alcohol.

Despite an occasional opinion to the contrary, researchers in the field seem convinced that television promotes smoking and drinking. But, of course, this conclusion is beyond the scope of the content analytic method and relies exclusively on belief in the validity and generalizability of social learning theory. Given this considerable leap of faith, it is especially important to assess the empirical evidence concerning the relationship between mass media exposure in general and television viewing in particular and smoking and drinking.

The evidence for a media–behavior link, at least in the case of alcohol, is equivocal. Studying male high school students, Tucker (1985) found a direct relationship between amount of television watching and drinking after controlling for demographics, such that heavy television watchers drank more than light or moderate television viewers. As if to confirm the fears of Wallack et al. (1987) regarding the imbalance between the frequency of televised drinking images and actual consumption, Gerbner and Gross (1976) reported that the responses of heavy television watchers to survey items tended toward the reality shown in the media as opposed to what exists in fact, a socializing process dubbed "mainstreaming" (Gerbner, Gross, Morgan, & Signorielli, 1980).

Contrary evidence was reported by Signorielli (1987) and Gerbner, Morgan, and Signorielli (1982), who found an inverse relationship between the amount of television viewing and alcohol consumption. However, demography was not controlled in these studies as it was in Tucker's. Chirco (1990) conducted an extensive analysis of media effects and social learning mechanisms and alcohol use using a nationally representative sample of high school seniors. Of the 13 regression analyses that included indices of television exposure, 12 found no relationship or an inverse one between the amount of viewing and alcohol consumption. Other aspects of social learning theory such as peer behavior and attitudes were consistently related to drinking.

Two final experiments are worth noting. Sobell et al. (1986) assigned normal drinkers, 96 male college students, to several experimental conditions defined by programming content (with or without alcohol scenes) and advertising type (beer, nonalcoholic beverage, food). No significant differences were noted in taste ratings of light beer or the amount consumed and commercial or programming content. However, when an at-risk group, 96 male alcoholics in treatment, was studied (Sobell, Sobell, Toneatto, & Leo, 1993) presence of alcohol cues in programming made the participants feel significantly less confident in their ability to resist drinking. No such loss of confidence was reported when the alcoholics viewed commercials prompting the investigators to speculate that the subjects, knowing ads are a form of consumptive communication, were forearmed and counterargued the selling message. With their defenses down, they were unprepared for alcohol cues in programming and were more apt to be affected.

CONSUMPTIVE COMMUNICATION—ADVERTISING

Like nonconsumptive communication, consumptive forms have been the subject of numerous content analyses. When compared with portrayals of alcohol and drinking in television programming, commercials for alcohol products are encountered infrequently. Perhaps the best estimate of the relative ratio of appearances is provided by Cafiso, Goodstadt, Garlington, and Sheppard (1982). Studying a composite week of all television programming, the investigators found nonconsumptive occurrences were six times more likely to be seen than consumptive ones, 0.62 versus 3.62 per hour. Further, ads for nonalcoholic beverages appeared 4.5 times more often, 2.82 times per hour, than ones for alcohol products. So although beverage images in programs disproportionately favor alcohol, commercials reverse the ratio showing soft drinks much more frequently. And finally, commercial depictions more accurately reflect the drinking preferences and practices of the viewing public.

Advertising for tobacco products in broadcast media was, of course, banned in 1971, which proved to be a boon for other media. Advertising expenditures in print media increased threefold immediately thereafter. In fact, tobacco is the second most heavily advertising product category in most media, following only the automotive category. While advertising for tobacco products may not be seen on television or heard on the radio, it is all but inescapable in the other media including print, outdoor, and direct mail.

Recent interest in the placement of tobacco advertising has centered on what appears to be industry efforts to circumvent the broadcast advertising ban. Particularly important in this regard are sports telecasts and manufacturer sponsorships of sport teams. Several investigators (Blum, 1991; Madden & Grube, 1994) have found that stadium and raceway signage are shown multiple times per program creating the potential for thousands of impressions per viewer. These findings are significant not only because brand names, logos, and slogans appear where they should be absent; what is doubly offensive to those who thought this battle was won is that the appearances are not accompanied by warning labels that would normally be required on ads. The latter charge has been leveled at other forms of promotional spending such as branded merchandise and clothing as well.

Other issues have surfaced around the placement and content of cigarette advertising. Of special concern is the apparent targeting of adolescents by placing ads in magazines with large audiences of young people or billboards in high adolescent traffic areas (Ammerman & Nolden, 1995). A number of studies (Minkler, Wallack, & Madden, 1987; Warner, 1985a; Warner & Goldenhar, 1989; Warner, Goldenhar, & McLaughlin, 1992) have found that advertising in magazines is associated with an avoidance or diminished coverage of smoking hazards. While others (Altman, Slater, Albright, & Maccoby, 1987; Cardador, Hazan, & Glantz, 1995) suggest cigarette advertising is used to allay or combat public health concerns or respond to smoking and health events such as the Surgeon General's Report (Warner, 1985b), counter-counteradvertising if you will.

A marketing prospective was added to the assessment of cigarette advertising content by Ringold and Calfee (1989). Sampling advertisements from 1926 to 1986, the investigators found health claims to be one of the most frequent themes in ads and that the claims emphasized the negative aspects of smoking (e.g., a product has less tar and hence is less harmful). Indeed, the authors stated manufacturers had an incentive to indirectly publicize smoking health hazards to promote their products as safer than alternatives, if not prevented from doing so by regulation, a conclusion that was, to say the least, controversial (see rejoinders by Cohen, 1989, and Pollay, 1989; reply to rejoinders, Ringold & Calfee, 1990; and re-reply, Cohen, 1992).

Despite the concerns about targeting youth, whether intentional or unintentional, the messages alcohol and tobacco ads carry or how the tobacco industry influences editorial content and combats antismoking, the fact remains that content analysis studies are not designed to determine media effects. They can describe the media environment, how often we are exposed to messages, who is exposed and what the messages are, but the behavioral implications of these findings are dependent on other methodologies. In this regard, the effects of advertising on both smoking and drinking can be discerned by examining the collective findings of experiments, survey-based quasi-experiments, econometric studies, and the effect of changes in advertising regulations.

The empirical evidence concerning the effect of advertising on alcohol use has been comprehensively reviewed by Fisher (1993). The major conclusions drawn from this review are:

1. There is no experimental evidence to suggest that exposure to alcohol ads, the number or type of ads, in laboratory or "real life" situations, is related to alcohol consumption.

2. Surveys of media exposure and drinking practices have shown a consistent, small, yet nonsignificant relationship between advertising, alcohol

consumption, and indicators of abuse. Specifically, advertising exposure accounted for 1–4% of the variance in consumption depending on the type of beverage and characteristics of the consumer, 0.2–1.2% of the variance in measures of intoxication, and 0.1–1.2% of the variance in other indicators of abuse.

3. Econometric studies have shown a rough 10:1 relationship between advertising and consumption such that a 10% increase in advertising is accompanied by a 1% increase in per capita consumption. However, the effects due to advertising were shown to dissipate across the system of alcoholic beverage options such that increases in consumption of one beverage, say beer, due to advertising reduced consumption of beverage substitutes, wine or spirits. The net effect is virtually no impact on total alcohol consumption and hence, according to the single distribution theory, there should be no concomitant increases in adverse societal outcomes.

4. There is no evidence to suggest that changes in regulations regarding permissible advertising, whether it is banned or allowed after having been banned, affects consumption.

Recent research is consistent with the above conclusions. For example, Lipsitz, Blake, Vincent, and Winters (1993) found no significant relationship between exposure to television beer commercials and alcohol expectancies. An econometric analysis of advertising, alcohol consumption, and mortality from alcohol-related disease in the United States from 1950 to 1990 found weak, nonsignificant relationships between advertising expenditures, per capita consumption, and mortality rates (Fisher & Cook, 1995). Like other studies, a 10% increase in advertising was associated with a 1% gain in consumption, and advertising accounted for small portions of the variance in consumption (<5%). Meanwhile, a quasi-experimental study of fifth- and sixth-graders (Grube & Wallack, 1994) identified a small relationship between advertising awareness and intention to drink as an adult. The magnitude of the effect, advertising awareness accounting for 2.26% of the variance in intentions, makes the result entirely consistent with other survey-based studies.

One of the problems with survey studies is that they assume but do not directly measure a temporal ordering of effects. It is never entirely clear if attention to ads precedes intentions to drink, if intention to drink raises interest in and attention to ads, or if both processes are operative and reinforcing. In this regard, an important longitudinal study was conducted in New Zealand by Connolly, Casswell, Zhang, and Silva (1994). The investigators correlated total television viewing, recall of alcohol appearances in entertainment programming, and commercials for alcohol products and moderation messages at ages 13 and 15 with alcohol consumption at age 18. Nonmedia variables were also measured, including socioeconomic status, occupation, and peer approval of drinking. Dependent variables examined were average amount of consumption, maximum amount consumed, and frequency of consumption of beer, wine, and spirits for males and females separately. The results of this study can be summarized as follows:

1. Of the 84 relationships between media exposure and advertising recall and consumption tested the vast majority, 89%, were nonsignificant.
2. Six of nine significant findings were associated with nonconsumptive media and alcohol use by females, specifically five of six tests of average hours of television watched per week at ages 13 and 15 were statistically significant as was one relationship between recall of entertainment appearances at age 13 and maximum amount consumed at age 18.
3. Number of alcohol commercials recalled by males at age 15 was significantly related to average amount and maximum amount of beer consumed at age 18.
4. Recall of moderation messages at ages 13 and 15 were unrelated to consumption at age 18 for either males or females.
5. All variables combined, including nonmedia variables, never accounted for more than 17% of the variance in drinking.

These findings argue against consistent or large media effects. They also imply nonconsumptive media are more significant in determining alcohol consumption by females, while the only consumptive media effects, if real, are highly specific to males for amount of beer consumed. The only truly pervasive finding of the study is that media, consumptive or nonconsumptive, do not influence the frequency or amount of alcoholic beverages consumed.

Before beginning the review of the evidence for advertising effects on tobacco use, it is worth reiterating a crucial distinction in how effects are evaluated. Because health problems attend any use of tobacco, even the smallest advertising effects can be viewed as consequential. Advertising effects that were not relevant to alcohol use, such as the reinforcement of behavior or the maintenance of demand at existing levels, are significant in the context of tobacco use.

There does not appear to be a great deal of support in the econometric literature for the notion that advertising affects demand for cigarettes. Recent studies of the U.S. from 1961 to 1990 (Franke, 1994; Wilcox & Vacker, 1992) did not find a significant relationship between advertising and cigarette consumption, expressed on a per capita or federal taxes paid basis. Similar null findings have been reported for South Korea from 1988 to 1992 (Wilcox, Tharp, & Yang, 1994), South Africa 1970 to 1989 (Reekie, 1994), and Spain 1964 to 1988 (Valdes, 1993). In contrast Chetwynd, Coope, Brodie, and Wells (1988) found a significant relationship between advertising and cigarette consumption in New Zealand from 1973 to 1985, a result that generated considerable comment but nonetheless appeared to bear up under reanalysis (see Boddewyn, 1989; Chetwynd, Brodie, & Harrison, 1989; Harrison, Chetwynd, & Brodie, 1989; Jackson & Ekelund, 1989; Joossens, 1989; Warner, 1990).

Literature reviews, meanwhile, present mixed conclusions about advertising effects. Simonich (1993) stated that 14 studies in the econometric literature found relations between advertising and cigarette consumption as opposed to 10 that did not. Advertising elasticities of demand for cigarettes were reported to range from .07 to .58 with an average elasticity of .21 (Raftery, 1989). The average elasticity suggests that a 10% increase in advertising would be associated with a 2.1% rise in cigarette consumption, double the usual elasticities reported for advertising and alcohol demand.

Cigarette consumption presents special problems that make the estimation of advertising effects difficult, moreover. In a critique of the field, Godfrey (1989) noted the need for double hurdle models, ones that take into account the probability of smoking first and then the effect of advertising on demand, as well as ones that take account of the habituating and addictive properties of the substance. The U.S. experience is also clouded by major media events, such as the Surgeon General's Report, policy changes like the broadcast advertising ban, and counteradvertising efforts, all of which, despite the efforts of investigators to control them, conspire to make the estimation of advertising effects difficult.

The notion that advertising and counteradvertising interact is supported by two studies that noted an evolution of advertising effects across time. A meta-analysis conducted by Andrews and Franke (1991) found that advertising elasticities were positive, .14, prior to 1970 and effectively zero thereafter. Seldon and Doroodian (1989) observed a steady decline in the magnitude of advertising elasticies in the U.S. from 1952 through 1984; elasticities declined from .25 to .09 over the period. Interestingly, the authors also presented evidence suggesting that health warnings reduced consumption and the industry responded by increasing advertising. Combined with previously cited content analyses this finding indicates that cigarette manufacturers combat health warnings with both the quantity and the content of advertising.

Historical analyses of advertising effects have identified relationships between the uptake of smoking and marketing campaigns for specific brands in the U.S. from 1890 to 1977 (Pierce & Gilpin, 1995) and for adolescent females from 1944 to 1988 (Pierce, Lee, & Gilpin, 1994). Smoking initiation rates by young males or females were found to increase if the group was targeted, while remaining the same for the nontargeted sex. These findings seem to confirm Godfrey's (1989) warning about using aggregate measures of consumption to estimate advertising elasticities, since advertising effects might be differential depending on age or sex. And indeed, these studies and a host of others suggest adolescents at the point of initiation may be especially susceptible to advertising.

Much of the belief in differential effects of advertising on young people are based on a body of research that shows strong associations between smoking involvement and awareness and appreciation of cigarette advertising. This literature is voluminous, and on the surface provides a strong prima facie case for advertising effects. Without attempting an exhaustive treatment of this literature, some of the major substantive findings are as follows: Smokers are twice as likely to correctly identify edited ads and slogans than are nonsmokers (Chapman & Fitzgerald, 1982); children as young as 12 apprehend the complex imagery in ads and hence perceive them much like adults do (Aitken, Leathar, & O'Hazan, 1985); smokers are more aware of ads and more knowledgeable about the brand imagery it contains (Aitken, Leathar, O'Hazan, & Squair, 1987); there is a nearly linear "dose–response" relationship between smoking and advertising recognition (Goldstein, Fischer, Richards, & Creten, 1987); smokers appreciate ads more and thus ads reinforce smoking (Aitken & Eadie, 1990); humorous ads appeal more to adolescents than adults (Hastings, Ryan, Teer, & MacKintosh, 1994); cartoon characters, namely Old Joe Camel, are much better at communicating with children than adults (Di Franza et al., 1991); susceptible nonsmokers like advertising more than do nonsusceptible nonsmokers (Unger, Johnson, & Rohrbach, 1995); receptivity to cigarette advertising is associated with susceptibility to smoking (Evans et al., 1995); and perhaps the most devastating conclusion of all, "by the age of 6 years, Old Joe [Camel] is as well recognized as Mickey Mouse" (Fischer, Schwartz, Richards, Goldstein, & Rojas, 1991).

From these data the authors conclude advertising affects young people and is a contributing factor to the onset of smoking. Although manufacturers may not intend to target children, advertising does influence their knowledge and attitudes. A recent report of the Surgeon General, *Preventing Tobacco Use Among Young People*, offered this summary of the evidence of a relation between advertising awareness, recognition, and appreciation and smoking:

> A substantial and growing body of scientific literature has been reported on young people's awareness of, and attitudes about, cigarette advertising and promotional activities. Considered together, these studies offer a compelling argument for the mediated relationship of cigarette advertising and adolescent smoking. (U.S. Department of Health and Human Services, 1994, p. 188)

The Surgeon General's Report outlined other potentially pejorative effects of advertising on adolescents, such as appealing to character traits that are associated with smoking uptake or giving a sense that smoking is more prevalent than it is and therefore normative.

The method used to draw these conclusions—survey analysis—provides room for alternative interpretations of the findings. As noted before with alcohol, smoking or intentions to smoke may increase awareness of advertising rather than advertising contributing to the uptake of smoking. And given that some of these investigators (notably Aitken and his colleagues) have made the same claims about advertising and alcohol use using the same methodology, the findings of Connolly et al.'s longitudinal study that showed few such relationships is perhaps sobering.

But here again, there are significant differences in the alcohol and tobacco literature. Botvin, Goldberg, Botvin, and Dusenburg (1993) found a significant relationship between advertising exposure and future intentions to smoke. Advertising accounting for 3.2% of the variability in smoking. Klitzner, Gruenewald, and Bamberger (1991) found evidence that both a selective exposure effect, those who had experimented with smoking were more apt to attend to ads, and effects attributable to exposure to cigarette advertising were operative. Additionally, two longitudinal studies indicate approval of advertising is associated with later smoking (Dobson, Woodward, & Leeder, 1992) and awareness of ads is associated with positive changes in intentions to smoke while lack of appreciation of ads is associated with negative changes in smoking intentions (Aitken, Eadie, Hastings, & Haywood, 1991). The last study should be interpreted cautiously given how few children changed intentions positively or negatively.

In sum, the literature indicates that advertising does influence smoking. While the effect of advertising on aggregate demand for cigarettes may be suspect, especially in recent years, elasticities are positive, often significant and on average twice the size of those reported for alcohol. A much clearer picture emerges when the adoption of smoking is considered. Historically, targeted marketing campaigns are associated with elevated and differential uptake rates among the target audience. Strong and persistent relationships between various measures of ad awareness, recognition, and appreciation smoking or intentions to smoke have been noted and in at least two cases these relationships appear to be predictive of uptake at later times. Lastly, it is worth noting again the burden of proof needed to conclude consequential advertising effects exist for tobacco are much less stringent than for alcohol. Even if the standard were not lower, the effects are stronger.

CONSUMPTIVE COMMUNICATION— COUNTERADVERTISING

The odds of encountering counteradvertising in the media, warning labels notwithstanding, are remote. On television, if advertisements for alcohol products are infrequent compared with nonconsumptive depictions, counteradvertisements are even scarcer still. Some estimates place the ratio of alcohol ads to antidrinking messages as high as 20 to 1. Antidrinking ads also tend to be shorter and appear in less favorable time slots than do alcohol ads. Counteradvertising, or as it is popularly known public service advertising, has all the earmarks of an uncoordinated and underfunded effort, the results of which are bound to reflect its comparative presence and placement.

The only consistent counteradvertising in public view are warning labels carried on packages and advertisings for alcohol and tobacco products. Despite the ubiquity of these messages, there is scant evidence to suggest they alter behavior. In the alcohol field, research indicates warning labels have no affect on consumers' alcohol risk ratings (Mayer, Smith, & Scammon, 1991; Scammon, Mayer, & Smith, 1991). Repeated exposure to warnings on beer advertisements was shown however to influence beliefs about benefits communicated in advertising (Slater & Domenich, 1995). Another study (MacKinnon, Pentz, & Stacy, 1993) reported an increase in awareness and memory of the labels but no change in use or beliefs about the risks associated with drinking a year after the alcohol labeling law went into effect.

There is some evidence that warning labels may have a polarizing effect among viewers, such that nondrinkers expressed less intention to drink after exposure while drinkers increased their intentions to drink (Bozinoff, Roth, & May, 1989). The polarizing effect was exacerbated if the warning label contained a high threat message with heavy drinkers seeming to consume in defiance of the warning (Bensley & Wu, 1991). It would appear then that warning labels have something of a paradoxical effect, actually strengthening the behavior among those susceptible to the problem.

In the tobacco arena, there is growing recognition that warning labels, although required since 1966, have done little to alter consumption patterns. Messages fatigue quickly and lose the little effectiveness they may have enjoyed at the outset. Rotating messages does not seem to ameliorate the problem. A fascinating study using eye tracking to observe how consumers read ads in practice determined that warnings were viewed only 8% of the time, 43.6% of those exposed never read the warning, and recognition of warning after exposure was not much better than chance (Fischer, Richards, Berman, & Krugman, 1989). It has even been suggested that advertisers construct commercials to draw attention away from warnings and thereby diminish their effectiveness.

If lack of effectiveness were not enough, warning labels proved to be a serendipitous blessing for the tobacco industry. As the Surgeon General's Report *Preventing Tobacco Use Among Young People* pointed out, "no one publicly anticipated that the display of a federally mandated warning would eventually shield tobacco manufacturers from product liability. Ironically, the tobacco industry has thus far been insulated from lawsuits by legislation it has resisted steadfastly since 1965" (U.S. Department of Health and Human Services, 1994, p. 261). Warning labels offer a humbling lesson that the best intended social legislation often goes awry.

But if the evidence suggests warning labels are ineffective, the reverse is true for mass media counteradvertising. The best illustration of the impact of counteradvertising, and its relative effectiveness versus advertising, was the media environment regarding smoking that existed in the 1960s. Part of this environment consisted of major medical announcements such as reports linking smoking and lung cancer or the first Surgeon General's Report and the attendant publicity. A more systematic and concerted effort was the antismoking ads that appeared as a result of the Federal Communications Commission Fairness Doctrine ruling. Warner (1977, 1981) estimated that the Surgeon General's Report alone cut cigarette consumption by 5%, while antismoking ads cut consumption 4% per year. All types of counteradvertising combined accounted for a 36.4% drop in per capita consumption.

Antismoking ads were effective despite being at a 3 to 1 disadvantage compared with product advertising. Estimates suggest that counteradvertising was 15 times more effective at preventing smoking than advertising was at promoting it. Given the one-third ratio of antismoking ads to product ads mandated by the Fairness Doctrine ruling, it has been calculated that the net effect of the media environment at the time was 5 to 1 for antismoking. It has even been suggested that cigarette manufacturers acquiesced to the broadcast advertising ban in recognition of the efficacy of counteradvertising efforts and as an opportunity to get antismoking ads off the air.

Indeed, the broadcast advertising ban proved to be a boon for the industry and another example of the social legislation producing contraintended results. Manufacturers saved enormous sums once designated for broadcast advertising and still had a variety of media options available. Not surprisingly, cigarette consumption rose immediately after the advertising ban, illustrating ex post facto the efficacy of antismoking ads as a demand depressant. Counteradvertising efforts were so effective a Health, Education and Welfare task force considered rescinding the advertising ban so the Fairness Doctrine could be reinstated and antismoking ads run again (Warner, 1979).

The antismoking campaign in the late 1960s was a pure example of counteradvertising, where an emphasis on the life-threatening consequences of use were used to curtail consumption. Images of well-known actors, terminally ill with lung cancer, giving impassioned appeals against smoking haunt the memory decades later. If anything, antismoking campaigns in recent years have eschewed a hardline health message, in favor of negative social consequences (e.g., bad breath, smelly clothes, or smoking is out of fashion), this despite recent evidence that health fear appeals are effective motivators (Quinn, Meenaghan, & Brannick, 1992).

Passage of Proposition 99 in California offered a recent experience with which to judge the efficacy of counteradvertising. Proposition 99 called for an increase in cigarette taxes from 10¢ to 35¢ a pack. Twenty percent of the incremental revenue collected was designated for use in antismoking education programs including mass media. Twenty-six million dollars was spent on the resulting multimedia campaign. A subsequent time series analysis of sales data (Hu, Sung, & Keeler, 1995a, 1995b) indicated both taxes and counteradvertising were effective in cutting sales, the former four times more effective in this regard. The elasticity for counteradvertising was estimated to be −.05, suggesting that a 10% increase in antismoking ads would decrease consumption by 0.5%, a statistically significant amount.

Counteradvertising, especially efforts directed at youth, are not without detractors, even among the staunchest antismoking activists. It has been argued, for example, that counteradvertising in California was effective in getting adults to quit but not in preventing adolescents from starting. Further, the emphasis on adolescent smoking diverts attention from other efforts. And finally, counteradvertising may have paradoxical effects among adolescents, the antismoking message being attractive to rebellious teens and thus providing an impetus to start smoking. Whatever the eventual policy outcome of this debate might be, the fact remains the Fairness Doctrine ruling and Proposition 99 demonstrated clearly counteradvertising, when deployed extensively and comprehensively, can decrease consumption of cigarettes.

ACKNOWLEDGMENTS

The author thanks Dr. Georges Bordage, Elizabeth Warstadt, Javeed Ismail, and Susan Warstadt for their help in the preparation of this chapter.

REFERENCES

Aitken, P., & Eadie, D. (1990). Reinforcing effects of cigarette advertising on under-age smoking. *British Journal of Addiction, 85,* 399–412.

Aitken, P., Eadie, D., Hastings, G., & Haywood, A. (1991). Predisposing effects of cigarette advertising on children's intentions to smoke when older. *British Journal of Addiction, 86,* 383–390.

Aitken, P., Leathar, D., & O'Hazan, F. (1985). Children's perceptions of advertisements for cigarettes. *Social Science & Medicine, 21,* 785–797.

Aitken, P., Leathar, D., O'Hazan, F., & Squair, S. (1987). Children's awareness of cigarette advertisements and brand imagery. *British Journal of Addiction, 82,* 615–622.

Altman, D., Slater, M., Albright, C., & Maccoby, N. (1987). How an unhealthy product is sold: Cigarette advertising in magazines, 1960–1985. *Journal of Communication, 37,* 95–106.

Ammerman, S., & Nolden, M. (1995). Neighborhood-based tobacco advertising targeting adolescents. *The Western Journal of Medicine, 162,* 514–518.

Andrews, R., & Franke, G. (1991). The determinants of cigarette consumption: A meta-analysis. *Journal of Public Policy & Marketing, 10*, 81–100.

Bandura, A. (1965). Influence of models' reinforcement contingencies on the acquisition of imitative responses. *Journal of Personality and Social Psychology, 1*, 589–595.

Bandura, A. (1977). *Social learning theory.* Englewood Cliffs, NJ: Prentice-Hall.

Bandura, A., Ross, D., & Ross, S. (1963). Imitation of film mediated aggressive models. *Journal of Abnormal and Social Psychology, 66*, 3–11.

Beckley, R., & Chalfant, H. (1979). Contrasting images of alcohol and drug use in country and rock music. *Journal of Alcohol and Drug Education, 25*, 44–51.

Bensley, L., & Wu, R. (1991). The role of psychological reactance in drinking following alcohol prevention messages. *Journal of Applied Social Psychology, 21*, 1111–1124.

Blum, A. (1991). The Marlboro Grand Prix: Circumvention of the television ban on tobacco advertising. *New England Journal of Medicine, 324*, 913–917.

Boddewyn, J. (1989). There is no convincing evidence for a relationship between cigarette advertising and consumption. *British Journal of Addiction, 84*, 1255–1261.

Botvin, G., Goldberg, C., Botvin, E., & Dusenburg, L. (1993). Smoking behavior of adolescents exposed to cigarette advertising. *Public Health Reports, 108*, 217–224.

Bozinoff, L., Roth, V., & May, C. (1989). Stages of involvement with drugs and alcohol: Analysis of effects of drug and alcohol abuse advertising. *Advances in Consumer Research, 16*, 215–220.

Breed, W., & De Foe, J. (1978). Bringing alcohol into the open. *Columbia Journalism Review, 17*, 18–19.

Cafiso, J., Goodstadt, M., Garlington, W., & Sheppard, M. (1982). Television portrayal of alcohol and other beverages. *Journal of Studies on Alcohol, 43*, 1232–1243.

Cardador, M., Hazan, A., & Glantz, S. (1995). Tobacco industry smokers' rights publication: A content analysis. *American Journal of Public Health, 85*, 1212–1217.

Chapman, S., & Fitzgerald, B. (1982). Brand preferences and advertising recall in adolescent smokers: Some implications for health prevention. *American Journal of Public Health, 72*, 491–494.

Chetwynd, F., Brodie, R., & Harrison, R. (1989). The influence of advertising on tobacco consumption: A reply to Boddewyn. *British Journal of Addiction, 84*, 1263–1265.

Chetwynd, F., Coope, P., Brodie, R., & Wells, E. (1988). Impact of cigarette advertising on aggregate demand for cigarettes in New Zealand. *British Journal of Addiction, 83*, 409–414.

Chirco, A. (1990). *An examination of stepwise regression models of adolescent alcohol and marijuana use with special attention to the television exposure—teen drinking issue.* Unpublished doctoral dissertation, Syracuse University, Syracuse, NY.

Cohen, J. (1989). Counting advertising assertions to assess regulatory policy: When it doesn't add up. *Journal of Public Policy & Marketing, 8*, 24–29.

Cohen, J. (1992). Research and policy issues in Ringold's and Calfee's treatment of cigarette health claims. *Journal of Public Policy & Marketing, 11*, 82–86.

Connolly, G., Casswell, S., Zhang, J., & Silva, P. (1994). Alcohol in the mass media and drinking by adolescents: A longitudinal study. *Addiction, 89*, 1255–1263.

Connors, G., & Alpher, V. (1989). Alcohol themes within country-western songs. *International Journal of Addiction, 24*, 445–451.

Cruz, J., & Wallack, L. (1986). Trends in tobacco use on television. *American Journal of Public Health, 76*, 689–699.

De Foe, J., Breed, W., & Breed, L. (1983). Drinking on television: A five-year study. *Journal of Drug Education, 13*, 25–38.

Diener, B. (1993). The frequency and content of alcohol and tobacco cues In daytime soap opera programs: Fall 1986 and Fall 1991. *Journal of Public Policy & Marketing, 12*, 252–257.

Di Franza, J., Richards, J., Paulman, P., Wolf-Gillespie, N., Fletcher, C., Jaffe, R., & Murray, D. (1991). RJR Nabisco's cartoon camel promotes Camel cigarettes to children. *Journal of the American Medical Association, 266*, 3149–3153.

Digby, J., & Digby, J. (Eds.). (1988). *Inspired by drink: An anthology*. New York: Morrow.

Dobson, A., Woodward, S., & Leeder, S. (1992). Tobacco smoking in response to cigarette advertising. *The Medical Journal of Australia, 156*, 815–816.

Evans, N., Farkas, A., Gilpin, E., Berry, C., & Pierce, J. (1995). Influence of tobacco marketing and exposure to smokers on adolescent susceptibility to smoking. *Journal of National Cancer Institute, 87*, 1538–1545.

Fernandez-Collado, C., & Greenberg, B., with Korzenny, F., & Atkin, C. (1978). Sexual intimacy and drug use in TV series. *Journal of Communications, 28*, 30–37.

Fischer, P., Richards, J., Berman, E., & Krugman, D. (1989). Recall and eye tracking study of adolescents viewing tobacco advertisements. *Journal of the American Medical Association, 261*, 84–89.

Fischer, P., Schwartz, M., Richards, J., Goldstein, A., & Rojas, T. (1991). Brand logo recognition by children aged 3 to 6 years. *Journal of the American Medical Association, 266*, 3145–3148.

Fisher, J. (1993). *Advertising, alcohol consumption, and abuse: A worldwide survey*. Westport, CT: Greenwood.

Fisher, J., & Cook, P. (1995). *Advertising, alcohol consumption, and mortality: An empirical investigation*. Westport, CT: Greenwood.

Franke, G. (1994). U.S. cigarette demand, 1961–1990: Econometric issues, evidence and implications. *Journal of Business Research, 30*, 33–41.

Futch, E., Lesman, S., & Geller, M. (1984). An analysis of alcohol portrayals on prime-time television. *The International Journal of the Addictions, 19*, 403–410.

Gerbner, G., & Gross, L. (1976). Living with television: The violence profile. *Journal of Communications, 26*, 172–199.

Gerbner, G., Gross, L., Morgan, M., & Signorielli, N. (1980). The "mainstreaming" of America: Violence profile no. 11. *Journal of Communications, 30*, 10–29.

Gerbner, G., Gross, L., Morgan, M., & Signorielli, N. (1981). Health and medicine on television. *New England Journal of Medicine, 305*, 901–904.

Gerbner, G., Morgan, M., & Signorielli, N. (1982). Programming health portrayals: What viewers see, say and do. In D. Pearl, L. Bouthilet, & J. Lazar (Eds.), *Television and behavior: Ten years of scientific progress and implications for the eighties* (Vol. 2, pp. 291–307). Washington, DC: U.S. Government Printing Office.

Godfrey, C. (1989). Factors influencing the consumption of alcohol and tobacco: The use and abuse of economic models. *British Journal of Addiction, 84*, 1123–1138.

Goldstein, A., Fischer, P., Richards, J., & Creten, D. (1987). Relationship between high school student smoking and recognition of cigarette advertisements. *Journal of Pediatrics, 110*, 488–491.

Greenberg, B. (1981). Smoking, drugging and drinking in top rated TV series. *Journal of Drug Education, 11*, 227–234.

Greenberg, B., Fernandez-Collado, C., Graef, D., Korzenny, F., & Atkin, C. (1979). Trends in use of alcohol and other substances on television. *Journal of Drug Education, 9*, 243–253.

Grube, J., & Wallack, L. (1994). Television beer advertising and drinking knowledge, beliefs and intentions among schoolchildren. *American Journal of Public Health, 84*, 254–259.

Hansen, A. (1986). The portrayal of alcohol on television. *Health Education Journal, 45*, 127–131.

Harrison, R., Chetwynd, J., & Brodie, R. (1989). The influence of advertising on tobacco consumption: A reply to Jackson & Ekelund. *British Journal of Addiction, 84*, 1251–1254.

Hastings, G., Ryan, H., Teer, P., & MacKintosh, A. (1994). Cigarette advertising and children's smoking: Why Reg was withdrawn. *British Medical Journal, 309*, 933–937.

Hazan, A., & Glantz, S. (1995). Current trends in tobacco use on prime-time fictional television. *American Journal of Public Health, 85*, 116–117.

Heilbronn, L. (1988). What does alcohol mean? Alcohol's use as a symbolic code. *Contemporary Drug Problems, 16*, 229–248.

Herd, D. (1983). Images of drinking: distortion or re-creation? In M. Grant & B. Ritson (Eds.), *Alcohol, the prevention debate* (pp. 97–104). London: Croom Helm.

Herd, D. (1986). Ideology, melodrama and the changing role of alcohol problems in American films. *Contemporary Drug Problems, 13,* 213–247.

Herd, D., & Room, R. (1982). Alcohol images in American film 1909–1960. *Drinking and Drug Practices Surveyor, 18,* 24–35.

Hu, T., Sung, H., & Keeler, T. (1995a). Reducing cigarette consumption in California: Tobacco taxes vs. an anti-smoking campaign. *American Journal of Public Health, 85,* 1218–1222.

Hu, T., Sung, H., & Keeler, T. (1995b). The state antismoking campaign and the industry response: The effects of advertising on cigarette consumption in California. *American Economic Review, 85,* 85–90.

Jackson, J., & Ekelund, R. (1989). The influence of advertising on tobacco consumption: Some problems with Chetwynd et al.'s analysis. *British Journal of Addiction, 84,* 1247–1250.

Joossens, L. (1989). The influence of advertising on tobacco consumption: Comments on Boddewyn & Chapman. *British Journal of Addiction, 84,* 1279–1281.

Klitzner, M., Gruenewald, P., & Bamberger, E. (1991). Cigarette advertising and adolescent experimentation with smoking. *British Journal of Addiction, 86,* 287–298.

Lipsitz, A., Blake, G., Vincent, E., & Winters, M. (1993). Another round for the brewers: Television ads and children's alcohol expectancies. *Journal of Applied Social Psychology, 23,* 439–450.

Lowery, S. (1980). Soap and booze in the afternoon: An analysis of the portrayals of alcohol use in daytime serials. *Journal of Studies on Alcohol, 41,* 829–838.

MacDonald, P. (1983). The "dope" on soaps. *Journal of Drug Education, 13,* 359–369.

MacDonald, P., & Estep, R. (1985). Prime time drug depictions. *Contemporary Drug Problems, 12,* 419–438.

MacKinnon, D., Pentz, M., & Stacy, A. (1993). The alcohol warning label and adolescents: The first year. *American Journal of Public Health, 83,* 585–587.

Madden, P., & Grube, J. (1994). The frequency and nature of alcohol and tobacco advertising in televised sports, 1990 through 1992. *American Journal of Public Health, 84,* 297–299.

Mayer, R., Smith, K., & Scammon, D. (1991). Evaluating the impact of alcohol warning labels. *Advances in Consumer Research, 18,* 706–714.

McEwen, W., & Hanneman, G. (1974). The depiction of drug use in television programming. *Journal of Drug Education, 4,* 281–243.

Minkler, M., Wallack, M., & Madden, P. (1987). Alcohol and cigarette advertising in Ms. Magazine. *Journal of Public Health Policy, 8,* 164–179.

Montagne, M. (1988). The influence of literary and philosophical accounts on drug taking. *Journal of Drug Issues, 18,* 229–244.

Noelke, G. (1986). Alcoholism in The Brothers Karamazov. *Counselor, 4,* 4–5, 14, 24–29.

Pierce, J., & Gilpin, E. (1995). A historical analysis of tobacco marketing and the uptake of smoking by youth in the United States: 1890–1977. *Health Psychology, 14,* 500–508.

Pierce, J., Lee, L., & Gilpin, E. (1994). Smoking initiation by adolescent girls, 1944 through 1988. *Journal of the American Medical Association, 271,* 608–611.

Pollay, R. (1989). Filters, flavors . . . flim-flam, too! On "health information" and policy implications in cigarette advertising. *Journal of Public Policy & Marketing, 8,* 30–39.

Quinn, V., Meenaghan, T., & Brannick, T. (1992). Fear appeals: Segmentation is the way to go. *International Journal of Advertising, 11,* 355–366.

Raftery, J. (1989). Advertising and smoking—a smoldering debate? *British Journal of Addiction, 84,* 1241–1246.

Reekie, W. (1994). Consumer's surplus and the demand for cigarettes. *Managerial and Decision Economics, 15,* 223–234.

Ringold, D., & Calfee, J. (1989). The informational content of cigarette advertising: 1926–1986. *Journal of Public Policy & Marketing, 8,* 1–23.

Ringold, D., & Calfee, J. (1990). What can we learn from the informational content of cigarette advertising: A reply and further analysis. *Journal of Public Policy & Marketing, 9*, 30–41.

Room, R. (1987). Alcoholism and alcoholics in U.S. films, 1945–1962: The party ends for the "Wet Generation." In P. Paakkanen & P. Sulkunen (Eds.), *Cultural studies on drinking problems: Report on a conference* (pp. 147–150). Helsinki: Social Research Institute of Alcohol Studies.

Room, R. (1988). The movies and the wettening of America: The media as amplifiers of cultural change. *British Journal of Addiction, 11*, 11–18.

Scammon, D., Mayer, R., & Smith, K. (1991). Alcohol warnings: How do you know when you have had one too many? *Journal of Public Policy & Marketing, 10*, 214–228.

Seldon, B., & Doroodian, K. (1989). A simultaneous model of cigarette advertising: Effects on demand and industry response to public policy. *The Review of Economics and Statistics, 71*, 673–677.

Signorielli, N. (1987). Drinking, sex and violence on television: The cultural indicators perspective. *Journal of Drug Education, 17*, 245–260.

Simonich, W. (1993). Banning tobacco advertising: Boon to industry? *Journal of the American Medical Association, 270*, 321–322.

Slater, M., & Domenich, M. (1995). Alcohol warnings in TV beer advertisements. *Journal of Studies on Alcohol, 56*, 361–367.

Sobell, L., Sobell, M., Riley, D., Klajner, F., Leo, G., Pavan D., & Cancilla, A. (1986). Effect of television programming and advertising on alcohol consumption in normal drinkers. *Journal of Studies on Alcohol, 47*, 333–340.

Sobell, L., Sobell, M., Toneatto, T., & Leo, G. (1993). Severely dependent alcohol abuses may be vulnerable to alcohol cues on television programs. *Journal of Studies on Alcohol, 54*, 85–91.

Tucker, L. (1985). Television's role regarding alcohol use among teenagers. *Adolescence, 20*, 593–598.

Unger, J., Johnson, C., & Rohrbach, L. (1995). Recognition and liking of tobacco and alcohol advertisements among adolescents: Relationships with susceptibility to substance abuse. *Preventive Medicine, 24*, 461–466.

U.S. Department of Health and Human Services. (1994). *Preventing tobacco use among young people: A report of the Surgeon General*. Atlanta: U.S. Department of Health and Human Services, Public Health Service, Centers for Disease Control and Prevention, National Center for Chronic Disease Prevention and Health Promotion, Office of Smoking and Health.

Valdes, B. (1993). Cigarette consumption in Spain: Empirical evidence and implications for health policy. *Applied Economics, 25*, 149–156.

Wallack, L., Breed, W., & Cruz, J. (1987). Alcohol on prime-time television. *Journal of Studies on Alcohol, 48*, 33–38.

Warner, K. (1977). The effects of the anti-smoking campaign on cigarette consumption. *American Journal of Public Health, 67*, 645–650.

Warner, K. (1979). Clearing the airwaves: The cigarette ad ban revisited. *Policy Analysis, 50*, 435–450.

Warner, K. (1981). Cigarette smoking in the 1970's: The impact of the anti-smoking campaign on consumption. *Science, 211*, 729–781.

Warner, K. (1985a). Cigarette advertising and media coverage of smoking and health. *New England Journal of Medicine, 312*, 384–388.

Warner, K. (1985b). Tobacco industry response to public health concern: A content analysis of cigarette ads. *Health Education Quarterly, 12*, 115–127.

Warner, K. (1990). Effects of cigarette advertising: Reply to Boddewyn. *British Journal of Addiction, 85*, 687–688.

Warner, K., & Goldenhar, L. (1989). The cigarette advertising broadcast ban and magazine coverage of smoking and health. *Journal of Public Health Policy, 10*, 32–42.

Warner, K., Goldenhar, L., & McLaughlin, C. (1992). Cigarette advertising and magazine coverage of the hazards of smoking: A statistical analysis. *New England Journal of Medicine, 326*, 305–309.

Waxer, P. (1992). Alcohol consumption in television programming in three English-speaking cultures. *Alcohol & Alcoholism, 27,* 195–200.

Wilcox, G., & Vacker, B. (1992). Cigarette advertising and consumption in the United States: 1961–1990. *International Journal of Advertising, 11,* 269–278.

Wilcox, G., Tharp, M., & Yang, K. (1994). Cigarette advertising and consumption in South Korea, 1988–1992. *International Journal of Advertising, 13,* 333–346.

Community Responses

Harold D. Holder
Prevention Research Center
Berkeley, California

The community is the new frontier for prevention of substance abuse problems. Previously, the national and state levels were the primary locations of efforts to reduce substance abuse. New prevention initiatives at the community level suggest that effective strategies will often be quite different from national or state policies, and they will require a different perspective.

Substance abuse is part of routine community life and must be considered in the context of the community, which is a dynamic and self-adapting system. To develop effective community-level interventions, prevention planners and policymakers must understand how various aspects of the community influence substance use and abuse, thereby contributing to alcohol and drug problems.

Substance abuse prevention interventions are actions, activities, efforts, or policies intended to reduce the future occurrence of substance abuse problems. The effects of interventions on alcohol and other drug-involved problems rarely are direct. Prevention interventions most often affect intermediate variables, which in turn affect the problem directly.

Most substance abuse prevention efforts organized at the local level fail to take into account the dynamic systems in which substance abuse problems exist. For this reason, most local prevention programs fail to affect substance abuse problems and have no effect or only a short-term effect (see Holder & Howard, 1992, concerning alcohol problems and Amsel, 1990, and Battjes, Leukefeld, & Amsel, 1990, on community approaches to intravenous drug use prevention).

This chapter presents a systems perspective on the community, a perspective that requires changes in community structure for effective long-term prevention. It reviews the new science of complexity, differentiates between catchment and a systems approach to prevention, describes a public health model within a systems approach, reviews local policy as a means to produce system changes, and reviews recent findings from one community-based prevention effort that employed a systems approach.

The use and abuse of alcohol and other drugs cannot be considered as isolated phenomena, independent of other forces acting on and within any community. A basic premise of a systems approach to alcohol and other drug-involved problems is that prevention strategies are most effective when focused on the community at large, rather than on specific individuals at risk.

COMPLEXITY, CHAOS, AND ADAPTIVE SYSTEMS

As scientific knowledge about substance abuse problems has accumulated, prevention researchers and policymakers have become increasingly aware that such problems depend upon simultaneous interactions of many factors. Many elements of the community system influence the use of alcohol and other drugs. Some aspects of substance abuse problems and processes may be understood in isolation, but knowledge of the larger picture is limited.

Western science has developed on the premise that the universe is governed by knowable "laws" that humans can discover by a process of reduction. The search for the basic building blocks of existence has been the foundation for much of biomedical and behavioral science in the study of addictions. As a result, the scientific base for much of substance abuse problem prevention also rests on a reductionist perspective. The site of the problem is believed to be the individual drinker who, as the result of specific factors that can be separately isolated and studied, consumes alcohol or other drugs in large quantities, sometimes in a compulsive and dependent fashion. A corollary to this premise is that the goal of prevention is to identify, sufficiently early, those individuals who drink in this fashion to prevent a natural progression to more and more destructive behavior.

Prevention practitioners are limited by the traditions of alcoholism and other drug treatment in which problems result from high-risk or developmentally inadequate (deviant) individuals. Thus, alcohol problems are caused by "flawed" people: alcoholics, addicts, dependent persons, poor people, those from broken families, incompletely socialized individuals, and psychologically damaged or genetically disadvantaged persons.

However, modern science has begun to incorporate the concept of "chaos," which is defined in physics as the result of starting two identical systems at the same time but observing different outcomes. In short, the results are not predetermined. This means that the mechanistic view of the natural world is being challenged, and we are confronted with the painful limitations of a mechanistic perspective on health problems in general, and substance abuse problems in particular.

Instead of continuing along deterministic, lawful paths, natural phenomena (including social and economic systems) may diverge from predicted or known pathways and transform into entirely new combinations or relationships. This adaptive complexity, written about in popular form by Waldrup (1992), is a new paradigm for physics, biology, economics, and other disciplines. The paradigm recognizes the adaptive, transformational, and unpredictable nature of complex systems.

This interest in unpredictability has given rise to a renewed interest in complex adaptive systems. A complex adaptive system is able to change specification, evolve, and transform itself into a new arrangement over time (Casti, 1992; Holland, 1975; Kauffman, 1991, 1992, 1995; Stonier & Yu, 1994). Adaptation refers to the ability or inherent nature of a system to accommodate unpredictable changes or disturbances, whether arising from within the system or from the external environment of the system. Clearly, adaptation is a fundamental attribute of all living organisms as well as an attribute of the social structures in which human beings live. It is the position of this author that the community in which substance use and abuse occurs is a complex adaptive system.

CATCHMENT AND SYSTEMS PERSPECTIVES ON ALCOHOL AND OTHER DRUGS IN THE COMMUNITY

Health problem prevention has commonly employed approaches that focus on individuals at risk. Such approaches are based on a "catchment area" perspective, in which a "community" is viewed as a collection of target groups with adverse behaviors or associated risks. Prevention is intended to reduce or eliminate these behaviors by finding the individuals at risk, then educating or serving them in an appropriate manner to reduce the identified individual risk.

Community-based approaches to substance abuse problem prevention are increasingly popular throughout the world. A community is often viewed simply as a set or collection of persons with adverse behaviors or associated risks with respect to substance abuse that the prevention is intended to reduce or eliminate. This catchment area perspective uses a straightforward model: find the persons at risk, or identify the risk factors that individuals may possess, then educate, treat, or serve them to reduce the individual risk to each person so identified. An example from community health illustrates this approach: If reduction of rates of breast cancer among, say, Latino women is the prevention goal, then encouraging regular breast examinations of all women living within one or more neighborhoods with concentrated Latino populations is a reasonable prevention strategy. Targeting the community may mean use of public service announcements in Spanish and English, neighborhood canvassing, and increased local medical resources. No particular changes in the social dynamics and behaviors of the community are proposed except those that make breast examination and mammograms available to the target population and those that change the awareness level of these women and, by implication, the values of all women and men in the catchment area about the protection of women's health.

As a further example, cirrhosis mortality might be an identified problem area in a low-income, transient neighborhood. The city or a local service organization would naturally target this neighborhood and seek to reduce the drinking levels of heavy chronic drinkers by establishing a recovery center. Adolescent use of alcohol and other drugs within a local middle school might also be targeted with strategies aimed at increasing resistance skills against peer pressure to drink in preadolescents, while developing alternative afterschool activities and school-based and family-focused education programs. This model would not affect community members not directly involved with the targeted at-risk populations.

Prevention planners using the catchment area approach select strategies that alter individual decisions and behavior or that provide direct services to individuals. Education-based activities, with social, physical, and economic reinforcement are favored, as are early identification and intervention with individual heavy, high-risk drinkers. Prevention efforts often include mass media announcements, focus groups, targeted communication, health promotion, health awareness, and physician education efforts. One-on-one and group treatment and counseling are also potential components. Most previous heart disease and cancer community prevention trials have employed some form of a catchment area approach. The targets of these trials have been well-defined states or conditions with which individual residents of a community can be accurately associated. For example, if heavy smoking is the target, then heavy smokers can be identified so that education programs for smoking reduction and cessation can be directed at them. Community heart disease projects make effective use of the link between diet, exercise, smoking, and genetics to assist individuals who are at risk from one or more of these factors in adjusting or moderating their behaviors.

The catchment area perspective has clear limitations in substance abuse problem prevention. Although it is true that heavy dependent users have the greatest individual risk rates for most alcohol problems, they are not collectively the largest at-risk group. Their absolute numbers are so small that they contribute only modestly to most aggregate problems. For example, infrequent and moderate users of alcohol, who are not currently nor likely ever to be dependent on alcohol, account for a greater number of alcohol-involved trauma such as auto crashes, falls, or drownings than do heavy dependent users (Edwards et al., 1994). Young people, in particular, account for a disproportionately large number of alcohol-related problem events, such as traffic crashes and accidental injuries. Most heavy addicted drinkers continue their drinking pattern throughout their lives and never incur an alcohol-involved traffic crash or encounter with the police. On the other hand, an 18-year-old with limited driving and drinking experience may cause a serious auto crash with only a small amount of alcohol in the blood system. Physical and cognitive impairment begins as soon as the body begins to metabolize ethanol. Impairment increases as more ethanol enters the blood, and the individual can become increasingly impaired over time as drinking continues. The rate of impairment is a function of such factors as alcohol experience and tolerance, body weight, amount of food consumed while drinking, and rate of alcohol intake.

A community systems approach to health problem prevention has been used less commonly, perhaps because the systems perspective is conceptually more complex than the catchment-area perspective. In this perspective, a "community" is viewed as a set of persons engaged in shared social, cultural, political, and economic processes. Prevention is intended to modify the system in an appropriate manner to reduce health problems identified in the community.

Within this systems perspective, substance abuse problems are outcomes of processes driven and sustained by the community at large. These processes potentially affect all members of the community, but they produce adverse effects more in some groups than in others. This is because individual and environmental factors contribute to disproportionate exposure or increased susceptibility of some groups. Prevention strategies focused on the community at large will be more effective than those focused on specific individuals at risk, because alcohol and other drug-involved problems are produced by the system, and are not simply attributable to a few maladapted individuals. Collective risk will be reduced through appropriate interventions affecting the community processes that influence substance use and abuse.

A community systems approach to prevention differs from approaches based on the catchment-area perspective in these important ways: (1) rather than addressing a single problem behavior or condition, it simultaneously considers a potentially wide-ranging set of problem behaviors; (2) rather than focusing on individuals at risk, it studies the community's entire population in concert; and (3) rather than basing prevention strategies on direct causal linkages, it suggests interventions that affect aspects of the behavioral environment and promote changes in decisions, thereby indirectly helping shift the behavior of the population away from problem-causing contexts.

In summary, the systems perspective on substance abuse problems is based upon the following premises:

- Substance abuse is the destructive or harmful use of alcohol and other drugs in any situation. Thus, substance abuse includes not only drinking by individuals who, because of their social, emotional, or genetic heritage, use alcohol and other drugs compulsively or without control, but also any drinking that potentially endangers the drinker or others.
- Alcohol and other drugs are mood-altering substances, and their inappropriate use entails high risk both to users and to others. Thus, alcohol and other drug use requires special attention on behalf of the public's well-being and safety.
- Misuse of alcohol and other drugs directly or indirectly affects all citizens in the community and is therefore a public health problem.
- Public health problems, by their very nature, are not limited to individuals, but form a part of the social system in which all members of the community live and work.
- Reducing the incidence of substance abuse problems requires intervention not only in individual lives but also in the overall system that produces these problems.

A systems approach to the community has stimulated new prevention strategies to modify system structures, environments, and contexts from which alcohol and other drug problems result. There are many public health and social problems that fit within a community systems perspective. For example, there is little evidence that youthful decisions about criminal behavior and the pursuit of "criminal careers" while still an adolescent are strictly the consequences of individual malfunctioning. Psychological, social, cultural, economic, and physical environmental factors can all play contributing roles in producing the young criminal. Efforts to date toward reducing youthful crime rates through individual-focused counseling and education or through law enforcement and the courts have not proven successful (Whitehead & Lab, 1989).

Aspects of systems strategies have been employed by community public health efforts such as heart disease and cancer prevention trials. For example, projects have persuaded restaurants to offer low-fat menu alternatives, to make low-salt food products available and prominently displayed in grocery stores, to get warning labels installed on the hazards of smoking at points of sale for cigarettes, and to increase the number of nonsmoking areas within public spaces and in the workplace. Some community health trials have employed public policy alternatives that mandate the availability of low-fat food alternatives or increase the retail price of cigarettes or legally restrict their availability by banning cigarette machines.

The community is a dynamic system. The system changes and adapts as new people enter and others leave; as alcoholic beverage marketing and promotion evolve; and as social and economic conditions, including employment and disposable income, change. No single prevention program, no matter how good, can sustain its impact, particularly if system-level changes are not accomplished (Holder & Wallack, 1986; Wallack, 1981). Even if high-risk individuals, such as alcoholics or drug addicts, were identified and somehow magically "fixed," but the system structure remained unchanged, then high-risk replacements naturally would be generated by the system.

THE PUBLIC HEALTH MODEL AND COMMUNITY-BASED PREVENTION

Within a community systems perspective, one can employ a public health model. The model provides a useful typology for characterizing community-based prevention approaches. The three elements of the public health model form an interacting triangle of host (alcohol and drug user), agent (alcohol and other drugs), and environment (drinking and drug use environment or context) (Giesbrecht et al., 1991).

Host approaches have enjoyed the greatest popularity of all community-based prevention. Such approaches are often directed at altering the decision-making behavior of drinkers or drug users (or delaying the initiation of alcohol and other drug use). The rationale for educational strategies directed at the host is that with sufficient information and personal support, better decisions will be made about such use.

Host educational strategies are generally of two types: (1) public educational programs using mass media, printed materials, and verbal information, such as information provided by health workers; and (2) targeted communication directed at a specific group, such as school children, pregnant mothers, and intravenous drug users (Hansen, 1993; Pentz et al., 1989).

Host educational strategies have many desirable attributes. Such strategies can often be used without opposition. They are "non-confrontive" in most cases, unless the information given runs counter to the cultural values and norms of the community (e.g., giving information on condom use as a protection against HIV infection in a primarily Catholic community that opposes condom use, or providing a needle exchange program as a means to reduce risk of HIV infection among intravenous drug users in a community that believes that needle exchange increases drug use).

For the most part, giving information is consistent with worldwide efforts to increase public awareness of health risks and personal preventive actions and decisions. Public educational campaigns have included giving information about the risks of any drug use to increase abstinence and to decrease the risks of heavy alcohol use or situational use, for example, in conjunction with driving.

Targeted group education usually customizes informational techniques to the population and the setting. As noted earlier, a popular community-based approach to targeted education is school-based education of children. Such education is designed to increase awareness of the risk of substance abuse, and, in some programs, to increase the resistance or ability of the students to resist peer pressure to drink or use drugs.

Agent strategies are those targeted at substances of abuse. There are both national and local law enforcement efforts to reduce the physical availability of illicit drugs. For alcohol, agent strategies have focused on restrictions on alcohol advertising and promotion at the local level, though such policies are also set at a national or state level in most countries. In the United States and Mexico, product warning labels have been mandated (Greenfield, Graves, & Kaskutas, 1992; Hankin et al., 1993; Hilton, 1992; Parker, Saltz, & Hennessy, 1994). In many states and provinces of the U.S. and Canada, local agent strategies have included warning labels at the point of purchase to complement the warning labels on the products themselves.

The third element of the public health model concerns the environment—that is, the drinking or drug-using context. This is the area of local policy that has generated considerable interest in recent years. Examples of local program efforts to alter system structures for alcohol problem prevention include:

1. Reducing alcoholic beverage availability through local zoning of outlets (Wittman, 1986; Wittman & Hilton, 1987).

2. Educating servers of alcohol to institute policies to reduce heavy consumption and reduce blood alcohol levels of patrons (McKnight, 1987; Russ & Geller, 1987; Saltz, 1987, 1989).

3. Changing the form of alcohol availability, such as sale of distilled spirits by the individual drink (Blose & Holder, 1987a, 1987b; Holder & Blose, 1987), or licensing private individuals to sell wine and distilled spirits by the bottle (Holder & Wagenaar, 1990; Wagenaar & Holder, 1991).

4. Increasing retail prices of alcoholic beverages (Cook & Tauchen, 1982; Hoadley, Fuchs, & Holder, 1984; Levy & Sheflin, 1983; Ornstein & Hanssens, 1983; Saffer & Grossman, 1987).

5. Reducing access to alcohol by young people through increased enforcement of the minimum purchase age (National Highway Traffic

Safety Administration, 1982; U.S. General Accounting Office, 1987; Wagenaar, 1983, 1986, 1987).

6. Establishing curfews to limit hours of alcohol sales to young people (Preusser, Williams, Lund, & Preusser, 1984).

7. Increasing local police enforcement of drinking and driving as a general deterrent (Ross, 1982; Voas & Hause, 1987).

8. Establishing random roadblocks for deterring drinking and driving (Homel, 1988; Voas, 1989).

9. Making loss of license mandatory and increasing punishment for any DUI conviction as a general deterrent (Vingilis, Blefgen, Lei, Sykora, & Mann, 1988; Williams et al., 1984).

A review of research changing the substance abuse environment can be found in Edwards et al. (1994) and Holder (1994b).

RATIONALE FOR ALCOHOL POLICY AT THE COMMUNITY LEVEL

Policy, as illustrated by some of the examples above, is conceived with organizational and community priorities and responses. A policy does not usually target a specific risk group but rather alters existing structures to reduce the potential risk of harm or of a social problem. For example, setting a minimum drinking age for alcohol is a state policy aimed at reducing access to alcohol by persons below a certain age and thus aimed at reducing alcohol problems in this age group.

While programs such as media campaigns, alcoholism and drug abuse recovery efforts, and school educational efforts have been popular in communities, policy as a tool for prevention at the local level has a relatively brief history. For the most part, local prevention strategies have been program-based, not policy-based (Greenfield & Zimmerman, 1993). However, there are examples of community efforts to use alcohol policy for affecting the drinking environment or the availability of alcohol (Casswell, Gilmore, Maguire, & Ransom, 1989; Giesbrecht & Ferris, 1993; Holder, 1992). Thus, there is a significant opportunity for exploration, design, implementation, and evaluation of local policy.

There are at least three positive features of locally applied policy for the prevention of substance abuse problems:

1. Research evidence: In general, policy, which usually addresses environmental strategies, has scientific evidence of effectiveness. Such policies include setting the retail price, availability of alcohol, location and type of

alcohol outlets including hours and days of sale, retail and social access to alcohol by young people, and enforcement and sanctions against high-risk alcohol use, such as drinking and driving (Edwards et al., 1994). Thus, policy approaches for alcohol problem prevention have a substantial base of science on which to rest.

2. Lower cost: There are few cases in which the actual cost of prevention programs or policies has been documented. However, on the average, local policies as they involve changes in rules and regulations or increased emphasis for existing activities are likely to be lower in cost than specially funded local prevention programs that require an additional investment in staff, materials, and other resources. For example, the cost of teacher and school administrator time, curriculum materials, and other costs for a school-based educational program likely exceed the cost of a local policy of reduced retail sales of alcohol to underage persons via such techniques as increased enforcement to prevent such sales by retail establishments. Raising the retail price of alcohol at a local level by imposing local special-purpose taxes generates increased revenue and, at the same time, is a low-cost prevention strategy.

3. Sustainability: Once implemented policies have a longer life than prevention programs that must be maintained and thus funded each year. For example, a policy of requiring training for alcoholic beverage servers through an existing adult education system has a longer potential effectiveness than a mass media campaign that must be planned, funded, and implemented each year. Even when the potential effectiveness of any policy decays over time due to lower compliance or lower regulation or enforcement, policies continue to have some sustaining effect, even without reinforcement. One example is the minimum drinking age. O'Malley and Wagenaar (1991) found that the effects on drinking and driving resulting from the increased minimum age were more sustained in states with higher drinking ages than in states with lower ages (18 to 19).

LOCAL POLICY GOALS: EXPERIENCES
FROM A COMMUNITY TRIALS PROJECT

There are a number of possible policies that can be implemented at the community level and have supporting scientific evidence of their potential effectiveness. An illustration of how local policies were actually developed and implemented is provided by a community prevention trials project at the Prevention Research Center in Berkeley, California. This program has as its goal the reduction of alcohol-involved injuries and death at the community level in three experimental communities, two in California and one in South Carolina. There was a matched control community for each experimental community (Holder, 1993).

The alcohol policies selected as prevention interventions for this project were grouped into four areas for convenience but have clear interactive and mutually supportive relationships. None of the policies is isolated from the specific effects of the others. The four policy areas implemented by local communities are described below:

1. Drinking and Driving—Establish highly visible drinking and driving enforcement.

The evidence of the effectiveness of DUI enforcement as a deterrent to drinking and driving, rather than a punishment, comes from a number of studies that have demonstrated that such behavior is reduced and the number of alcohol-involved crashes is decreased (Homel, 1988; Ross, 1982; Voas & Hause, 1987). The evidence is clear that the perceived risk of detection of drinking and driving is a primary intervening variable. Thus, community members should be informed about increased enforcement and have it confirmed in direct experience with frequent enforcement checkpoints. This policy requires a policy commitment within local law enforcement to carry out frequent and highly visible DUI enforcement checks. Routine DUI enforcement must become a high priority among competing law enforcement activities. The second aspect of this policy is continuous mass media attention. For instance, news media are encouraged to report on the increased DUI enforcement and the new DUI detection capability of local law enforcement via advanced officer training and the use of new technology for detecting drinking drivers (e.g., passive BAC sensors).

2. Responsible Beverage Service—Establish alcohol serving practices for bars and restaurants that will reduce the level and frequency of alcohol impairment by customers.

The evidence about this policy comes from studies of the reduction in alcohol-involved traffic crashes from mandatory server training (Holder & Wagenaar, 1994) and controlled studies in local communities (Saltz, 1987, 1993). Studies have shown that licensed establishments with an alcohol serving policy that (a) encourages servers to intervene with customers who are at risk of becoming intoxicated, and (b) discourages high-volume consumption, results in customers leaving with lower levels of alcohol impairment. A responsible beverage serving policy of a bar or restaurant can also be reinforced when local government requires server training (e.g., via zoning or business licensing requirements) and when local police enforce laws against service to intoxicated patrons (McKnight & Streff, 1994).

3. Underage Drinking—Establish retail sales practices and limit youthful social events to reduce drinking by underage persons.

The evidence of the effectiveness of an enforced higher minimum age of alcohol purchase comes from studies of higher ages of purchasers and reduced alcohol consumption and alcohol-involved traffic crashes (O'Malley & Wagenaar, 1991; Wagenaar, 1987). Local policies can include a routine sales practice by on- and off-premise alcohol outlets of age identification and refusal of sales to underage persons. Such a local policy approach can be reinforced by parent, adult, and law enforcement practice of actual sales to underage persons. Other local policy alternatives include parent and law enforcement checks on alcohol availability at youthful social events. The first policy can be reinforced via local requirements (business license or zoning), training of sales clerks for age identification, and law enforcement checks about such sales, such as using "sting operations." The second policy can be reinforced, for example, by a local keg registration ordinance that registers the name of the person who rented a beer keg used at a social event in which underage persons were drinking. The policy can also be supported by parental and other adult mobilization and training concerning enforcement of drinking practices at social events in which underage persons are present.

4. Alcohol Retail Access—Reduce density of alcohol outlets and their concentration in certain areas of a community.

The evidence to support this policy comes from studies of the relationship of alcohol availability, alcohol consumption, and alcohol problems. Some of these studies have examined changes in forms of alcohol availability (Blose & Holder, 1987b; Holder & Blose, 1987; Makela, 1980) and density of alcohol outlets by population or geography (Godfrey, 1988; Gruenewald, Ponicki, & Holder, 1993; Watts & Rabow, 1983; Wilkinson, 1987). This policy is created by local land use planning and zoning capabilities that, when available by state law, enable communities to establish local limits on the number of outlets in certain areas of the community (or the entire community), distances between outlets, as well as distances from schools and churches and other locations and alcohol outlets.

WHAT HAS BEEN LEARNED ABOUT LOCAL POLICY

The following are observations on community-wide prevention efforts. Educational strategies have produced only limited evidence of effectiveness. Some (but not all) school-based projects that reported some success in delaying onset of alcohol and drug use (Hansen, 1993; Moskowitz, 1989; Pentz et al., 1989) have concurrently employed parental and community participation. More consistent findings are needed to scientifically establish the potential of school-based projects. There is no evidence that mass media campaigns alone can change or prevent alcohol- or drug-using behavior. Such campaigns can increase awareness of a problem, but alone they are not sufficient to reduce the problem.

Media advocacy is a newly developed aspect of the purposeful use of the mass media (Wallack, 1989, 1990). Previously, mass communication was based upon planned and purposeful employment of the mass media—for example, public service announcements on radio and TV, and billboards. These are often professionally developed campaigns with a defined campaign life. The effects, if any, rapidly decay following the end of the campaign.

Media advocacy, on the other hand, refers to a much larger use of the news media to bring attention to a local alcohol or drug problem, to identify the policy options or preferred option for response to the problem, and eventually to effect a policy change. In such an approach, there is no ability or attempt to manage the news or to get preset materials such as press releases published. Rather, this is a creative approach of bringing local data, issues, and problems to the attention of the community and its leadership as well as lending support to preferred policy options (Holder, 1994a).

As Edwards et al. (1994) have shown, the research evidence on environmental approaches to prevention of alcohol problems is strong enough to provide a solid, scientific basis for implementing such approaches at the local level. Environmental approaches include changes in retail prices; limiting hours and days of sale; enforcement of minimum drinking ages; and location and density of alcohol outlets. For problems related to other drugs, community approaches to mobilize community leadership in developing drug abuse prevention show promise (Johnson et al., 1990). For illicit drugs, there is limited scientific evaluation of the effectiveness of interdiction strategies to reduce local availability. Evidence on limiting local alcohol availability suggests that reducing local drug availability could reduce drug use. More research is needed.

RECOMMENDATIONS FOR FUTURE COMMUNITY PREVENTION EFFORTS

As a complex adaptive system, a community will adjust to any efforts to change conditions within the system. Thus, local prevention programs that target specific high-risk individuals are unlikely to have any long-term effects; the system will adapt and continue to produce individuals and problems as before. This is especially true if no structural changes occur.

The field of community-level alcohol and other drug prevention cannot be described by a series of scientifically documented successes. The primary focus on educational and target group strategies has not yielded much evidence of effectiveness in reducing substance abuse. There have been few community efforts to alter community-system environments and contents that give rise to problems. Thus, it has been "business as usual" for communities in terms of substance abuse and associated problems. It is the position of this chapter that different approaches and perspectives are needed in the future.

The following are recommendations to increase the effectiveness of future community prevention efforts for substance abuse:

1. Consider alcohol and other drug problems as outputs of the community system. Seek to understand the structures that give rise to problems as a means to identify potential system-level interventions.

2. Use the best scientific evidence in designing and implementing community strategies. Community excitement and enthusiasm for any community-based strategy is necessary for successful local programs, but this is not enough. While educational efforts are often highly visible and usually quite popular with citizens, there is little evidence that they alone have any effectiveness in reducing problems.

3. Mixed, complementary system strategies are more likely to be effective in reducing community-wide alcohol and drug problems than are single, even intensive strategies. Synergism, or mutually reinforcing prevention strategies, hold more promise for long-term, sustained effectiveness than do special, time-limited programs.

4. Existing governmental capabilities should be favored over specially funded initiatives. Community policies can produce structural changes that are more likely to reduce alcohol problems than are specially funded prevention programs, and perhaps local drug problems as well, but there is no current research evidence available at this writing. Whenever policies are implemented and maintained by existing governmental enforcement and planning capabilities, such policies have a greater opportunity to achieve long-term effects. Funded prevention programs, even if successful, require annual funding to maintain stability.

Community-based prevention of substance abuse problems is a challenge for the 21st century. Such prevention can increase the ownership of the effort by local people and place the effort at the point that is closest to the action. However, without a consideration of the entire community system and without solid scientific evidence on which to base the design of prevention efforts, community-level prevention efforts are not very likely to be effective.

REFERENCES

Amsel, Z. (1990). Introducing the concept "Community Prevention." In C. G. Leukefeld, R. J. Battjes, & Z. Amsel (Eds.), *AIDS and intravenous drug use: Future directions for community-based prevention research* (NIDA Research Monograph 93, pp. vii–xiv). Rockville, MD: National Institute on Drug Abuse.

Battjes, R. J., Leukefeld, C. G., & Amsel, Z. (1990). Community prevention efforts to reduce the spread of AIDS associated with intravenous drug abuse. In C. G. Leukefeld, R. J. Battjes, & Z. Amsel (Eds.), *AIDS and intravenous drug use: Future directions for community-based prevention research* (NIDA Research Monograph 93, pp. 288–299). Rockville, MD: National Institute on Drug Abuse.

Blose, J. O., & Holder, H. D. (1987a). Liquor-by-the-drink and alcohol-related traffic crashes: A natural experiment using time-series analysis. *Journal of Studies on Alcohol, 48,* 52–60.

Blose, J. O., & Holder, H. D. (1987b). Public availability of distilled spirits: Structural and reported consumption changes associated with liquor-by-the-drink. *Journal of Studies on Alcohol, 48,* 371–379.

Casswell, S., Gilmore, L., Maguire, V., & Ransom, R. (1989). Changes in public support for alcohol policies following a community-based campaign. *British Journal of Addiction, 84,* 515–522.

Casti, J. L. (1992). *Reality rules.* New York: Wiley.

Cook, P. J., & Tauchen, G. (1982). The effect of liquor taxes on heavy drinking. *Bell Journal of Economics, 13,* 379–390.

Edwards, G., Anderson, P., Babor, T. F., Casswell, S., Ferrence, R., Giesbrecht, N., Godfrey, C., Holder, H. D., Lemmens, P., Mäkelä, K., Midanik, L. T., Norström, T., Österberg, E., Romelsjö, A., Room, R., Simpura, J., & Skog, O.-J. (Eds.). (1994). *Alcohol policy and the public good.* New York: Oxford University Press.

Giesbrecht, N., & Ferris, J. (1993). Community-based research initiatives in prevention. *Addiction 88,* 83S–93S.

Giesbrecht, N., et al. (1991, June). *Community action research projects: Integrating community interests and research agenda in multicomponent initiatives.* Paper presented at the 36th International Institute on the Prevention and Treatment of Alcoholism, Stockholm, Sweden.

Godfrey, C. (1988). Licensing and the demand for alcohol. *Applied Economics, 20,* 1541–1558.

Greenfield, T. K., Graves, K. L., & Kaskutas, L. A. (1992, March). *Do alcohol warning labels work? Research findings.* Paper presented at Alcohol Policy VIII, National Association for Public Health Policy, Washington, DC.

Greenfield, T. K., & Zimmerman, R. (Eds.). (1993). *Experiences with community action projects: New research in the prevention of alcohol and other drug problems* (CSAP Prevention Monograph 14). Rockville, MD: USDHHS, Center for Substance Abuse Prevention.

Gruenewald, P. J., Ponicki, W. B., & Holder, H. D. (1993). The relationship of outlet densities to alcohol consumption: A time series cross-sectional analysis. *Alcoholism: Clinical and Experimental Research, 17,* 38–47.

Hankin, J. R., Sloan, J. J., Firestone, I. J., Ager, J. W., Sokol, R. J., & Martier, S. S. (1993). A time series analysis of the impact of the alcohol warning label on antenatal drinking. *Alcoholism: Clinical and Experimental Research, 17,* 284–289.

Hansen, W. B. (1993). School-based alcohol prevention programs. *Alcohol Health & Research World, 17,* 54–60.

Hilton, M. E. (1992, May–June). *Perspectives and prospects in warning label research.* Paper presented at the 18th Annual Alcohol Epidemiology Symposium, Toronto, Ontario, Canada.

Hoadley, J. F., Fuchs, B. C., & Holder, H. D. (1984). The effect of alcohol beverage restrictions on consumption: A 25-year longitudinal analysis. *American Journal of Drug and Alcohol Abuse, 10,* 375–401.

Holder, H. D. (1992). Chapter 2: What is a community and what are implications for prevention trials for reducing alcohol problems and Chapter 14: Undertaking a community prevention trial to reduce alcohol problems: Translating theoretical models into action. In H. D. Holder & J. M. Howard (Eds.), *Community prevention trials for alcohol problems: Methodological issues* (pp. 15–33 and 227–243). Westport, CT: Praeger.

Holder, H. D. (1993). Prevention of alcohol-related accidents in the community. *Addiction, 88,* 1003–1012.

Holder, H. D. (1994a). Mass communication as an essential aspect of community prevention to reduce alcohol-involved traffic crashes. *Alcohol, Drugs, and Driving, 10,* 1–14.

Holder, H. D. (1994b). Public health approaches to the reduction of alcohol problems. *Substance Abuse, 15,* 123–138.

Holder, H. D., & Blose, J. O. (1987). Impact of changes in distilled spirits availability on apparent consumption: A time series analysis of liquor-by-the-drink. *British Journal of Addiction, 82,* 623–631.

Holder, H. D., & Howard, J. M. (Eds.). (1992). *Community prevention trials for alcohol problems: Methodological issues.* Westport, CT: Praeger.

Holder, H. D., & Wagenaar, A. C. (1990). Effects of the elimination of a state monopoly on distilled spirits; retail sales: A time-series analysis of Iowa. *British Journal of Addiction, 85,* 1615–1625.

Holder, H. D., & Wagenaar, A. C. (1994). Mandated server training and the reduction of alcohol-involved traffic crashes: A time series analysis in the state of Oregon. *Accident Analysis & Prevention, 26,* 89–94.

Holder, H. D., & Wallack, L. (1986). Contemporary perspectives for preventing alcohol problems: An empirically-derived model. *Journal of Public Health Policy, 7,* 324–339.

Holland, J. H. (1975). *Adaptation in natural and artificial systems.* Ann Arbor: University of Michigan Press.

Homel, R. (1988). *Policing and punishing the drinking driver: A study of general and specific deterrence.* New York: Springer-Verlag.

Johnson, C. A., Pentz, M. A., Weber, M. D., Dwyer, J. H., Baer, N., MacKinnon, D. P., Hansen, W. B., & Flay, B. R. (1990). Relative effectiveness of comprehensive community programming for drug abuse prevention with high-risk and low-risk adolescents. *Journal of Consulting and Clinical Psychology, 58,* 447–456.

Kauffman, S. A. (1991, August). Antichaos and adaptation. *Scientific American,* 78–84.

Kauffman, S. A. (1992). *Origins of order: Self-organization and selection in evolution.* Oxford: Oxford University Press.

Kauffman, S. A. (1995). *At home in the universe.* New York: Oxford University Press.

Levy, D., & Sheflin, N. (1983). New evidence on controlling alcohol use through price. *Journal of Studies on Alcohol, 44,* 929–937.

Makela, K. (1980). Differential effects of restricting the supply of alcohol: Studies of a strike in Finnish liquor stores. *Journal of Drug Issues, 10,* 131–144.

McKnight, A. J. (1987). *Development and field test of a responsible alcohol service program. Volume I: Research findings* (Report No. DOT HA 807 221). Washington, DC: U.S. Department of Transportation, National Highway Traffic Safety Administration.

McKnight, A. J., & Streff, F. M. (1994). The effect of enforcement upon service of alcohol to intoxicated patrons of bars and restaurants. *Accident Analysis and Prevention, 26,* 19–88.

Moskowitz, J. (1989). The primary prevention of alcohol problems: A critical review of the research literature. *Journal of Studies on Alcohol, 50,* 54–88.

National Highway Traffic Safety Administration. (1982). *Evaluation of minimum drinking age laws using the National Electronic Injury Surveillance System.* Washington, DC: Author.

O'Malley, P. M., & Wagenaar, A. C. (1991). Effects of minimum drinking age laws on alcohol use, related behaviors and traffic crash involvement among American youth: 1976–1987. *Journal of Studies on Alcohol, 52,* 478–491.

Ornstein, S. K., & Hanssens, D. M. (1983). *Alcohol control laws and the consumption of distilled spirits and beer* (working paper). Los Angeles: University of California, Research Program in Competition and Business Policy, Graduate School of Management.

Parker, R. N., Saltz, R. F., & Hennessy, M. (1994). The impact of alcohol beverage container warning labels on alcohol-impaired drivers, drinking drivers and the general population in Northern California. *Addiction, 89,* 1639–1651.

Pentz, M. A., Dwyer, J. H., MacKinnon, D. P., Flay, B. R., Hansen, W. B., Wang, E. Y. I., & Johnson, C. A. (1989). A multicommunity trial for primary prevention of adolescent drug abuse: Effects on drug use prevalence. *Journal of the American Medical Association, 261,* 3259–3266.

Preusser, D. F., Williams, A. R., Zador, P. L., & Blomberg, R. D. (1984). The effect of curfew laws on motor vehicle crashes. *Law and Policy, 6,* 115–128.

Ross, H. L. (1982). *Deterring the drinking driver: Legal policy and social control.* Lexington, MA: Heath.

Russ, N. W., & Geller, E. S. (1987). Training bar personnel to prevent drunk driving: A field evaluation. *American Journal of Public Health, 77,* 952–954.

Saffer, H., & Grossman, M. (1987). Beer taxes, the legal drinking age, and youth motor vehicle fatalities. *Journal of Legal Studies, 16,* 351–374.

Saltz, R. F. (1987). The roles of bars and restaurants in preventing alcohol-impaired driving: An evaluation of server intervention. *Evaluation and Health Professions, 10,* 5–27.

Saltz, R. F. (1989). Research needs and opportunities in server intervention programs. *Health Education Quarterly, 16,* 429–438.

Saltz, R. F. (1993). The introduction of dram shop legislation in the United States and the advent of server training. *Addiction, 88,* 95S–203S.

Stonier, R. J., & Yu, X. H. (Eds.). (1994). *Complex systems: Mechanism of adaptation.* Amsterdam/Oxford/Washington, DC: IOS Press.

U.S. General Accounting Office. (1987). *Drinking-age laws: An evaluation synthesis of their impact on highway safety.* Report to the Chairman, Subcommittee on Investigations and Oversight, Committee on Public Works and Transportation, House of Representatives. Washington, DC: U.S. Superintendent of Documents.

Vingilis, E., Blefgen, H., Lei, H., Sykora, K., & Mann, R. (1988). An evaluation of the deterrent impact on Ontario's 12-hour license suspension law. *Accident Analysis and Prevention, 20,* 9–17.

Voas, R. B. (1989). *Sobriety check points, an evaluation.* Paper presented at the 11th Triannual Meeting of the International Committee on Alcohol, Drugs, and Traffic Safety, Chicago, IL.

Voas, R. B., & Hause, J. M. (1987). Deterring the drinking driver: The Stockton experience. *Accident Analysis and Prevention, 19,* 81–90.

Wagenaar, A. (1983). *Alcohol, young drivers, and traffic accidents: Effects of minimum-age laws.* Lexington, MA: Lexington.

Wagenaar, A. C. (1986). Preventing highway crashes by raising the legal minimum age for drinking: The Michigan experience six years later. *Journal of Safety Research, 17,* 101–109.

Wagenaar, A. C. (1987). Effects of minimum drinking age on alcohol-related traffic crashes: The Michigan experience five years later. In H. D. Holder (Ed.), *Control issues in alcohol abuse prevention: Strategies for states and communities* (pp. 119–131). Greenwich, CT: JAI Press.

Wagenaar, A. C., & Holder, H. D. (1991). A change from public to private sale of wine: Results from natural experiments in Iowa and West Virginia. *Journal of Studies on Alcohol, 52,* 162–173.

Waldrup, M. M. (1992). *Complexity: The emerging science at the edge of order and chaos.* New York: Simon & Schuster.

Wallack, L. (1981). Mass media campaigns: The odds against finding behavior change. *Health Education Quarterly, 8,* 209–260.

Wallack, L. (1989). Mass media and health promotion: A critical perspective. In R. Rice & C. Atkin (Eds.), *Public communication campaigns.* Newbury Park, CA: Sage.

Wallack, L. (1990). Two approaches to health promotion in the mass media. *World Health Forum, 11*, 143–164.

Watts, R. K., & Rabow, J. (1983). Alcohol availability and alcohol-related problems in 213 California cities. *Alcoholism: Clinical and Experimental Research, 7*, 47–58.

Whitehead, J. T., & Lab, S. P. (1989). A meta-analysis of juvenile correctional treatment. *Journal of Research in Crime and Delinquency, 26*, 276–295.

Wilkinson, J. T. (1987). Reducing drunken driving: Which policies are most effective? *Southern Economic Journal, 54*, 322–334.

Williams, A., Lund, A., & Preusser, D. (1984). *Night driving curfews in New York and Louisiana*. Washington, DC: Insurance Institute for Highway Safety.

Wittman, F. (1986). Regulation of availability as a focus for community-level prevention planning. In A. Cox & N. Giesbrecht (Eds.), *Prevention, alcohol and the environment—Issues, constituencies, and strategies*. Toronto: The Addiction Research Foundation.

Wittman, F., & Hilton, M. (1987). Uses of planning and zoning ordinances to regulate alcohol outlets in California cities. In H. D. Holder (Ed.), *Control issues in alcohol abuse prevention: Strategies for states and communities* (pp. 337–366). Greenwich, CT: JAI Press.

INTERVENTION: PRIMARY AND SECONDARY PREVENTION

16

Prevention in Schools

Gilbert J. Botvin
Institute for Prevention Research
Cornell University Medical College

Recent national survey data indicate that the decade-long decline in substance abuse that took place throughout most of the 1980s has not only been reversed, but that adolescent substance abuse has increased markedly since 1992. The problem is particularly keen among junior and senior high school youth, where there has been a sharp increase in marijuana use among 8th, 10th, and 12th graders as well as an increase for all three grade levels in the use of cigarettes, stimulants, LSD, and inhalants (Johnston, O'Malley, & Bachman, 1995). For marijuana, lifetime use has nearly tripled since 1992 among 8th graders, has nearly doubled for 10th graders, and has increased by 50% among 12th graders.

These trends highlight the importance of developing effective approaches to substance abuse prevention. The quest for effective preventive interventions has taken more than two decades. Most efforts to identify effective prevention approaches have achieved only a limited degree of success and many have failed completely. However, over the past decade, the arduous task of developing and testing potentially effective substance abuse prevention approaches has begun to bear some fruit. During this time, mounting empirical evidence from a growing number of carefully designed and methodologically sophisticated research studies clearly indicates that at least some approaches to substance abuse prevention work. The purpose of this chapter is to provide a brief overview of what is currently known about the effectiveness of substance abuse prevention efforts in school settings. The primary focus is on approaches that have been subjected to careful evaluation using acceptable scientific methods and where results have been published in peer-reviewed journals.

THE IMPORTANCE OF SCHOOL-BASED PREVENTION APPROACHES

Although substance abuse prevention efforts have been developed and tested in a variety of settings, the vast majority of prevention research has been conducted in schools. Schools are natural sites for both implementing and testing prevention programs targeted at children and adolescents. Schools provide easy access to large numbers of individuals who are the logical targets of prevention efforts. They also provide the kind of well-structured setting necessary for conducting methodologically rigorous evaluation research studies. Moreover, despite their traditional educational mission, schools in most states are generally required to provide their students with programs in health education and tobacco, alcohol, and drug education. And while there has been periodic debate concerning whether schools should be asked to deal with the health and social problems confronting today's students, many educators have come to the realization that problems such as substance abuse can seriously hinder the attainment of educational objectives.

Substance abuse has come to be seen as both a health problem and as a barrier to educational achievement. As a consequence, the U.S. Department of Education has included drug-free schools as one of its goals for improving the quality of education in America. And, considering substance abuse within the broader concern of adolescent health, a major report on the education of young adolescents by the Carnegie Council on Adolescent Development, *Turning Points: Preparing American Youth for the Twenty-first Century* (Task Force on Education of Young Adolescents, 1989), recommends that "schools should be environments for health promotion" and concludes that "the education and health of young adolescents must be inextricably linked." Clearly, health promotion in general and substance abuse prevention in particular are not only appropriate activities for the school setting, but are vitally important to the healthy physical, emotional, and educational development of our nation's youth.

THE EMPIRICAL UNDERPINNINGS OF SCHOOL-BASED PREVENTION EFFORTS

Over the past decade and a half, substance abuse prevention studies have proceeded through several phases from small-scale pilot studies designed to test the acceptability, feasibility, and preliminary efficacy of promising approaches to large-scale randomized field trials designed to provide the strongest possible evidence that a particular prevention method worked. Three distinguishing features of the best contemporary prevention research are that the most promising approaches are based on an understanding of what is known about the etiology of substance abuse; that they are conceptualized within a theoretical framework; and that they have been subjected to empirical testing using appropriate research methods. While all three are critically important, the most fundamental element of any prevention program is an approach that is based on an understanding of the etiology of substance abuse.

Etiologic Factors

Understanding the causes of substance abuse and its developmental progression are important because together they offer essential information concerning the nature and timing of potentially effective prevention approaches. Considerable research has been conducted over the past 20 years concerning the etiology of substance abuse. Surprisingly, many prevention efforts appear to have been developed without any recognition of this literature. Despite the fact that etiologic research shows that substance abuse is the result of a multivariate mix of factors, the most ubiquitous prevention approaches, until recently, were those that focused on providing students with factual information about various drugs and their pharmacologic effects, methods of using drugs, and the adverse consequences of using drugs.

The existing empirical evidence clearly indicates that substance abuse is caused by the complex interaction of a number of different etiologic factors including knowledge, attitudes, social, personality, pharmacological, biological, and developmental factors (Baumrind & Moselle, 1985; Blum & Richards, 1979; Jessor & Jessor, 1977; Jones & Battjes, 1985; Kandel, 1978; Meyer & Mirin, 1979; Newcomb & Bentler, 1988; Wechsler, 1976). The most promising prevention approaches not only take into account the complex etiology of substance abuse, but recognize the important role that social factors play in promoting the initiation of substance use. Friends and family members (Barnes & Welte, 1986; Gfroerer, 1987; Kandel, 1985; Krosnick & Judd, 1982) as well as the media (Tye, Warner, & Glantz, 1987; Whelan, 1984) exert powerful influences during childhood and early adolescence that can promote and sustain substance abuse. Individuals who are unaware of the adverse consequences of using drugs and have positive attitudes toward drug use are at increased risk of becoming substance abusers (Krosnick & Judd, 1982; Smith & Fogg, 1978) as are individuals who see substance use as being a highly normative behavior (Chassin, Presson, Sherman, Corty, & Olshavsky, 1984).

Psychological characteristics such as low self-esteem, self-confidence, self-satisfaction, social confidence, assertiveness, personal control, and self-efficacy have been found to be associated with substance abuse (Dielman, Leech, Lorenger, & Horvath, 1984; Weir, 1968). Substance abusers have also been found to be more anxious, impulsive, rebellious, impatient to acquire adult status, and in need of more social approval than nonusers (Jessor & Jessor, 1977; Jones & Battjes, 1985). The clinical literature suggests that individuals with a specific psychiatric condition (e.g., anxiety, depression) may use particular substances as a way of alleviating the symptoms associated with those conditions (Millman & Botvin, 1983). For example, highly anxious individuals may have found that alcohol or other depressants help decrease their anxiety, and may use one or more depressants to regulating their feelings of anxiety.

While the pharmacology of commonly abused drugs varies considerably, virtually all produce effects that are highly reinforcing and result in physical or psychological dependence. For tobacco, alcohol, and most illicit drugs, tolerance develops quickly, leading to increased dosages and an increased frequency of use. Once a pattern of dependent use has been established, termination of use produces dysphoric feelings and physical withdrawal symptoms.

Over the years, it has become clear that for most individuals drug use is part of a general syndrome or lifestyle reflecting a particular value orientation and involving other problem behaviors (Jessor & Jessor, 1982). Drug use not only tends to involve the use of multiple psychoactive substances, but also is associated with poor academic performance and antisocial behaviors such as aggressiveness, lying, stealing, and cheating (Demone, 1973; Jessor & Jessor, 1972; Newcomb & Bentler, 1986; Wechsler & Thum, 1973).

Onset and Developmental Progression

The onset of substance abuse typically begins with the use of one or more "gateway" substances. The three major gateway substances are tobacco (most commonly cigarettes), alcohol, and marijuana. In recent years, inhalants (e.g., glue, the gas from aerosol cans) have been added to the list of gateway substances. Experimentation with drugs nearly always occurs in social situations, followed later by use in both social and solitary situations. After a brief period of experimentation, many individuals develop patterns of drug use characterized by both psychological and physiological dependence. The initial social and psychological motivations for using drugs eventually yield to one driven increasingly by pharmacological factors (Meyer & Mirin, 1979; Ray, 1974). Moreover, drug use tends to follow a logical and predictable progression (Hamburg, Kraemer, & Jahnke, 1975; Kandel, 1978). Most individuals begin by using alcohol and tobacco, progressing later to the use of marijuana.

Linking Etiology to Intervention

The knowledge base that has developed over the years concerning the etiology of substance abuse indicates that substance abuse is not caused by a single etiologic factor. Instead, there are many different factors that appear to interact with one another to produce a complex risk equation. This makes prevention much more difficult because instead of identifying a single cause and developing an intervention to target it, interventions must target multiple risk and protective factors. As indicated above, research on the etiology of substance abuse suggests that to be effective, prevention programs targeting children and adolescents must impact on social factors as well as knowledge, attitudes, norms, skills, and personality. Information concerning the age of onset and developmental progression suggests that interventions should target individuals by at least the beginning of the adolescent period (middle or junior high school), although how early prevention efforts should begin is as yet unclear. Another implication from the etiology literature for prevention is that prevention programs should target the gateway substances of tobacco, alcohol, and marijuana. The recent increase in inhalant use and its potential role as a form of gateway drug suggests that it should also be the focus of prevention efforts. Understanding the etiology of substance abuse also makes it easy to recognize why some prevention approaches have not succeeded.

TYPES OF SCHOOL INTERVENTIONS

Before discussing the various approaches to substance abuse prevention that have been developed for implementation in schools and the evaluation research supporting their efficacy, a few general comments about school interventions are in order. These interventions include: classroom interventions, school-wide activities, policy interventions, and interventions designed to restructure the school environment.

Classroom Interventions

Most evaluation research has focused on classroom-level prevention approaches. These approaches by their very nature are typically universal interventions, in that they are designed to involve all of the students in a particular class or grade level regardless of their potential risk of becoming a substance user. Unlike selective interventions, no effort is made to identify high-risk individuals. Universal interventions have the advantage of avoiding logistical problems associated with selective interventions as well as possibly stigmatizing individuals with the label of being "high-risk" or "at risk" or even worse. The disadvantage of universal interventions is that they may either be inefficient—by utilizing intervention resources for individuals who are highly unlikely to develop a problem with drugs—or ineffective—by failing to provide high-risk individuals with the level of intervention required to assist the most difficult-to-reach adolescents.

Classroom interventions are generally conceptualized as curricula and are frequently formalized with student objectives, lesson plans, specific content, and classroom activities. These interventions are often taught by regular classroom teachers, but they can also be taught by peer leaders, college students, substance abuse prevention specialists, health educators, or other health professionals. Classroom interventions can either be implemented as a separate curriculum module or infused into the regular academic curriculum.

School-Wide Activities

School-wide intervention activities may take the form of assembly programs, poster contests, periodic announcements over the school PA system, or displays in the halls or cafeteria. Although prevention programs of this kind are common, researchers have generally avoided relying on school-wide prevention activities as the primary mode of intervention. These approaches are regarded as being more useful for increasing awareness of the problem of substance abuse than preventing it. They offer only minimal intervention with little realistic potential for having an impact on the complex combination of factors leading individuals to use drugs.

School Policy

Formulating new school policies or modifying existing ones can be a powerful source of change. With respect to substance abuse prevention, policy interventions are designed to have an impact on tobacco, alcohol, and illicit drug use by changing the rules or regulations governing the behavior of students, school personnel, and visitors. It is unlikely that changing school policies about using drugs will totally eliminate or prevent substance abuse. However, it does have value as a means of emphasizing the importance of the substance abuse problem, helping to establish antidrug norms, and eliminating substance use on school property and at school functions such as sporting events, dances, or school trips. Policy interventions have been widely used for dealing with the use of alcohol and tobacco. These policies are then monitored and enforced in the same manner as other school policies, with offenders being punished with anything ranging from warnings or detention for first offenses to suspension or even expulsion.

In the case of cigarette smoking, for example, school policies have been designed to either restrict cigarette smoking or to curtail it entirely. Over the past decade, the number of schools throughout the country with explicit policies governing the use of tobacco have grown considerably. It is possible for restrictive smoking policies to gain considerable support and acceptance, as witnessed by developments during the early 1990s in the state of Minnesota, where tobacco-free policies for students, staff, and visitors increased from 3 to 361 school districts (representing 83% of all school districts in the state). Although there has been relatively little research documenting the effectiveness of these policies on behavior, evidence does exist showing that school policies can make a difference, particularly if they include a combination of smoking restrictions and prevention programs (Pentz, Brannon, et al., 1989).

Restructuring the School

Restructuring the school is another approach suggested by some (Comer, 1985; Felner & Adan, 1988). While school restructuring or reorganization efforts have not been motivated by an interest in preventing substance abuse, they are worth considering because of their potential for both decreasing risk factors associated with substance abuse (e.g., low school bonding and school failure) and providing a more conducive environment for conducting substance abuse prevention programs. The rationale behind efforts to restructure schools is that schools need to be organized in a way that supports the developmental and educational needs of today's children and adolescents. Perhaps the best known among these restructuring efforts is that suggested by Comer (1985). From the point of substance abuse prevention, restructuring efforts have the potential for making the school more student-friendly and for enhancing school bonding and school attachment, and reducing school failure. Comer's approach involved a multidisciplinary intervention team working together with school personnel, parents, and students. The team set goals, met regularly, established new school policies, and modified the system of school governance in an effort to facilitate more positive interactions between school staff and parents and to better meet the health, social, emotional, and educational needs of their students. Although substance abuse prevention was not an explicit goal of these efforts, they have been documented to dramatically reduce behavioral problems as well as improving academic performance, parent–teacher relations, and school bonding.

Some experts have even suggested more significant structural changes (Task Force on Education of Young Adolescents, 1989). These include dividing large schools into smaller communities for learning to facilitate sustained individual attention, utilizing cooperative learning and other techniques for ensuring success for all students, vesting in teachers and principals the authority to transform their own schools promoting positive interactions between school staff and parents, fostering alliances between schools and community organizations in educating students and providing community service opportunities, and providing teachers with a stronger background in adolescent development to increase their understanding of the emerging needs of young adolescents.

SCHOOL-BASED APPROACHES FOR PREVENTING SUBSTANCE ABUSE

Most of the research on substance abuse prevention has involved testing interventions in school settings. Most of this research has involved testing interventions within the classroom (usually in the form of a curriculum). These school-based substance abuse prevention efforts can be divided into four general approaches: (1) information dissemination approaches, (2) affective education approaches, (3) social influences approaches, and (4) competence enhancement approaches. Although the first two substance abuse prevention approaches will be discussed briefly, the main emphasis of this chapter will be on the last two approaches, as the available evidence indicates that they are the most promising.

Information Dissemination

Information dissemination approaches attempt to promote substance abuse prevention by imparting health information and in many cases also rely on the use of fear-arousal methods. Evaluation studies have consistently shown that these approaches are ineffective (Dorn & Thompson, 1976; Goodstadt, 1974; Kinder, Pape, & Walfish, 1980; Richards, 1969; Schaps, Bartolo, Moskowitz, Palley, & Churgin, 1981; Swisher & Hoffman, 1975). While results indicate that they can increase knowledge and sometimes change attitudes toward substance use, these approaches have not reduced substance abuse. Although limited, there is even some evidence to suggest that this approach may lead to *increased* substance use, possibly because it may serve to stimulate curiosity (Mason, 1973; Swisher, Crawford, Goldstein, & Yura, 1971). While developmentally appropriate and personally relevant health information has a place in substance abuse prevention programs, it is clear that information alone is not effective.

Affective Education

Rather than focusing on information, affective education approaches have attempted to prevent substance abuse by promoting affective development. Affective education approaches focus on increasing self-understanding and acceptance through activities such as values clarifications and responsible decision making; improving interpersonal relations by fostering effective communication, peer counseling, and assertiveness; and increasing students' abilities to fulfill their basic needs through existing social institutions (Swisher, 1979). Evaluation studies testing the effectiveness of affective education approaches have been as discouraging as evaluations of informational approaches. Although affective education approaches have, in some instances, been able to demonstrate an impact on one or more of the correlates of substance abuse, they have not been able to impact on behavior (Kearney & Hines, 1980; Kim, 1988).

Social Influence

Toward the end of the 1970s, Evans and his colleagues developed and tested a smoking prevention approach that was a major departure from previous approaches to tobacco, alcohol, and substance abuse prevention. Unlike prevention approaches relying on information dissemination, fear arousal, or affective education, this approach focused on the social and psychological factors believed to be involved in the initiation of cigarette smoking (Evans, 1976; Evans et al., 1978).

Psychological Inoculation

The prevention approach developed by Evans was based on persuasive communications theory and a concept called psychological inoculation (McGuire, 1964, 1968). Psychological inoculation is analogous to that of inoculation used in infectious disease prevention. Persuasive communications designed to alter attitudes, beliefs, and behavior are conceptualized as the psychosocial analogue of germs. To prevent "infection" it is necessary to expose the individual to a weak dose of those germs in a way that facilitates the development of "antibodies" and thereby increases resistance to any future exposure to persuasive messages in their more virulent form. From the perspective of psychological inoculation, cigarette smoking is conceptualized as being the result of social influences (persuasive messages) to smoke from peers and the media, which are either direct (i.e., offers to smoke from other adolescents or cigarette advertising) or indirect (i.e., exposure to high-status role models who smoke). If adolescents are likely to be ridiculed for refusing to try cigarettes, they can be exposed to that kind of pressure in small doses and provided with the necessary skills for countering it.

Consistent with this, the intervention developed by Evans was designed to make students aware of the various social pressures to smoke that they would be likely to encounter as they progressed through junior high school. It also included demonstrations of techniques for effectively resisting various pressures to smoke, periodic assessment of smoking with feedback to students to correct the misconception that smoking was a highly normative behavior, and information about the immediate physiological effects of smoking. Results showed that the treatment group had 50% fewer smokers than the control condition (Evans et al., 1978).

Teaching Drug-Resistance Skills

Variations on the social influence model have been developed and tested by a number of research teams over the years (Arkin, Roemhild, Johnson, Luepker, & Murray, 1981; Donaldson, Graham, & Hansen, 1994; Ellickson & Bell, 1990; Hurd et al., 1980; Luepker, Johnson, Murray, & Pechacek, 1983; McAlister, Perry, & Maccoby, 1979; Perry, Killen, Slinkard, & McAlister, 1983; Snow, Tebes, Arthur, & Tapasak, 1992; Sussman, Dent, Stacy, & Sun, 1993; Telch, Killen, McAlister, Perry, & Maccoby, 1982). While these interventions were designed to increase awareness of the various social influences to use drugs, they placed much greater emphasis on teaching specific skills for effectively resisting both peer and media pressures than the original social influence model developed by Evans. Several names have been used for these approaches including the broad term "social influence approach" (because they target the social influences promoting substance use), "refusal skills training" (because a central feature of these programs is that they teach how to say "no" to drug use offers), and "drug resistance skills training."

Resistance skills training approaches are based on a conceptual model stressing the fundamental importance of social factors in promoting the initiation of drug use among adolescents. These influences come from the family, peers, and the mass media. As Bandura (1977) has indicated, all social influences are themselves a product of the interaction between individual learning histories and forces in both the community and the larger society. On the individual level, influences related to specific behaviors arise from learned expectations and skills regarding those behaviors. For example, individuals may smoke because they expect immediate positive outcomes such as increased alertness, relief from anxiety, or enhanced social status. Logically, it would appear reasonable that individuals would choose not to smoke if they did not expect to receive rewarding consequences or if they had the ability to resist specific social pressures to smoke. Expectations and skills are learned both from observation and from direct experience.

Resistance skills training approaches generally teach students how to recognize, handle, or avoid situations in which they will have a high likelihood of experiencing peer pressure to use drugs. Students are not only taught what to say in response to a peer pressure situation, but also how to say it in the most effective way possible.

Using Peer Leaders

An important component of many prevention approaches based on the social influence model is the use of peer leaders as program providers. These peer leaders are typically older students (e.g., 10th graders might serve as peer leaders for 7th graders). In some cases, the peer leaders have been the same age as the participants and may even have been from the same class. The rationale for using peer leaders is that peers often appear to have higher credibility with adolescents than do adults. Peer leaders are useful as discussion leaders, non-drug-using role models, and can facilitate skills training by demonstrating the drug-refusal skills being taught in these prevention programs.

Correcting Normative Expectations

Studies show that adolescents typically overestimate the prevalence of smoking, drinking, and the use of certain drugs (Fishbein, 1977). Therefore, correcting normative expectations has been included as another important component of social influence approaches. Efforts to modify or correct normative expectations has involved providing students with information concerning the prevalence rates of drug use among their peers. This has been accomplished by providing participating students with national survey data so that they can compare their own estimates with the actual prevalence rates. Another approach is for the students participating in the prevention program to organize and conduct classroom or school-wide surveys of drug use themselves. Finally, social influence prevention programs have also typically included a component designed to increase students' awareness of the techniques used by advertisers to promote the sale of tobacco products or alcoholic beverages and to teach techniques for formulating counterarguments to the messages utilized by advertisers.

Personal and Social Skills Training

Considerable prevention research has also been conducted with a prevention model that teaches general personal and social skills either alone (Caplan et al., 1992) or in combination with components of the social resistance skills model (Botvin, Baker, Botvin, Filazzola, & Millman, 1984; Botvin, Baker, Filazzola, & Botvin, 1990; Botvin, Baker, Renick, Filazzola, & Botvin, 1984; Botvin & Eng, 1980; Botvin, Eng, & Williams, 1980; Botvin, Renick, & Baker, 1983; Gilchrist & Schinke, 1983; Pentz, 1983; Schinke, 1984; Schinke & Gilchrist, 1983; Schinke & Gilchrist, 1984). These approaches, also known as competence enhancement approaches, are more comprehensive than either information dissemination, affective education approaches, or social influence approaches. Moreover, unlike affective education approaches, which rely on experiential classroom activities, these approaches emphasize the use of proven cognitive/behavioral skills training methods. They are based on social learning theory (Bandura, 1977) and problem behavior theory (Jessor & Jessor, 1977). Substance abuse is conceptualized as a socially learned and functional behavior, resulting from the interplay of social and personal factors. Substance use behavior is learned through modeling and reinforcement and is influenced by cognition, attitudes, and beliefs.

Personal and social skills training prevention approaches typically teach two or more of the following: (1) general problem-solving and decision-making skills, (2) general cognitive skills for resisting interpersonal or media influences, (3) skills for increasing self-control and self-esteem, (4) adaptive coping strategies for relieving stress and anxiety through the use of cognitive coping skills or behavioral relaxation techniques, (5) general social skills, and (6) general assertive skills. These skills are taught using a combination of instruction, demonstration, feedback, reinforcement, behavioral rehearsal (practice during class), and extended practice through behavioral homework assignments.

Personal and social skills training programs have as their primary aim enhancing general competence by teaching the kind of skills for coping with life that will have a relatively broad application. In contrast to the social influence approaches, which are designed to teach information, norms, and refusal skills with a problem-specific focus, personal and social skills training programs emphasize the application of general skills to situations directly related to substance use and abuse (e.g., the application of general assertive skills to situations involving peer pressure to smoke, drink, or use drugs). These same skills can be used for dealing with the many challenges confronting adolescents in their everyday lives, including but not limited to drug use.

Evidence from one study suggests that broad-based competence enhancement approaches may not be effective unless they also contain some resistance skills training material (Caplan et al., 1992). This may be necessary both because such material includes a focus on antidrug norms and helps students apply generic personal and social skills to situations related specifically to the prevention of substance abuse. Thus, the most effective prevention approaches appear to be those that combine the features of the problem-specific social influence model and the broader competence enhancement model.

Most of the prevention studies using this approach that have been conducted thus far have focused on 7th graders. However, some studies have been conducted with 6th graders (Kreutter, Gewirtz, Davenny, & Love, 1991) and one was conducted with 8th, 9th, and 10th graders (Botvin, Eng, & Williams, 1980). Program length has ranged from as few as 7 sessions to as many as 20 sessions. Some of these prevention programs were conducted at a rate of one class session per week, while others were conducted at a rate of two or more classes per week. Most of the studies conducted so far have used adults as the primary program providers. In some cases these adults were teachers; in other cases they were outside health professionals (project staff members, graduate students, social workers). Some studies have included booster sessions as a means of preserving initial prevention effects.

Age of Participants

Research concerning the etiology of substance abuse and adolescent development indicates that a critical time for experimentation with tobacco, alcohol, and illicit drugs occurs at the beginning of adolescence. For this reason, most of the substance abuse prevention research studies have involved middle or junior high school students. The primary year of intervention for these studies has generally been the 7th grade. However, some studies have included students as young as 4th, 5th, and 6th graders (Donaldson, Graham, & Hansen, 1994; Donaldson, Graham, Piccinin, & Hansen, 1995; Flynn et al., 1992; Shope, Dielman, Butchart, & Campanelli, 1992). While there is general agreement that at least some of the risk factors for substance abuse may have their roots in early childhood (arguing for beginning interventions at a young age), a major concern of prevention researchers testing the efficacy of one or more intervention approaches is the fact that base rates of drug use are typically quite low prior to adolescence. In order to adequately test the impact of prevention programs on drug use it is necessary to select an age range that not only makes sense from an intervention perspective, but also is old enough to include individuals who are likely to begin using drugs in sufficient numbers for researchers to detect statistically significant differences between treatment and control groups. Generally speaking, the base rates of even the most prevalent forms of drug use are too low prior to 7th grade for meaningful prevention research.

FINDINGS FROM EVALUATION STUDIES

Preventing Cigarette Smoking

Both the social influence and the competence enhancement approaches have produced reductions (relative to controls) in cigarette smoking. The effectiveness of social influences approaches has been documented in a number of studies. The results of these studies show that they are able to reduce the rate of smoking by between 35% and 45% after the initial intervention. Most of these prevention studies have focused primarily on preventing the onset of cigarette smoking—that is, preventing the transition from nonsmoking to smoking. The results reported range from reductions of 30% to 40% in the proportion of individuals beginning to smoke (comparing the proportion of new smokers in the experimental group with that of the control group). Several studies have demonstrated reductions in the overall prevalence of cigarette smoking among the participating students both for experimental smoking (less than one cigarette per week) and for regular smoking (one or more cigarettes per week). In these studies, the impact on the prevalence of regular smoking has typically been in the 40% to 50% range. Although most studies assessing the impact of these prevention approaches on tobacco use have focused on cigarette smoking, the social influence approach has also been found to reduce smokeless tobacco use (Sussman et al., 1993).

Evaluation studies testing competence enhancement approaches have also demonstrated significant behavioral effects on cigarette smoking. These studies have demonstrated that generic skills approaches to substance abuse prevention can produce reductions in new experimental smoking ranging from 40% to 75%. Data from two studies with a promising program called *Life Skills Training* (Botvin & Eng, 1982; Botvin, Renick, & Baker, 1983) demonstrated reductions ranging from 56% to 66% in the proportion of pretest nonsmokers becoming regular smokers at the 1-year follow-up without additional booster sessions. With booster sessions these reductions have been as high as 87% (Botvin, Renick, & Baker, 1983). Moreover, initial reductions of an equal magnitude have also been reported for regular smoking (Botvin & Eng, 1982; Botvin, Renick, & Baker, 1983).

Preventing Alcohol and Marijuana Use

Although the majority of the evaluation studies with social influence and competence enhancement approaches has focused primarily on cigarette smoking, a number of studies has also examined the extent to which these prevention approaches had an impact on other substances. In keeping with efforts to target gateway substances, the next logical step in evaluating the efficacy of these prevention approaches was with alcohol and marijuana. Studies testing the efficacy of the social influence approach on alcohol and marijuana have reported reductions of roughly the same magnitude as for cigarette smoking (Ellickson & Bell, 1990; McAlister, Perry, Killen, Slinkard, & Maccoby, 1980; Shope et al., 1992). Several studies also provide evidence for the efficacy of the competence enhancement approach on the use of alcohol (Botvin, Baker, Botvin, Filazzola, & Millman, 1984; Botvin, Baker, Dusenbury, Tortu, & Botvin, 1990; Botvin, Baker, Renick, et al., 1984; Epstein, Botvin, Diaz, & Schinke, 1995; Pentz, 1983) and marijuana (Botvin, Baker, Botvin, et al., 1984; Botvin, Baker, Dusenbury, et al., 1990; Epstein, Botvin, Diaz, Toth, & Schinke, 1995). In general, prevention effects have been the strongest for cigarette smoking and marijuana use. Effects have been the weakest and the most inconsistent across studies with respect to alcohol use.

Long-Term Effects

Arguably one of the most important issues concerning the effectiveness of current substance abuse prevention approaches is the durability of effects over time. Follow-up studies using school-based approaches indicate that the positive behavioral effects of these prevention approaches are evident for up to 3 years after the conclusion of these programs for cigarette smoking (Luepker et al., 1983; McAlister et al., 1980; Sussman et al., 1993; Telch et al., 1982) and multicomponent studies have found prevention effects for up to 7 years (Perry & Kelder, 1992). However, despite these impressive effects, the results of most long-term follow-up studies of school-based approaches indicate that prevention effects are typically not maintained (Bell, Ellickson, & Harrison, 1993; Ellickson, Bell, & McGuigan, 1993; Flay et al., 1989; Murray, Davis-Hearn, Goldman, Pirie, & Luepker, 1988). As a consequence, some have concluded that school-based prevention approaches may simply not be powerful enough to produce lasting prevention effects (Dryfoos, 1993). On the other hand, others have argued that the prevention approaches tested in these studies may have had deficiencies that undermined their long-term effectiveness (Resnicow & Botvin, 1993).

The failure to find long-term prevention effects may have to do with factors related to either the type of intervention tested in these studies or the way these interventions were implemented. The absence of long-term prevention effects in some studies should not be taken as an indictment of all school-based prevention programs. Some of the reasons why durable prevention effects may not have been produced in several long-term follow-up studies are because (1) the length of the intervention may have been too short (i.e., the prevention approach was effective, but the initial prevention "dosage" was too low to produce a long-term effect), (2) booster sessions were either inadequate or not included (i.e., the prevention approach was effective, but it eroded over time because of the absence or inadequacy of ongoing intervention), (3) the intervention was not implemented with enough fidelity to the intervention model (i.e., the correct prevention approach was used, but it was implemented incompletely, improperly, or both), or (4) the intervention was based on a faulty assumptions, was incomplete, or was otherwise deficient (i.e., the prevention approach was ineffective).

Long-term follow-up data from one of the largest school-based substance abuse prevention studies ever conducted found reductions in smoking, alcohol, and marijuana use 6 years after the initial baseline assessment

(Botvin, Baker, Dusenbury, Botvin, & Diaz, 1995). This randomized, controlled, field trial involved nearly 6,000 7th graders from 56 public schools in New York State. After random assignment to prevention and control conditions, students in the prevention condition received the LST program during the 7th grade (15 prevention sessions) with booster sessions in the 8th grade (10 sessions) and 9th grade (5 sessions). No intervention was provided during grades 10 to 12. Follow-up data were collected by survey in class, by mail, or by telephone at the end of the 12th grade and beyond for those students not available for the school survey. The prevalence of cigarette smoking, alcohol use, and marijuana use for the students in the prevention condition was up to 44% lower than for controls. Significant reductions (relative to controls) of up to 66% were also found with respect to the prevalence of polydrug use (students using all three gateway drugs) during the past week. The results of this study suggest that, to be effective, school-based interventions need to be more comprehensive and have a stronger initial dosage than most studies using the social influence have had. Prevention programs also need to include at least two additional years of (booster) intervention and be implemented in a manner that is faithful to the underlying intervention model.

Prevention With Minority Youth

By and large, prevention research has been limited to predominantly White, middle-class, suburban populations. Racial and ethnic minority youth have been underserved with respect to prevention services and underrepresented in prevention evaluation studies. Relatively little is known concerning the etiology of substance abuse among minority youth. However, existing evidence indicates that there is substantial overlap in the factors promoting and maintaining drug use among different populations (Bettes, Dusenbury, Kerner, James-Ortiz, & Botvin, 1990; Botvin et al., 1993; Botvin, Epstein, Schinke, & Diaz, 1994; Botvin, Goldberg, Botvin, & Dusenbury, 1993; Epstein, Dusenbury, Botvin, & Diaz, 1994). This suggests that prevention approaches found to be effective with one population should also be effective with others. Over the past decade, this hypothesis has been tested in a number of studies. Although some may argue that separate and distinct intervention approaches are necessary to prevent substance abuse with various racial and ethnic minority populations in recognition of the unique characteristics of these populations, most of these studies have tested the generalizability of prevention approaches previously found to be effective with White youth.

Studies testing the efficacy of a competence enhancement approach called *Life Skills Training* have shown that it is effective in decreasing drug use, intentions to use drugs, and risk factors associated with drug use. Qualitative research with parents, teachers, and students found high acceptance and perceived utility for this prevention approach among Black and Hispanic populations. Where appropriate, the language, examples, and behavioral rehearsal scenarios were modified to increase cultural sensitivity and relevance to each of the target populations. But no modifications were made to the underlying prevention approach, which focused on teaching generic personal and social skills, antidrug use norms, drug-refusal skills, and prevention-related knowledge and information.

Most of the research with minority youth has been directed at cigarette smoking. These studies have consistently shown that the *Life Skills Training* approach can decrease cigarette smoking (relative to controls) for inner-city Hispanic youth (Botvin, Dusenbury, Baker, James-Ortiz, & Kerner, 1989; Botvin et al., 1992) and African American youth (Botvin et al., 1989; Botvin & Cardwell, 1992). Follow-up data with Hispanic youth have demonstrated the continued presence of lower levels of cigarette smoking up to the end of the 10th grade (Botvin, Schinke, Epstein, & Diaz, 1994). The results of several recent studies with minority youth show that school-based substance abuse prevention approaches such as *Life Skills Training* are also able to reduce alcohol and marijuana use (Botvin, Schinke, Epstein, & Diaz, 1994; Botvin, Schinke, Epstein, Diaz, & Botvin, 1995), and that tailoring the intervention to the culture of the target population can enhance its effectiveness (Botvin, Schinke, Epstein, Diaz, & Botvin, 1995).

Efficacy of Different Program Providers

Considerable variation exists among the individuals responsible for implementing school-based substance abuse prevention programs. Some programs have been implemented by college students, others by members of the research project staff, and still others have used classroom teachers to implement the prevention programs. It has generally been assumed that peer leaders play an important role in social influence approaches. Same age or older peer leaders have been included in nearly all of the studies testing social influence approaches and in some of the studies testing the personal and social skills training approaches. In general, evidence supports the use of peer leaders for this type of prevention strategy (Arkin et al., 1981; Perry et al., 1983).

Although peer leaders have been used successfully to varying degrees in these programs, they usually assist adult program providers and have specific and well-defined roles. The primary providers in most of these studies have been either members of the research project staff or teachers. There is also evidence to suggest that peer-led programs may not be uniformly effective for all students. For example, the results of one study suggest that, while boys and girls may be equally affected by social influence programs when conducted by teachers, girls may be more influenced by peer-led programs than boys (Fisher, Armstrong & deKler, 1983).

Research studies with competence enhancement approaches have shown that they can be successfully implemented by project staff, peer leaders, and classroom teachers (Botvin & Botvin, 1992). However, not all adult program providers are equally effective (Botvin, Baker, Filazzola, & Botvin, 1990). Additional research is needed to identify the characteristics of the most effective providers as well as the optimal match between the characteristics of providers and prevention program participants.

On the other end of the program provider spectrum from programs using peer leaders is Project DARE, which is conducted by police officers. DARE is without a doubt one of the best-known applications of the social influence model. Project DARE (Drug Abuse Resistance Education) was initially developed by the Los Angeles Police Department, based on research conducted at the University of Southern California. The fact that it has been embraced by police departments throughout the country has provided a natural dissemination system throughout the country unparalleled by other prevention programs. Having a prevention program that is implemented by police officers and supported by law enforcement agencies around the country makes DARE unique. This has no doubt contributed to its adoption by a large number of schools. According to news accounts, DARE is said to be used in approximately 60% of the elementary school classrooms in America.

Yet, despite its acknowledged success in promoting an awareness of substance abuse and gaining adoption by more schools across the country than any other program, DARE has been plagued by disappointing evaluation results and a surprising amount of negative news coverage. According to a major meta-analysis of studies evaluating the DARE program, it is less effective than other social influence approaches and has produced only minimal effects on substance use behavior (Ennett, Tobler, Ringwalt, & Flewelling, 1994). Since DARE has much in common with other prevention approaches based on the social influence model, its poor evaluation results are difficult to explain. In view of the fact that the main difference between similar programs showing reductions in substance use and DARE is the program provider, a logical conclusion is that the absence of strong prevention effects may be related more to the program provider than the program itself. The rationale for using peer leaders as program providers has been that peers have greater credibility regarding lifestyle issues than parents, teachers, or other adults who are viewed as authority figures during a developmental period when individuals—particularly those who are at greatest risk for engaging in deviant behaviors—are increasingly likely to rebel against authority figures. Since a police officer is the ultimate symbol of authority in our society, it is reasonable to expect them to have lower credibility with high-risk children and adolescents and, correspondingly, to be less effective as a substance abuse prevention program provider. Still, because the effectiveness of police officers as program providers has not been directly tested, it remains an open question in need of empirical clarification.

Intervention Components and Their Efficacy

Contemporary substance abuse prevention programs contain a variety of components. Progress has clearly been made toward identifying effective prevention approaches. Yet little is known concerning the extent to which different intervention components contribute to substance abuse prevention. In order to increase our understanding of why the most effective interventions work, as well as to facilitate the development of more effective interventions, it is necessary to identify the relative efficacy of specific program components. This may not only prove helpful in guiding practitioners concerning the "active ingredients" or essential elements in prevention programs, but may also enable program developers to identify nonessential components and decrease the length of interventions, thereby increasing the likelihood of utilization by schools. Effective substance abuse prevention programs may work because of a few key components or they may be the result of the synergistic interactions of all program components.

While there is a paucity of knowledge about the relative effectiveness of various intervention components, some studies have addressed this issue. For example, many prevention approaches based on the social influence model have included a public commitment component; however, at least one study suggests that this component may not contribute to the effectiveness of these programs (Hurd et al., 1980). Similarly, many of these programs have used films or videotapes similar to those initially developed by Evans and his colleagues (Evans et al., 1978). However, it is not yet clear what type of media material is the most effective or the extent to which it is necessary as a component. In addition to studies testing the effectiveness of approaches in school settings, studies have also tested this intervention approach along with media (Flynn et al., 1992), parent (Rohrbach, Hodgson, Broder, & Montgomery, 1994), or media and parent (Pentz, Dwyer, et al., 1989; Perry, Kelder, Murray, & Klepp, 1992) components. These studies indicate that the inclusion of additional intervention components produces stronger prevention effects than the school-based intervention alone.

SUMMARY AND CONCLUSION

This chapter has focused on substance abuse prevention efforts in school settings. Schools are a natural and convenient site for conducting substance abuse prevention programs. Increasingly, educators are coming to recognize that promoting health and preventing substance abuse are vitally important both to the general well-being of their students and to the achievement of their primary educational objectives. Substance abuse prevention approaches that rely on providing students with information about the adverse consequences of using drugs have consistently been found to be ineffective—when the standard of effectiveness is deterring substance use. Similarly, efforts to promote affective development through unfocused, experiential activities have also been found to be ineffective.

The only prevention approaches that have been demonstrated to effectively impact on substance use behavior are those that teach junior high school students social resistance skills and antidrug norms, either alone or in combination with teaching generic personal and social skills. Both approaches emphasize skills training and de-emphasize the provision of information concerning the adverse health consequences of substance use. These approaches have been shown to work with different program providers and different target populations, including racial and ethnic minority youth. Despite generally impressive initial prevention effects, it is evident that without booster sessions these effects decay over time. Thus, to produce lasting prevention effects, it is necessary to have ongoing prevention activities throughout early adolescent years and perhaps until the end of high school.

The field of substance abuse prevention has advanced considerably in the past decade and a half. Yet, despite the promise offered by existing school-based approaches, additional research is needed to further refine current prevention models in order to optimize their effectiveness and increase our understanding of how they work. However, evidence now exists from a number of rigorously designed evaluation studies that specific school-based prevention models are effective. It is now incumbent upon health care professionals, educators, community leaders, and policymakers to move expeditiously toward wide dissemination and utilization of these approaches. It is equally important for private and governmental agencies to provide adequate funding for the important research necessary to further refine existing prevention models and to increase our understanding of the causes of substance abuse.

REFERENCES

Arkin, R. M., Roemhild, H. J., Johnson, C. A., Luepker, R. V., & Murray, D. M. (1981). The Minnesota smoking prevention program: A seventh grade health curriculum supplement. *Journal of School Health, 51,* 616–661.

Bandura, A. (1977). *Social learning theory.* Englewood Cliffs, NJ: Prentice-Hall.

Barnes, G. M., & Welte, J. W. (1986). Patterns and predictors of alcohol use among 7–12th grade students in New York State. *Journal of Studies on Alcohol, 47,* 53–62.

Baumrind, D., & Moselle, K. A. (1985). A developmental perspective on adolescent drug abuse. *Advances in Alcohol and Substance Abuse, 4*, 41–67.

Bell, R. M., Ellickson, P. L., & Harrison, E. R. (1993). Do drug prevention effects persist into high school? *Preventive Medicine, 22*, 463–483.

Bettes, B. A., Dusenbury, L., Kerner, J., James-Ortiz, S., & Botvin, G. J. (1990). Ethnicity and psychosocial factors in alcohol and tobacco use in adolescence. *Child Development, 61*, 557–565.

Blum, R., & Richards, L. (1979). Youthful drug use. In R. I. Dupont, A. Goldstein, & J. O'Donnell (Eds.), *Handbook on drug abuse (National Institute on Drug Abuse)* (pp. 257–267). Washington, DC: Government Printing Office.

Botvin, G. J., Baker, E., Botvin, E. M., Dusenbury, L., Cardwell, J., & Diaz, T. (1993). Factors promoting cigarette smoking among black youth: A causal modeling approach. *Addictive Behaviors, 18*, 397–405.

Botvin, G. J., Baker, E., Botvin, E. M., Filazzola, A. D., & Millman, R. B. (1984). Alcohol abuse prevention through the development of personal and social competence: A pilot study. *Journal of Studies on Alcohol, 45*, 550–552.

Botvin, G. J., Baker, E., Dusenbury, L. D., Botvin, E. M., & Diaz, T. (1995). Long-term follow-up results of a randomized drug abuse prevention trial in a White middle-class population. *Journal of the American Medical Association, 273*, 1106–1112.

Botvin, G. J., Baker, E., Dusenbury, L., Tortu, S., & Botvin, E. M. (1990). Preventing adolescent drug abuse through a multimodal cognitive-behavioral approach: Results of a 3-year study. *Journal of Consulting and Clinical Psychology, 58*, 437–446.

Botvin, G. J., Baker, E., Filazzola, A., & Botvin, E. M. (1990). A cognitive-behavioral approach to substance abuse prevention: A one-year follow-up. *Addictive Behaviors, 15*, 47–63.

Botvin, G. J., Baker, E., Renick, N. L., Filazzola, A. D., & Botvin, E. M. (1984). A cognitive-behavioral approach to substance abuse prevention. *Addictive Behaviors, 9*, 137–147.

Botvin, G. J., Batson, H. W., Witts-Vitale, S., Bess, V., Baker, E., & Dusenbury, L. (1989). A psychosocial approach to smoking prevention for urban black youth. *Public Health Reports, 104*, 573–582.

Botvin, G. J., & Botvin, E. M. (1992). Adolescent tobacco, alcohol, and drug abuse: Prevention strategies, empirical findings, and assessment issues. *Journal of Development and Behavioral Pediatrics, 13*, 290–301.

Botvin, G. J., & Cardwell, J. (1992). Primary prevention (smoking) of cancer in black populations. *Final Report to National Cancer Institute (NCI)* (grant contract number N01-CN-6508). Cornell University Medical College, Ithaca, NY.

Botvin, G. J., Dusenbury, L., Baker, E., James-Ortiz, S., Botvin, E. M., & Kerner, J. (1992). Smoking prevention among urban minority youth: Assessing effects on outcome and mediating variables. *Health Psychology, 11*, 290–299.

Botvin, G. J., Dusenbury, L., Baker, E., James-Ortiz, S., & Kerner, J. (1989). A skills training approach to smoking prevention among Hispanic youth. *Journal of Behavioral Medicine, 12*, 279–296.

Botvin, G. J., & Eng, A. (1980). A comprehensive school-based smoking prevention program. *Journal of School Health, 50*, 209–213.

Botvin, G. J., & Eng, A. (1982). The efficacy of a multicomponent approach to the prevention of cigarette smoking. *Preventive Medicine, 11*, 199–211.

Botvin, G. J., Eng, A., & Williams, C. L. (1980). Preventing the onset of cigarette smoking through life skills training. *Preventive Medicine, 9*, 135–143.

Botvin, G. J., Epstein, J. A., Schinke, S. P., & Diaz, T. (1994). Predictors of cigarette smoking among inner-city minority youth. *Developmental and Behavioral Pediatrics, 15*, 67–73.

Botvin, G. J., Goldberg, C. J., Botvin, E. M., & Dusenbury, L. (1993). Smoking behavior of adolescents exposed to cigarette advertising. *Public Health Reports, 108*, 217–224.

Botvin, G. J., Renick, N., & Baker, E. (1983). The effects of scheduling format and booster sessions on a broad-spectrum psychosocial approach to smoking prevention. *Journal of Behavioral Medicine, 6*, 359–379.

Botvin, G. J., Schinke, S. P., Epstein, J. A., & Diaz, T. (1994). The effectiveness of culturally-focused & generic skills training approaches to alcohol and drug abuse prevention among minority youth. *Psychology of Addictive Behaviors, 8*, 116–127.

Botvin, G. J., Schinke, S. P., Epstein, J. A., Diaz, T., & Botvin, E. M. (1995). Effectiveness of culturally focused and generic skills training approaches to alcohol and drug abuse prevention among minority adolescents: Two-year follow-up results. *Psychology of Addictive Behaviors, 9*, 183–194.

Caplan, M., Weissberg, R. P., Grober, J. S., Sivo, P., Grady, K., & Jacoby, C. (1992). Social competence promotion with inner-city and suburban young adolescents: Effects on social adjustment and alcohol use. *Journal of Consulting and Clinical Psychology, 60*, 56–63.

Chassin, L., Presson, C. C., Sherman, S. J., Corty, E., & Olshavsky, R. W. (1984). Predicting the onset of cigarette smoking in adolescents: A longitudinal study. *Journal of Applied Social Psychology, 14*, 224–243.

Comer, J. P. (1985). The Yale–New Haven Primary Prevention Project: A follow-up study. *Journal of the American Academy of Child Psychiatry, 24*, 154–160.

Demone, H. W. (1973). The nonuse and abuse of alcohol by the male adolescent. In M. Chafetz (Ed.), *Proceedings of the Second Annual Alcoholism Conference* (DHEW Publication No. HSM 73-9083) (pp. 24–32). Washington, D.C.: Government Printing Office.

Dielman, T. E., Leech, S. L., Lorenger, A. T., & Horvath, W. J. (1984). Health locus of control and self-esteem as related to adolescent health behavior and intentions. *Adolescence, 19*, 935–950.

Donaldson, S. I., Graham, J. W., & Hansen, W. B. (1994). Testing the generalizability of intervening mechanism theories: Understanding the effects of adolescent drug use prevention interventions. *Journal of Behavioral Medicine, 17*, 195–216.

Donaldson, S. I., Graham, J. W., Piccinin, A. M., & Hansen, W. B. (1995). Resistance skills training and onset of alcohol use: Evidence for beneficial and potentially harmful effects in public schools and in private catholic schools. *Health Psychology, 14*, 291–300.

Dorn, N., & Thompson, A. (1976). Evaluation of drug education in the longer term is not an optional extra. *Community Health, 7*, 154–161.

Dryfoos, J. G. (1993). Common components of successful interventions with high-risk youth. In N. J. Bell & R. W. Bell (Eds.), *Adolescent risk taking* (pp. 131–147). Newbury Park, CA: Sage.

Ellickson, P. L., & Bell, R. M. (1990). Prospects for preventing drug abuse among young adolescents. *Rand Publication Series*.

Ellickson, P. L., Bell, R. M., & McGuigan, K. (1993). Preventing adolescent drug use: Long term results of a junior high program. *American Journal of Public Health, 83*, 856–861.

Ennett, S. T., Tobler, N. S., Ringwalt, C. L., & Flewelling, R. L. (1994). How effective is drug abuse resistance education? A meta-analysis of project DARE outcome evaluations. *American Journal of Public Health, 84*, 1394–1401.

Epstein, J. A., Botvin, G. J., Diaz, T., & Schinke, S. P. (1995). The role of social factors and individual characteristics in promoting alcohol among inner-city minority youth. *Journal of Studies on Alcohol, 56*, 39–46.

Epstein, J. A., Botvin, G. J., Diaz, T., Toth, V., & Schinke, S. P. (1995). Social and personal factors in marijuana use and intentions to use drugs among inner city minority youth. *Journal of Developmental and Behavioral Pediatrics, 16*, 14–20.

Epstein, J. A., Dusenbury, L., Botvin, G. J., & Diaz, T. (1994). Determinants of intentions of junior high school students to become sexually active and use condoms: Implications for reduction and prevention of AIDS risk. *Psychological Reports, 75*, 1043–1053.

Evans, R. I. (1976). Smoking in children: Developing a social psychological strategy of deterrence. *Preventive Medicine, 5*, 122–127.

Evans, R. I., Rozelle, R. M., Mittlemark, M. B., Hansen, W. B., Bane, A. L., & Havis, J. (1978). Deterring the onset of smoking in children: Knowledge of immediate physiological effects and coping with peer pressure, media pressure, and parent modeling. *Journal of Applied Social Psychology, 8*, 126–135.

Felner, R. D., & Adan, A. M. (1988). The School Transitional Environment Project: An ecological intervention and evaluation. In R. H. Price, E. L. Cowen, R. P. Lorion, & J. Ramos-McKay (Eds.), *14 ounces of prevention: A casebook for practitioners* (pp. 111–122). Washington, DC: American Psychological Association.

Fishbein, M. (1977). Consumer beliefs and behavior with respect to cigarette smoking: A critical analysis of the public literature. In Anonymous (Ed.), *Federal Trade Commission Report to Congress pursuant to the Public Health Cigarette Smoking Act of 1976*. Washington, DC: Government Printing Office.

Fisher, D. A., Armstrong, B. K., & deKler, N. H. (1983). *A randomized-controlled trial of education for prevention of smoking in 12 year-old children*. Paper presented at the Fifth World Conference on Smoking and Health, Winnipeg, Canada.

Flay, B. R., Keopke, D., Thomson, S. J., Santi, S., Best, J. A., & Brown, K. S. (1989). Long-term follow-up of the first Waterloo smoking prevention trial. *American Journal of Public Health, 79*, 1371–1376.

Flynn, B. S., Worden, J. K., Secker-Walker, S., Badger, G. J., Geller, B. M., & Costanza, M. C. (1992). Prevention of cigarette smoking through mass media intervention and school programs. *American Journal of Public Health, 82*, 827–834.

Gfroerer, J. (1987). Correlation between drug use by teenagers and drug use by other family members. *American Journal of Drug and Alcohol Abuse, 13*, 95–108.

Gilchrist, L. D., & Schinke, S. P. (1983). Self-control skills for smoking prevention. In P. F. Engstrom, P. Anderson, & L. E. Mortenson (Eds.), *Advances in cancer control* (pp. 125–130). New York: Alan R. Liss.

Goodstadt, M. S. (1974). Myths and methodology in drug education: A critical review of the research evidence. In M. Goodstadt (Ed.), *Research on methods and programs of drug education*. Toronto: Alcoholism and Drug Addiction Research Foundation of Toronto.

Hamburg, B. A., Kraemer, H. C., & Jahnke, W. (1975). A hierarchy of drug use in adolescence: Behavioral and attitudinal correlates of substantial drug use. *American Journal of Psychiatry, 132*, 1155–1163.

Hurd, P., Johnson, C. A., Pechacek, T., Bast, C. P., Jacobs, D., & Luepker, R. (1980). Prevention of cigarette smoking in 7th grade students. *Journal of Behavioral Medicine, 3*, 15–28.

Jessor, R., & Jessor, S. L. (1972). On becoming a drinker: Social-psychological aspects of an adolescent transition. In Anonymous (Ed.), *Annual of the New York Academy of Sciences* (197th ed., pp. 199–213). New York: New York Academy of Sciences.

Jessor, R., & Jessor, S. L. (1977). *Problem behavior and psychosocial development: A longitudinal study of youth*. New York: Academic Press.

Jessor, R., & Jessor, S. L. (1982). Critical issues in research on adolescent health promotion. In T. Coates, A. Peterson, & C. Perry (Eds.), *Promoting adolescent health: A dialogue on research and practice* (pp. 447–465). New York: Academic Press.

Johnston, L. D., O'Malley, P. M., & Bachman, J. G. (1995). *National survey results on drug use from the Monitoring the Future Study, 1975–1994, Vol. I: Secondary school students*. Washinton, DC: U.S. Department of Health and Human Services.

Jones, C. L., & Battjes, R. J. (1985). *Etiology of drug abuse: Implications for prevention. NIDA Research Monograph No. 56*. Washington, DC: Government Printing Office.

Kandel, D. (1985). On processes of peer influences in adolescent drug use: A developmental perspective. *Advances in Alcohol and Substance Abuse, 3*(4), 139–163.

Kandel, D. B. (1978). Convergences in prospective longitudinal surveys of drug use in normal populations. In D. B. Kandel (Ed.), *Longitudinal research on drug use: Empirical findings and methodological issues* (pp. 3–38). Washington, DC: Hemisphere (Halsted-Wiley).

Kearney, A. L., & Hines, M. H. (1980). Evaluation of the effectiveness of a drug prevention education program. *Journal of Drug Education, 10*, 127–134.

Kim, S. (1988). A short- and long-term evaluation of "Here's Looking at You." II. *Journal of Drug Education, 18*, 235–242.

Kinder, B. N., Pape, N. E., & Walfish, S. (1980). Drug and alcohol education programs: A review of outcome studies. *International Journal of the Addictions, 15*, 1035–1054.

Kreutter, K. J., Gewirtz, H., Davenny, J. E., & Love, C. (1991). Drug and alcohol prevention project for sixth-graders: First-year findings. *Adolescence, 26*, 287–292.

Krosnick, J. A., & Judd, C. M. (1982). Transitions in social influence at adolescence: Who induces cigarette smoking? *Developmental Psychology, 18*, 359–368.

Luepker, R. V., Johnson, C. A., Murray, D. M., & Pechacek, T. F. (1983). Prevention of cigarette smoking: Three year follow-up of educational programs for youth. *Journal of Behavioral Medicine, 6*, 53–61.

Mason, M. L. (1973). Drug education effects. *Dissertation Abstract, 34*(4-B), 418.

McAlister, A., Perry, C., & Maccoby, N. (1979). Adolescent smoking: Onset and prevention. *Pediatrics, 63*, 650–658.

McAlister, A., Perry, C. L., Killen, J., Slinkard, L. A., & Maccoby, N. (1980). Pilot study of smoking, alcohol, and drug abuse prevention. *American Journal of Public Health, 70*, 719–721.

McGuire, W. J. (1964). Inducing resistance to persuasion: Some contemporary approaches. In L. Berkowitz (Ed.), *Advances in experimental social psychology* (pp. 192–227). New York: Academic Press.

McGuire, W. J. (1968). The nature of attitudes and attitude change. In G. Lindzey & E. Aronson (Eds.), *Handbook of social psychology* (pp. 136–314). Reading, MA: Addison-Wesley.

Meyer, R. E., & Mirin, S. M. (1979). *The heroin stimulus: Implications for a theory of addiction*. New York: Plenum.

Millman, R. B., & Botvin, G. J. (1983). Substance use, abuse, and dependence. In M. D. Levine, W. B. Carey, A. C. Crocker, & R. T. Gross (Eds.), *Developmental-behavioral pediatrics* (pp. 683–708). Philadelphia: Saunders.

Murray, D. M., Davis-Hearn, M., Goldman, A. I., Pirie, P., & Luepker, R. V. (1988). Four and five year follow-up results from four seventh-grade smoking prevention strategies. *Journal of Behavioral Medicine, 11*, 395–405.

Newcomb, M. D., & Bentler, P. M. (1986). Drug use, educational aspirations, and work force involvement: The transition from adolescence to young adulthood. *American Journal of Community Psychology, 14*, 303–321.

Newcomb, M. D., & Bentler, P. M. (1988). *Consequences of adolescent drug use: Impact on the lives of young adults*. Thousand Oaks, CA: Sage.

Page, P. M. (1989). Shyness as a risk factor for adolescent substance use. *Journal of School Health, 59*, 432–435.

Pentz, M. A. (1983). Prevention of adolescent substance abuse through social skill development. In T. J. Glynn, C. G. Leukefeld, & J. B. Ludford (Eds.), *Preventing adolescent drug abuse: Intervention strategies NIDA Research Monograph No. 47* (pp. 195–232). Washington, DC: Government Printing Office.

Pentz, M. A., Brannon, B. R., Charlin, V. L., Barrett, E. J., MacKinnon, D. P., & Flay, B. R. (1989). The power of policy: The relationship of smoking policy to adolescent smoking. *American Journal of Public Health, 79*, 857–862.

Pentz, M. A., Dwyer, J. H., MacKinnon, D. P., Flay, B. R., Hansen, W. B., Wang, E. Y., & Johnson, C. A. (1989). A multicommunity trial for primary prevention of adolescent drug abuse. Effects on drug prevalence. *Journal of American Medical Association, 261*, 3259–3266.

Perry, C., Killen, J., Slinkard, L. A., & McAlister, A. L. (1983). Peer teaching and smoking prevention among junior high students. *Adolescence, 9*, 277–281.

Perry, C. L., & Kelder, S. H. (1992). Models for effective prevention. *Journal of Adolescent Health, 13*, 355–363.

Perry, C. L., Kelder, S. H., Murray, D. M., & Klepp, K. I. (1992). Community-wide smoking prevention: Long-term outcomes of the Minnesota heart health program and the class of 1989 study. *American Journal of Public Health, 82,* 1210–1216.

Ray, O. S. (1974). *Drugs, society, and human behavior.* St. Louis: Mosby.

Resnicow, K., & Botvin, G. J. (1993). School-based substance use prevention programs: Why do effects decay? *Preventive Medicine, 22,* 484–490.

Richards, L. G. (1969). *Government programs and psychological principals in drug abuse prevention.* Paper presented at the annual convention of the American Psychological Association, Washington, DC.

Rohrbach, L. A., Hodgson, C. S., Broder, B. I., & Montgomery, S. B. (1994). Parental participation in drug abuse prevention: Results from the Midwestern Prevention Project. Special issue: Preventing alcohol abuse among adolescents: Preintervention and intervention research. *Journal of Research on Adolescence, 4,* 295–317.

Schaps, E., Bartolo, R. D., Moskowitz, J., Palley, C. S., & Churgin, S. (1981). A review of 127 drug abuse prevention program evaluations. *Journal of Drug Issues, 11,* 17–43.

Schinke, S. P. (1984). Preventing teenage pregnancy. In M. Hersen, R. M. Eisler, & P. M. Miller (Eds.), *Progress in behavior modification* (16th ed., pp. 31–63). New York: Academic Press.

Schinke, S. P., & Gilchrist, L. D. (1983). Primary prevention of tobacco smoking. *Journal of School Health, 53,* 416–419.

Schinke, S. P., & Gilchrist, L. D. (1984). Preventing cigarette smoking with youth. *Journal of Primary Prevention, 5,* 48–56.

Shope, J. T., Dielman, T. E., Butchart, A. T., & Campanelli, P. C. (1992). An elementary school-based alcohol misuse prevention program: A follow-up evaluation. *Journal of Studies on Alcohol, 53,* 106–121.

Smith, G. N., & Fogg, C. P. (1978). Psychological predictors of early use, late use, and non-use of marijuana among teenage students. In D. B. Kandel (Ed.), *Longitudinal research on drug use: Empirical findings and methodological issues.* Washington, DC: Hemisphere-Wiley.

Snow, D. L., Tebes, J. K., Arthur, M. W., & Tapasak, R. C. (1992). Two-year follow-up of a social-cognitive intervention to prevent substance use. *Journal of Drug Education, 22,* 101–114.

Sussman, S., Dent, C. W., Stacy, A. W., & Sun, P. (1993). Project towards no tobacco use: 1-year behavior outcomes. *American Journal of Public Health, 83,* 1245–1250.

Swisher, J. D. (1979). Prevention issues. In R. I. Dupont, A. Goldstein, & J. O'Donnell (Eds.), *Handbook on drug abuse* (pp. 49–62). Washington, DC: National Institute on Drug Abuse.

Swisher, J. D., Crawford, J. L., Goldstein, R., & Yura, M. (1971). Drug education: Pushing or preventing? *Peabody Journal of Education, 49,* 68–75.

Swisher, J. D., & Hoffman, A. (1975). Information: The irrelevant variable in drug education. In B. W. Corder, R. A. Smith, & J. D. Swisher (Eds.), *Drug abuse prevention: Perspectives and approaches for educators* (pp. 49–62). Dubuque, IA: Brown.

Task Force on Education of Young Adolescents. (1989). *Turning points: Preparing American youth for the 21st century.* Washington, DC: Carnegie Council on Adolescent Development.

Telch, M. J., Killen, J. D., McAlister, A. L., Perry, C. L., & Maccoby, N. (1982). Long-term follow-up of a pilot project on smoking prevention with adolescents. *Journal of Behavioral Medicine, 5,* 1–8.

Tye, J., Warner, K., & Glantz, S. (1987). Tobacco advertising and consumption: Evidence of a causal relationship. *Journal of Public Health Policy,* 492–507.

Wechsler, H. (1976). Alcohol intoxication and drug use among teenagers. *Journal of Studies on Alcohol, 37,* 1672–1677.

Wechsler, H., & Thum, D. (1973). Alcohol and drug use among teenagers: A questionnaire study. In M. Chafetz (Ed.), *Proceedings of the Second Annual Alcoholism Conference* (pp. 33–46). Washington, DC: Government Printing Office.

Weir, W. R. (1968). A program of alcohol education and counseling for high school students with and without a family alcohol problem. *Dissertation Abstract,* 28(11-A), 4454–4455.

Whelan, E. M. (1984). *A smoking gun: How the tobacco industry gets away with murder.* Philadelphia: Stickley.

Prevention in the Workplace

Paul M. Roman
University of Georgia

Terry C. Blum
Georgia Institute of Technology

The American workplace has great potential for both the primary and the secondary prevention of substance abuse. Most adult Americans are employed, and they work in settings that are characterized by employment rules and personnel policies. These structures allow for a number of different preventive interventions.

The effects of substance abuse on productivity would seem to make the workplace a high-priority emphasis for controlling this problem. Generally speaking, this has not been the case. While the employed problem drinker was a primary target of initiatives at the founding of the National Institute on Alcohol Abuse and Alcoholism (NIAAA), and while a great deal of progress in workplace programming has marked the past two decades, use of the workplace as an intervention site remains a somewhat marginal concern for the professional and occupational groups traditionally focused on substance abuse prevention.

Understanding barriers to the planning and implementation of workplace prevention efforts is an important concern of this chapter. First, however, it is important to provide a context by examining the range of strategies that have been developed that can be appropriately placed under the rubric of prevention. The scope of these activities may be more extensive than many observers would typically assume.

The most prominent intervention is the employee assistance program (EAP), a set of techniques encapsulated in varying policies and procedures that has diffused widely since the early 1970s (Blum & Roman, 1995). EAPs have become well known in the communities of substance abuse problem practitioners, and have important functions as the sources of clients for substance abuse treatment programs. It is likely that many assume EAPs to be the single worksite-based device for addressing issues in substance abuse.

EAPs are in many ways a paradigmatic illustration of secondary prevention. The strategy rests upon techniques of early identification of substance abuse, and there is great promise as well as established success in the effectiveness of early identification in producing motivation for change that can be accomplished through short-term treatment. (For a review, see Blum & Roman, 1995.) Counseling or treatment is a central part of EAP design, but as such, EAPs should deliver neither counseling nor treatment. Because they deal with problems at some stage of development, EAPs cannot be appropriately classified as primary prevention, despite the attractiveness of such claims in the contemporary context of limiting treatment. Their identity with the ambiguous area of secondary prevention may in part explain the marginality of worksite foci to the broader substance abuse problem field.

There are, however, several workplace strategies for primary prevention. These include prohibition and direct employee education, and other related strategies for changing behavior. Two other strategies can also be included under the rubric of prevention, but they intermingle concepts of primary, secondary, and tertiary prevention: peer intervention and "member" assistance programs, and efforts to assure employment of persons with substance abuse problems.

WORKPLACE PROHIBITION OF PSYCHOACTIVE SUBSTANCE USE

Among the several primary prevention strategies in the workplace, foremost is the presence of alcohol prohibition rules in nearly all workplaces. With the emergence of attention to illegal drugs, these were added to prohibition policy statements about 25 years ago. While these norms are so well institutionalized that they often escape recognition, alcohol and work have not always been segregated. Drinking breaks and on-the-job drinking were historically part of many occupational settings, and it has been observed that the provision of alcohol by employers was in some instances an accepted "right" of employment (Ames, 1989). While the explanation of America's partially successful temperance movement is typically traced to class conflicts and embedded pressures to preserve the status quo (Gusfield, 1963), it is clear that the industrial revolution and capitalist economic growth in 19th and early 20th century America probably contributed as much if not more to the acceptance of limitations on alcohol consumption (Clark, 1976; Rumbarger, 1989). This emphasis led directly to workplace prohibition.

While reams of pages have been written about the failure of alcohol prohibition in American history, the successful implementation and institutionalization of such prohibition in the workplace is easily and typically overlooked. Because of this neglect, and because of the almost total adoption of prohibition practices, there is essentially no research on the impact or effectiveness of the strategy.

While a recent study suggests that the extent of on-the-job drinking is far higher than is often assumed to be the case (Ames & Delaney, 1992), one can only speculate on the possibilities of high accident and injury rates were drinking allowed in combination with many of the machine technologies of today as well as those of the recent past. It would appear that the typical investment of resources in worksite prohibition are minimal, suggesting that prevention of even a small number of injurious events would render such investment cost-effective. But we know essentially nothing about the differential efficacy of the most widespread and time-honored workplace strategy of primary prevention aimed at employees' alcohol-related behaviors.

DIRECT PRIMARY PREVENTION STRATEGIES

Primary prevention remains a highly valued goal for interventionists. Its role in worksite programming can be broken into four categories: research with etiological intentions, workplace educational efforts, screening, and a residual category of health promotion and screening.

Social Etiology

There is a tradition, largely based in sociology, of locating workplace factors that have causal linkages to undesirable outcomes among employees. These include various job-related attitudes such as job satisfaction, alienation, and job commitment, and have also included a number of behavioral outcomes such as psychiatric impairment and substance abuse. The extensive literature in the latter category is typified by work by Cooper, Russell, and Frone (1990), Greenberg and Grunberg (1995), Martin and Roman (1996), and Parker and Farmer (1988).

Most recent instances of this work use job-related attitudes as mediators between adverse work conditions and substance abuse behaviors. While rarely explicit in these writings, the implications are definitely salient to primary prevention. Presumably if the noxious factors were removed, there would be positive increments in job attitudes as well as reductions in substance abuse behaviors. Missing in such formulations, however, are suggested strategies for implementing such changes in the workplace, many of which are structured by technology as well as by institutionalized patterns of management. Thus, from the perspective of primary prevention, these efforts are at best suggestive.

Education and Training

More recently, there have been reports of efforts at direct change of employee drinking and related behaviors. Unlike the previous research tradition, these studies are not grounded in ideas about how the workplace might be changed in order to prevent drinking problems, but instead operate from a fundamental educational model. Using relatively small study samples, Cook, Back, and Trudeau (1996) and Shain, Suurvali, and Boutilier (1986) demonstrated that workplace educational programs are associated with reduced drinking among employees. Stoltzfus and Benson (1994) conducted a pilot program in a manufacturing plant of 3M Corporation with a goal of informing employees about company policy, altering the company culture relative to substance abuse, and reducing drinking among employees. Unlike many such studies, these researchers used an experimental design. They found that their threefold strategy of supervisory training, employee training, and peer helper program produced statistically significant impacts in the desired directions around all three goals.

To qualify these findings somewhat, the Shain group reported that the educational program in their study workplaces was not associated with change in heavy drinkers but was associated with change in moderate drinkers. Further, Stoltzfus and Benson (1994) point out that the absolute rates of change found in their study were not great.

Such findings should be placed in the unusual context of the workplace. In the workplace, a single employee with a drinking problem can produce costs far in excess of that employee's wages, or the training investment that the company may have placed in the person. Potent examples of such impacts may include impaired judgments, mistakes in production, or damage to customer relations. Such an outcome could occur among moderate drinkers who, "on a lark," may have drank heavily the previous evening or drank during a workday lunch. The "prevented" events are not patterned, systematic, or necessarily visible. Thus an attempted experimental comparison of their incidence relative to a particular intervention might likely show little change.

Of significance is that an experimental impact can be produced in a natural workplace setting with such seemingly mundane inputs as training. There is a high potential for cost-effectiveness, which, unfortunately, may be very difficult to document. The implementation of such training likely will be restricted to those workplaces where progressive managers see the logic of hidden outcomes that are prevented through these interventions. In any event, such program implementation requires persuading managers of the value of investing employee training time around the subject of drinking in the face of pressures for training employees on topics more visibly linked to ongoing organizational performance.

Testing

Urine testing has been validated as a method of identifying job applicants who have used certain illegal drugs in the recent past (Macdonald & Roman, 1995). The appropriateness or effectiveness of drug screening as a primary prevention strategy has been the subject of much discussion and debate. Despite the furor, the majority of workplaces have adopted such policies, and their implementation has generally proceeded smoothly. Somewhat parallel to workplace prohibition, this strategy enjoys wide adoption, but rarely has been subjected to anything like a rigorous evaluation.

At issue is whether pre-employment screening identifies persons with drug problems; if it does, a second question arises about the propriety of simply turning these persons back into the community. Persons with problems may be identified in the applicant population, but rarely is anything done to direct such persons toward assistance. Indeed it is likely that few applicants who are found positive are made aware of this reason for their not being hired. There is no evidence that pre-employment drug screening reduces the rate of drug problems that are subsequently identified in workplaces. Oft-cited data indicating that positive pre-employment screens have declined only describes the behavior of job applicants, not the efficacy of pre-employment screening.

As a prevention strategy, random drug screening of current employees raises nearly all of the same issues as pre-employment screening, because it involves the same technology that neither identifies drug abusers nor performance impairment. Random screening is, however, a highly charged social ceremony, demonstrating both the evils of illegal drugs as well as the power of management, an excellent example of management as symbolic action (Pfeffer, 1981).

Screening done for cause fits more closely with traditional workplace intervention approaches, and is very commonly accompanied by referral to an EAP for assistance, but often with the condition that such an offer of help will not be repeated. By definition, for-cause screening is linked to a performance problem, which may involve accidents or injury. As a strategy, it is definitely a dimension of secondary prevention in that it identifies an existing problem and usually attempts some form of intervention.

Alcohol testing is currently mandated by U.S. Department of Transportation regulations, particularly following accidents. This is not an innovation, for many workplaces, as part of their "rules of conduct" or "fitness for duty" regulations, have reserved the right to test employees for the presence of alcohol either upon suspicion of intoxication or after an accident or other disruptive incident. However, there is yet to be developed a pre-employment test that would provide the employer with any reasonable assurance that an applicant has an alcohol problem. Such technology is being pursued, but prospects for successful development of a practical alcohol screening application are unknown. Were this to happen, it would have dramatic implications for other preventive interventions.

Health Promotion

Beyond these educational, behavior change, and screening strategies, another approach is currently of only minor consequence as a primary prevention strategy. There has been some suggestion that health promotion and wellness programs have potential effectiveness in the prevention of substance abuse problems. When health problems such as obesity, high blood pressure, or gastric problems are identified in some form of health-risk appraisal that is administered at the worksite, an agent with medical authority might suggest reduction in drinking as a means of alleviating the primary symptom. There is yet to be evidence of the widespread use or impact of such a strategy on employee drinking. Alternatively, it is possible that employees undertaking exercise programs or other health-oriented leisure activities might change their drinking behavior because of its lack of fit with their new regimen. Again, while such an intervention seems like a possibility, evidence of its implementation is lacking.

PEER AND MEMBER ASSISTANCE PROGRAMS

Since the 1970s, a range of professions encompassing medicine, law, dentistry, psychology, and nursing have reported activities among their members oriented toward resolving problems of alcohol abuse and alcoholism through peer intervention programs. Two intertwined rationales underlie such programs.

First, most professionals are not part of a typical employment relationship; they often have considerable autonomy in determining work hours, techniques, and other aspects of work styles. Indeed, independence of performance often marks highly creative or heroic accomplishments among professionals. A second feature is a strong sense of community such that members of a professional group tend to protect one another from external confrontations, interventions, or criticism. This relates to the first feature: to the extent that supervision of professionals occurs at all, it is typically one member of a profession supervising other members.

With these characteristics of work, typical organization-based interventions directed toward the substance abuse problems of professionals would have a low likelihood of effectiveness. It would be expected that professionals' problematic performance would be at a level of low visibility, that the power of professionals would make them highly resistant to any form of confrontation, and that professionals would readily cover up for each other.

However, it is likely that if anyone is aware of a professional's drinking problem, it is likely another professional. Given the distribution of power and the mode of governance within the professions, there is also a reasonable likelihood that professionals would pay attention to one another. Further, an aspect of the community of interest is that the deviance, misbehavior, or malpractice of one professional may have a widespread and adverse impact on professional peers. Finally, because most professions are certified or licensed through boards composed of professional peers, the profession itself may be in a unique position to threaten sanctions against nonconforming members.

It is these ingredients that are said to make up a peer intervention program for professionals. Such programs reportedly exist in a great number of locations, generally lodged in the local or statewide association of a particular professional group. The peer intervention programs are operated and governed by members of the profession, sometimes by members who have recovered from their own substance abuse.

As might be expected however, these groups do not readily admit outsiders to carry out objective research studies on the profession, particularly potentially threatening aspects such as the patterns of substance abuse among physicians or attorneys. Given what has been described about the nature of professional power and how it is maintained, this is certainly not surprising. Thus, while there are a number of reports of the success of these programs, they are prepared by the program operatives or by others with a clear vested interest in the program's success. Therefore, while professional peer intervention programs are widespread, practically nothing is known about them in terms of objective scientific data.

There is an important second category of peer interventions. A research group at Cornell University has been examining member assistance programs in labor unions for more than a decade. In a first set of studies (summarized in Sonnenstuhl, 1996), the focus was on a small, independent union with an intense drinking culture that included on-the-job drinking. Through the slow introduction of a union-based program to provide recovery assistance to alcoholic union members (a program manned by a union member who was a recovering alcoholic), a gradual transformation of the workplace drinking culture emerged, with acceptance of recovery and abstinence as chosen lifestyles, and diminution of the near-universal pressure to drink with work peers both on and off the job. This was a dramatic example of a change in what appeared to be deeply entrenched drinking norms, and the study is suggestive of the potential for preventive impact through workplace interventions directed toward cultural change.

A second set of studies by the Cornell group (Bacharach, Bamberger, & Sonnenstuhl, 1994) focused on member assistance programs with broader ranges of coverage. They examined programs in the railroad industry and one organized by the flight attendants in commercial air transportation. The research findings were almost uniformly positive regarding the impact of these programs. While there was no means for comparing the relative efficacy of these member assistance programs with management-based EAPs, it is clear that from an absolute basis, the programs had an impact on the substance abuse of union members across these wide-ranging settings within the transportation industry.

The focus on a single type of industry and the lack of comparison with other types of strategies are obvious limitations of this research. The applicability of the findings is also constricted by the relative small proportion of the labor force that is unionized and the apparent continuing decline of this coverage. The findings are of considerable importance, and offer an important addition to ongoing evaluations of traditional, management-based EAPs.

Many prognosticators see the American workplace moving more toward a model of peer organization, accompanied by a decline in traditional patterns of top-down hierarchical management. This generic model includes many features of participative management and collective responsibility within the rank and file. Should this transformation prove to be true, the model of a peer or member assistance program may have considerable applicability for dealing with employees' substance abuse. Perhaps its most attractive feature is its operation outside traditional definitions of authority, power, and accompanying opportunities for coercion and threat. Such features appear as parallel descriptions of what have been accepted for several decades as successful models of alcoholism treatment and sobriety maintenance.

On the other hand, we are still in the dark regarding the actual dynamics and effectiveness of peer intervention programs within groups of relatively affluent and powerful professionals. To some extent, the research on member assistance programs tends to have a working-class orientation. While the Cornell group's work offers an abundance of insights, it is remarkably uncritical, offering virtually no descriptions of program dysfunctions, problematic incidents, or unsuccessful outcomes. Peer intervention is not without its potential difficulties. By defining and implementing actions toward deviant behavior within an informal and undocumented framework, potential abuses may be greater than when power is implemented through a bureaucratic hierarchy. While bureaucracy remains as a negative connotation, many of its features that openly define authority, procedure, and rules offer opportunities for equitable treatment and for lodging grievances to seek justice when these definitions are breached.

In sum, peer and member intervention programs are important new frontiers for addressing substance abuse among employed people. A good research and conceptual foundation has been launched with studies of member assistance programs, indicating that their success and potential are very real.

ASSURING EMPLOYMENT OF PERSONS WITH SUBSTANCE ABUSE PROBLEMS

In the triad of primary, secondary, and tertiary prevention, least attention is paid to the last. The concept is centered around avoiding permanent losses through disability and impairments that preclude full social participation. Central in such social participation is employment. Most treatment evaluations affirm that employment is probably the single most important predictor of long-term success following substance abuse treatment. Thus, it may be important to promote interventions that increase the likelihood of employment of treated or recovering substance abusers for the purpose of tertiary prevention.

It is perhaps curious that very little attention has been paid to assuring the employment of treated and recovering substance abusers. While rarely discussed, it is clear that the design of EAPs anticipate this problem by trying to assure that a gap in employment does not occur.

As a socially stigmatized group, there is no doubt that treated and recovering alcoholics are targets of discrimination in the hiring process. In part this is due to the social construction of alcoholism that the alcoholism interventionists themselves have produced. This dilemma is evident in the compulsive use of the term "recovering" rather than "recovered" to describe sober alcoholics. This substitution occurred sometime in the 1970s, whereas the term "recovered" had seemed to enjoy a degree of prior institutional acceptance. Apparently it is assumed that "recovering" emphasizes the growth that may continue in "working" the AA program or other therapeutic regimens. It may also signal to alcoholics that they are "one drink away" from a relapse, reflecting the context of requiring total abstinence as the sole route to dealing with the disease of alcoholism.

These ideological and therapeutic intentions likely create considerable confusion for the employer, especially when coupled with the message "alcoholism is a disease like any other." There can be little doubt that employers are encouraged to expect relapse and unpredictability on the part of persons labeled as alcoholic, with these being clearly problematic in many if not most workplaces. It is unfair to assume that employer gatekeeping reduces employment of alcoholics against the wishes of the rank-and-file workforce. Similar doubts and ambivalence exists among potential co-workers and supervisors. Although there is clearly an increase in levels of social acceptance of alcoholism as a legitimate disease (permitting roles paralleling the treatment of those suffering from other diseases), data clearly indicate that substantial proportions of the general public are ambivalent toward or socially reject alcoholic persons (Blum, Roman, & Bennett, 1989).

One of the few documents developed to persuade employers about the value of hiring persons with alcohol or drug problems is remarkably counter-persuasive (National Institute on Drug Abuse, 1983). The "four important reasons" for hiring such persons include that they "may" prove to be better-than-average employees, that it is illegal to discriminate against them, that hiring may give the employer access to government tax credits, and finally, that refusing to hire such persons does not guarantee that the company does not already have employees with alcohol and drug problems on the payroll, and that hiring a treated person could encourage these other employees to seek treatment. It is difficult to see how these arguments could do anything but affirm negative attitudes toward such hiring.

The landscape in regard to such hiring may be changing, however (Bruyere, 1996). The Americans with Disabilities Act (ADA) specifically proscribes discrimination against persons with alcohol or drug problems. The legislative provisions reflect the ambivalence and confusion that is created by the several ideological stances of the interventionists that were discussed above. The most clearcut categories of protected individuals under this section of the legislation are persons who have formerly been in treatment programs, who indicate that they have a history of substance abuse in the past, and those who are currently in a treatment program and performing successfully. Those who are currently using illegal drugs are not protected by the legislation. The most ambiguous group that is subject to protection includes persons with a current or past history of alcohol problems who are currently using alcohol, assuming that they are able to perform the essential requirements of the job.

There are yet no accumulated data on the impact of ADA provisions on the hiring of treated, recovering, or possibly active alcoholics. Rather than centering on hiring issues, much of the action around ADA is concerned with dismissal of employees. It is quite clear that employers may face litigation if they discipline or dismiss employees with alcohol or drug problems who are actively trying pursue treatment or rehabilitation (i.e., those who clearly do not accept their problem and want to do something about it). These implications bolster the importance of EAPs.

EMPLOYEE ASSISTANCE PROGRAMS

History

Part of the core of EAPs goes back to the 1940s (Trice & Schonbrunn, 1981). Led by the example of the medical director of the DuPont Corporation, workplace physicians used the emerging fellowship of Alcoholics Anonymous to bring alcoholic employees back to levels of effective performance through AA participation.

The actions these physicians took were indirect, however. The resulting program involved extending "12-Step" work into a quasi-professional mode. Through some form of mutual acquaintance, employees in several major work organizations who were AA members were recruited by company physicians to penetrate their organization's alcoholic population. Their jobs were to convince relatively visible alcoholic employees to affiliate with AA, and then foster and sustain these work peers' AA affiliation through continuing workplace follow-up. It is important to recognize that this innovation typically occurred with the support and sponsorship of a nonalcoholic company-employed physician, often the corporate medical director. This endorsement was a critical vehicle for carrying the AA modality (and ultimately, support for formal alcoholism treatment) into the workplace.

This genre of industrial alcoholism programming became formalized in several dozen more worksites over the next two decades. Despite the simplicity of the concept as an approach to dealing with the otherwise unresolved problem of workplace alcoholism, the idea did not really catch on.

All of this changed rather dramatically with the establishment and funding of the National Institute on Alcohol Abuse and Alcoholism (NIAAA) in 1970 (Roman, 1981). NIAAA adopted workplace programming as a major priority, part of a larger effort to mainstream the treatment of alcohol problems into the overall health care system (Roman & Blum, 1987). A new and different programming model emerged, partly as a step toward mainstreaming, and partly as a result of the general bewilderment among NIAAA staff and their consultants over the slowness of the model's diffusion over the previous decades.

Core Technology

The key components and core technology of EAPs (Blum & Roman, 1989; Roman, 1988) can be summarized in four categories of techniques or strategies. These assure maximum impact of EAPs that include a clear focus on substance abuse. To a considerable extent, these categories embody the technical program standards advanced by the national association of EAP providers, the Employee Assistance Professionals Association.

First, there should be a written policy clearly based on job performance. Such a statement should include the notion that employees' behaviors are significant to the employer to the extent that these behaviors impinge on job performance. EAP policy does not supersede in any way preexisting rules of conduct or fitness for duty policies. Supervisors' responsibility is to document events of performance problems, with an eye toward an eventual confrontation if these accumulate

Second, the EAP should be appropriately staffed with experts in substance abuse and be directly and immediately accessible to supervisors and employees. The EAP coordinator should be integrated into the workplace, so that supervisors and employees respect his/her knowledge of the workplace. The coordinator should be readily available to provide consultative assistance to supervisors on how to appropriately deal with employees suspected to have EAP-relevant problems.

Third, supervisors, employees, and union representatives should be aware of and supportive of the use of the strategy of constructive confrontation. When documented evidence of performance problems have accumulated beyond guidelines of acceptable work behavior, and the employee does not volunteer to participate in guided behavioral change, constructive confrontation is implemented. Constructive confrontation is centered on the evidence of performance problems, and presents disciplinary steps that will be taken unless performance is improved. The context includes the supportive assistance of the company to suspend discipline if the employee will undertake counseling or treatment.

Fourth, the EAP coordinator should link employees with appropriate resources for assistance with substance abuse and other problems, engage in case management through the treatment period, and implement long-term follow-up based in the workplace. Resources are selected on the basis of established effectiveness, and referrals should be consistent with employees' particular health insurance coverage and with employees' job demands and career contingencies. The linkage is not a suggestion or recommendation, but the EAP coordinator is directly involved in linkage and monitors compliance. Further, the coordinator participates in re-entry and involves supervisors as appropriate, generates post-treatment support linkage, and engages in work-based supportive follow-up for 36 months or longer.

Effectiveness

It is foolhardy to make blanket statements about the effectiveness of EAPs in dealing with employee substance abuse, because "success" has so many possible contingencies. First, there is often confusion as to whether EAP goals are centered upon clinical improvement or job performance improvement. These two outcomes are far from perfectly correlated; the remission of symptoms does not necessarily assure that the employee will be able to perform adequately on the job. Employers often do not address the question of the specific goals of their company's program. While it can be argued that the employer may benefit from an employee's clinical improvement as well as from the employee's return to effective work performance, such a blending of goals does not give the EAP appropriate direction. Likewise, such vagueness can make the EAP vulnerable to subsequent program evaluations focused upon "hard" work-based program outcomes.

Second, well-designed EAPs can produce poorer-than-expected results when one or more key techniques of EAP practice are missing. Often these missing components are the nonclinical strategies that must be in place for EAPs to realize their full potential with employees troubled by substance abuse. These include the absence of sound training of supervisors in the nature and goals of the EAP, what the supervisor should and should not do when facing a suspected employee substance abuse problem, and how to access EAP services. In some otherwise well-designed programs, there may be a high degree of social distance and low social visibility between members of the workforce and the EAP functionaries they need to access in order to obtain assistance. Another common example of a missing element is the absence of consistent follow-up after an employed individual has undergone some form of intervention and counseling and has returned to the job. Data indicate that EAP functioning may be significantly impeded, especially with employed persons with substance abuse, when follow-up is not consistently implemented (Foote & Erfurt, 1991).

In addition to unclear goals and missing EAP components, a third issue is that EAP effectiveness may also be impacted by the interventions and treatments that are made available to employees. It should be clear that while EAPs are deeply involved with directing employed persons toward interventions and toward treatments, EAPs are not treatment delivery systems. EAP personnel should be equipped to select the most appropriate treatment, direct an employed client toward that treatment, and conduct routine follow-up after return to the job. But since EAPs cannot deliver treatment, their success is contingent upon the kinds of treatment that are available in the community or accessible through the employer's health care plan. There is a strong belief that treatment ineffectiveness is more likely associated with EAPs that are heavily controlled in their treatment referrals by managed care contractors. While refusing access to adequate care would be expected to have an adverse effect on outcomes among employed persons with substance abuse problems, this has not yet been documented.

An extensive review of both published and unpublished studies of EAP effectiveness produced overwhelming consensus that they work, using generalized criteria of return on investment in the program (Blum & Roman, 1995). Such conclusions are somewhat risky when standards for effective EAPs are not adequately diffused or enforced. Despite current notions that EAP designs vary greatly, much of the apparent differences are cosmetic as far as program effectiveness is concerned. There is a core of EAP techniques that must be present. In the most general terms, there is clear evidence that there is no substitute for ongoing and consistent attention to the employee's motivation to recover his or her full level of functioning.

BARRIERS TO THE DEVELOPMENT
OF WORKPLACE INTERVENTIONS

At the opening of the chapter, we alluded to the relative marginality of attention to the workplace within the larger complex of preventive programming to deal with substance abuse. This also describes a major barrier structured into worksite perceptions, namely the lack of salience of substance abuse issues to the ongoing concerns of the workplace.

Of course, substance abuse programming in any major social institution such as a workplace, a school, or a church should not be that institution's primary concern. Likely it should not even be on the short list of organizational priorities. But unlike schools and religious institutions where "soft" socioemotional types of activities are primary, the subcultural theme of the workplace is "hard" and instrumental: getting the work out, being at the top of the competitive ladder, and putting first things first.

While there is no doubt that a vast number of social issues have worked their way into workplace attention, managerial concern, and ultimately institutionalized programming, this does not mean that new concerns defined as social issues are welcomed with open arms. Instead, the reaction is more likely "Enough already!" Thus a key hurdle that must be overcome in drawing employers' attention to substance abuse issues is establishing salience in terms of the direct and indirect costs rendered to both productivity and human resources, as well as the disruption produced by such behaviors.

A second principal barrier to the types of worksite programming that have been described here is gaining both employers' and employees' attention to substance abuse. The legal status of alcohol and its use by a majority of both employers and employees is a built-in pressure toward a generalized pattern of normalization of apparent alcohol problems; there is not a high degree of social distance between workplace personnel and alcohol problems, which has been shown to lead to a generalized reluctance to take action toward such problems (Trice & Belasco, 1968). Thus it is critical to draw attention away from the actual problems and toward the various and sundry consequences of the problematic behaviors, nearly all of which cause disruption and exact significant costs from workplace operation.

A third major barrier is embedded in the tremendous societal attention that has been drawn to the distribution and use of illegal drugs. This concern has certainly extended to the workplace, and is manifest in remarkably large investments in drug-testing programs, despite the clear evidence of the limited efficacy of such strategies (Macdonald & Roman, 1995). There are a variety of complex reasons why employers and the workplace in general have been drawn into strong concerns and concerted efforts to deal with suspected drug problems among employees (Roman & Blum, 1995).

In complex and contradictory ways, alcohol and drug issues are linked in the public mind, the orientations of managers and workers, as well as in the clinical reality of the overlap of patterns of use and abuse (cf. Blum et al., 1989). But in direct contrast to alcohol, most employers and employees sense great social distance between themselves and the use of illegal drugs, manifest in a high level of readiness to act. While it is possible that some of the attention to illegal drugs in the workplace has had positive "spillover" effects on alcohol-related programming, these effects are minimal compared to the symbolic contrasts that are generated between alcohol and illegal drugs. Resources to deal with substance abuse in the workplace are certainly limited, having increased from being virtually nonexistent several decades ago.

Thus, attention to workplace alcohol problems is muted by programming and what may be largely symbolic managerial actions (Pfeffer, 1981) toward illegal drug issues. Beyond the stretching of resources is the simple sense that the workplace is "doing something" about substance abuse issues through its attention to drug problems. Within the framework of the differential senses of social distance, the energies devoted to drugs may help keep alcohol issues out of sight and out of mind, relatively speaking.

A fourth barrier lies in the mainstreaming of alcohol problems that is implicit in the design of EAPs. As mentioned, EAPs were designed to blunt the image of dealing with workplace alcohol problems, and to shift the focus away from the problems themselves to the salient consequences they produce in the workplace. The mechanisms for assuring this were first to train supervisors to identify and refer to EAP staff particular types of employees whose performance had slipped below par for no discernible reason associated with job conditions; and second, to encourage self-referral to EAP staff of employees who perceived that they had problems that were affecting their job performance.

Both of these mechanisms served to draw attention away from alcohol problems. Unless it was specifically emphasized in specially designed training, the mode of supervisory identification offered no counterpressures to supervisors' expected orientation away from subordinates who they suspected might have alcohol problems. Through these means, the mechanism obliquely encouraged referral of those whose suspected conditions did not carry the stigma or emotional charge of substance abuse. In the case of self-referral, where opportunities for employee training were not likely, employees were actually encouraged to self-identify those problems that were least likely to stigmatize them. Within the clinical lore of alcohol problem treatment, it is certainly possible that a problem drinker who had hit bottom would self-refer, but such behavior is hardly to be expected among those who, within the design of an EAP, are supposed to be in the category of early identification.

Lest the impression be left that these flaws were intractably built into the EAP model, it is clear that some carefully designed and implemented supervisory training curricula included both an emphasis on the costliness of the employee troubled by alcohol or drugs, and strategic guidance about constructive confrontation as vital for motivating the employee with substance abuse problems. But from a purist perspective, there is a rather blatant contradiction in emphasizing the identification of a particular problem category while urging that supervisory attention be focused solely upon job performance issues.

Thus, the key to the success in sustaining an emphasis on employee substance abuse problems is access to consultation from an EAP operative who is competent in dealing with these problems, while sustaining the basic program principles of the EAP. This brings attention to a third potential weakness beyond the referral process itself, namely EAP structures that did not offer access to consultation with an EAP expert, or where such consultation might not include expertise about substance abuse.

These problems were endemic to some externally contracted EAPs, where neither the EAP providers or their organizational clients had particular interests in reaching employees with substance abuse problems, but were interested in the overall "help" mode that was presented by the EAP concept. This returns us to the first and primary barrier to workplace programming, drawing employers' and employees' attention to substance abuse. Thus, while it is evident that much progress has been made in implementing workplace interventions that are effective, many barriers remain for sustaining the gains that have been made as well as for further diffusion.

WORKPLACE-RELATED PREVENTION RESEARCH

While some programmatic concepts enjoy a wide reception because of the intrinsic attraction of their "logic" at the time they are introduced, a sound research foundation ultimately becomes indispensable for sustaining the momentum of any innovation and assuring its institutionalization. Research studies confirm the value of a particular intervention, specify an intervention's strong and weak points, and especially provide for its fine-tuning when it is implemented in varied populations.

Research related to workplace substance abuse programming has developed slowly and sporadically. Although an effort to institutionalize such research was represented by the presence of an Occupational Programs Branch in NIAAA during its first decade, the demise of this branch in reorganization left worksite programming and research without the potency of an organizational base for research and development. Research related to these issues has been funded, with applications being reviewed in the contexts of epidemiology, prevention strategies, and treatment. More recently the potential has developed within the National Institutes of Health for the funding of such studies under the rubric of health services research.

Several recent and ongoing studies point to possibilities of primary prevention of substance abuse at the worksite. One study, building on a long tradition of research on the consequences of worker alienation, confirmed a direct linkage between alienation and the likelihood of problem drinking among blue-collar workers (Greenberg & Grunberg, 1995). A program of research on workplace harassment has revealed direct connections between problematic drinking behavior and experiences of sexual harassment in a professional socialization setting (Richman, 1992). Another recent study used a substantial sample of different worksites to examine patterns of managerial and worker drinking behavior. Data from the study indicate that managerial drinking behavior is directly tied to the cultural characteristics of work settings (Howland et al., 1996). The spillover effects of drinking that serves to cope with job-related stresses were demonstrated in a new study (Martin & Roman, 1996). Finally, a recent analysis looked beyond the workplace to examine the dynamics of drinking with co-workers away from the worksite. This study revealed that data collections that look only at job-related drinking and their connections to job conditions and interactions will underestimate the contributions of work linkages to drinking behavior (Martin, Roman, & Blum, 1996).

In addition to these publications, each of these cited groups has ongoing research studies, looking, for example, at the relationships between employees' drinking behavior and a range of independent variables: worksite downsizing, participative management and workgroup reorganization, cross- national managerial styles, instrumental social support at work, and a range of harassment behaviors extending beyond sexual harassment. Thus, the upcoming decade should be marked by considerable new knowledge about the workplace roots and consequences of employee substance abuse.

ACKNOWLEDGMENTS

The authors gratefully acknowledge support from Grant No. R01-DA-07417 from the National Institute on Drug Abuse and Grant No. R01-AA-10130 from the National Institute on Alcohol Abuse and Alcoholism.

REFERENCES

Ames, G. (1989). Alcohol related movements and their effects on drinking policies in American workplaces: An historical review. *Journal of Drug Issues, 19,* 489–510.

Ames, G., & Delaney, W. (1992). Minimization of workplace alcohol problems: The supervisor's role. *Alcoholism: Clinical and Experimental Research, 16,* 180–189.

Bacharach, S. B., Bamberger, P., & Sonnenstuhl, W. (1994). *Member assistance programs in the workplace.* Ithaca, NY: ILR Press of Cornell University Press, ILR Bulletin No. 69.

Blum, T. C., & Roman, P. (1989). Employee assistance and human resources management. In K. Rowland & G. Ferris (Eds.), *Research in personnel and human resources management* (Vol. 7, pp. 258–312). Greenwich, CT: JAI Press.

Blum, T. C., & Roman, P. (1995). *The cost effectiveness and preventive implications of employee assistance programs.* Washington, DC: Substance Abuse and Mental Health Administration, Center on Substance Abuse Prevention Monograph 5.

Blum, T. C., Roman, P., & Bennett, N. (1989). Public images of alcoholism: Data from a Georgia survey. *Journal of Studies on Alcohol, 50,* 5–14.

Bruyere, S. M. (1996). *Employing and accommodating individuals with histories of alcohol or drug abuse.* Ithaca, NY: ILR Program on Employment and Disability, Cornell University.

Clark, N. S. (1976). *Deliver us from evil.* New York: Norton.

Cook, R. F., Back, A., & Trudeau, J. (1996). Preventing alcohol use problems among blue collar workers: A field test of the Working People Program. *Substance Use and Misuse, 31,* 255–275.

Cooper, M. L., Russell, M., & Frone, M. (1990). Work stress and alcohol effects: A test of stress-induced drinking. *Journal of Health and Social Behavior, 31,* 260–276.

Foote, A., & Erfurt, J. (1991). Effects of EAP followup on prevention of relapse among substance abuse clients. *Journal of Studies on Alcohol, 52,* 241–248.

Greenberg, E. S., & Grunberg, L. (1995). Work alienation and problem drinking behavior. *Journal of Health and Social Behavior, 36,* 83–106.

Gusfield, J. (1963). *Symbolic crusade.* Urbana: University of Illinois Press.

Howland, J., Mangione, T., Kuhlthau, K., Bell, N., Heeran, T., Lee, M., & Levine, S. (1996). Worksite variation in managerial drinking. *Addiction, 91,* 1007–1017.

Macdonald, S., & Roman, P. (Eds.). (1995). *Drug testing in the workplace.* New York: Plenum.

Martin, J. K., & Roman, P. (1996). Job satisfaction, job reward characteristics and employees' problem drinking behaviors. *Work and Occupations, 23,* 4–25.

Martin, J. K., Roman, P., & Blum, T. (1996). Job stress, drinking networks, and social support at work: A comprehensive model of employees' problem drinking behaviors. *Sociological Quarterly, 37,* 579–599.

National Institute on Drug Abuse. (1983). *Employer's guide to the employment of former drug and alcohol abusers.* Washington, DC: Department of Health and Human Services Publication No. ADM-83-1292.

Parker, D. A., & Farmer, G. (1988). The epidemiology of alcohol abuse among employed men and women. In M. Galanter (Ed.), *Recent developments in alcoholism* (Vol. 6, pp. 113–130). New York: Plenum.

Pfeffer, J. (1981). Management as symbolic action. In L. Cummings & B. Staw (Eds.), *Research in organizational behavior* (Vol. 3, pp. 11–52). Greenwich, CT: JAI Press.

Richman, J. (1992). Occupational stress, psychological vulnerability and alcohol related problems over time in future physicians. *Alcoholism: Clinical and Experimental Research, 16,* 166–171.

Roman, P. (1981). From employee alcoholism to employee assistance: An analysis of the de-emphasis on prevention and on alcoholism problems in work-based programs. *Journal of Studies on Alcohol, 42,* 244–272.

Roman, P. (1988). Growth and transformation in workplace alcoholism programming. In M. Galanter (Ed.), *Recent developments in alcoholism* (Vol 6, pp. 131–158). New York: Plenum.

Roman, P., & Blum, T. (1987). Notes on the new epidemiology of alcoholism in the USA. *Journal of Drug Issues, 11*, 321–332.

Roman, P., & Blum, T. (1995). Employers. In R. H. Coombs & D. Ziedonis (Eds.), *Handbook of drug abuse prevention* (pp. 139–158). Englewood Cliffs, NJ: Prentice-Hall.

Rumbarger, J. J. (1989). *Power, profits and prohibition: Alcohol reform and the industrializing of America, 1800–1930*. Albany: State University of New York Press.

Shain, M., Suurvali, H., & Boutilier, M. (1986). *Healthier workers: Health promotion and employee assistance programs*. Lexington, MA: Heath.

Sonnenstuhl, W. J. (1996). *Working sober*. Ithaca, NY: ILR Press of Cornell University Press.

Stoltzfus, J. A., & Benson, P. (1994). The 3M alcohol and other drug prevention program. *Journal of Primary Prevention, 15*, 147–159.

Trice, H. M., & Belasco, J. (1968). Supervisory training about alcoholics and other problem employees: A controlled evaluation. *Journal of Studies on Alcohol, 29*, 392–398.

Trice, H. M., & Schonbrunn, M. (1981). A history of job-based alcoholism programs, 1900–1955. *Journal of Drug Issues, 11*, 171–198.

18

Prevention in the Community

Mary Ann Pentz

Institute for Health Promotion and Disease Prevention Research,
University of Southern California

Based on 1988 estimates, alcohol and drug abuse costs the American public over $144 billion per year in treatment, crime, lost work time, accidents, and related morbidity and mortality (Rice, Kelman, Miller, & Dunmeyer, 1990; Rice, Max, Novotony, Schultz, & Hodgson, 1992). Controlling substance abuse and its related costs to society starts with youth. Unfortunately, after several years of slight decline shown in youth tobacco, alcohol, and marijuana use during the last half of the 1980s, tobacco and marijuana use are again increasing among youth at the rate of 1% to 2% per year, and heavy alcohol use (as indexed by reported drunkenness) has not changed (Johnston, 1995). These statistics suggest that youth continue to experiment with drugs and may progress to abuse levels even more rapidly than in previous years, despite prevention efforts that have received continuous federal funding since the 1980 U.S. Anti–Drug Abuse Act (Bukoski, 1990). The logical question raised by these trends is: What is wrong with our current prevention efforts?

EFFECTIVENESS OF PREVENTION PROGRAMS: SCHOOL VERSUS COMMUNITY

To date, the majority of prevention efforts have taken the form of school-based educational programs. The most effective programs focus on counteracting social pressures to use drugs; incorporate interactive social learning methods such as modeling, role-playing, and group discussion; and include standardized teacher training, periodic booster sessions, and home-work activities with parents (Botvin, Baker, Dusenbury, Botvin, & Diaz, 1995; Pentz, 1994a; Tobler, 1992). These programs have achieved 20% to 60% or more net reductions in tobacco and marijuana use, and lesser reductions in alcohol use (Botvin et al., 1995; Pentz, 1994a). The reductions are typically calculated as the difference in rates of drug use increase between program and control groups, divided by the control group rate of increase, rather than as absolute differences in the proportion of drug users (Pentz, 1994a). While these effects seem substantial, they tend to concentrate on occasional use rates such as average monthly use rather than the heavy or regular use rates that are typically associated with substance abuse morbidity (Rice et al., 1992). The effects also dissipate 1 to 4 years after the program has ended (Pentz, 1995b; Tobler, 1992). One exception is a life-skills training program that showed maintenance of effects at 5-year follow-up on monthly tobacco use, and on monthly and regular use of alcohol and marijuana (Botvin et al., 1995). This program was more comprehensive than most school pro-grams, incorporating 30 sessions over a 3-year period. Another exception showed strong effects on weekly tobacco use through the end of the inter-vention period, which included continuous school and mass media program-ming across 4 years (Jason, Ji, Anes, & Birkhead, 1991).

The loss of prevention effects from most school programs over time may be associated with several factors that constitute limitations to implement-ing school-based prevention programs in isolation of or independent of other efforts. One limitation is that prevention programs compete with regular academic subject areas for teaching time and resources; the result may be the delivery of an abbreviated prevention program that does not provide students with adequate exposure to prevention skills. Another is that schools vary from year to year in their commitment to implementing prevention programs; the commitment tends to vary as a function of pro-gram novelty and whether the school district or an outside source provides funding for program delivery (Farquhar, Fortman, Maccoby, et al., 1984; Pentz, 1994a). A third limitation is that the prevention principles taught in school programs are not sufficiently disseminated to the extracurricular settings that constitute the greater community. The likely result is that the school program has no impact on changing one of the strongest predictors of youth substance use: social norms (Hansen, 1992). A fourth limitation is that schools are mandated to change knowledge but not behavior; a possible result is that over time, schools may gravitate toward teaching more didac-tic, knowledge-based programs rather than the skills-based programs that have shown effects on changing substance use behavior (Tobler, 1992).

Given the limitations of school-based prevention programs, it would seem logical to expand prevention efforts to the larger community in ways that would compensate for these limitations. There are several practical advantages to complementing a school-based prevention program with community prevention activities or programs. First, the community represents a larger pool of prevention activities and resources to draw on than a school with its limited, competing academic agendas. This pool also offers more variety to sustain the novelty of drug prevention programs. Second, including the community is likely to increase support of and thus regular commitment to implementing school-based programs. That is, the greater the community's understanding of what and why prevention programs are taught in schools, and how effective programs may decrease the prevalence of drug use, violence, and delinquency in the community, the more likely the community will increase its support of such programs in the form of volunteer time, monitoring public places, and money. Third, efforts that include the community could potentially reach a larger audience than just school-attending youth—for example, community leaders whose work affects youth in out-of-school settings, and young adults who serve as role models for youth. Fourth, involving the community capitalizes on expertise and influences that enable youth to practice substance use avoidance behavior and value activities not involving substance use. For example, business leaders could model marketing or job-hunting skills for youth; community leaders who direct youth service agencies could develop leisure-time programs to continue resistance skills training taught in school.

Compared to school-based programs, community-based drug prevention programs are a fairly recent phenomenon, one that has proliferated since the mid-1980s and has only begun yielding results since the early 1990s. Most of these community programs vary considerably in their interpretation of what constitutes a drug prevention program and in their relationship to school programs. For example, the Kaiser Family Health Foundation's community prevention initiative and the Robert Wood Johnson Foundation's Fighting Back program have funded small to moderate-sized communities to coordinate drug prevention and treatment services that are individually tailored to meet the needs of each specific community; the emphasis is on service networking and referral rather than linking with school-based programs (Pentz, 1994b). The Center for Substance Abuse Prevention (CSAP)'s Community Partnership grants fund communities to build coalitions among existing agencies, schools, and groups related to drug abuse prevention, with the intent to streamline the delivery of prevention services and reduce duplication (Johnson, Amatetti, Funkhoser, & Johnson, 1988). At least five programs developed from individual research projects or collaborative trials have integrated school prevention programs with one or more additional community programs or strategies that were evaluated in quasi-experimental designs involving mass media, community organizations for drug abuse prevention, and parent programs (Bowen, Kinns, & Orlandi, 1995; Jason et al., 1991; Kelder, Perry, & Klepp, 1993; Murray et al., 1992; Pentz, 1994a).

Results from community-based prevention programs vary, partially because of a lack of standardization of what constitutes a "community" program, and partially because of differences in the methodologies used to evaluate programs. For example, the CSAP and Robert Wood Johnson Foundation grants focused on evaluating the process of coalition-building, service networking, and community leader communication. Process evaluations of programs funded by these grants suggest that they were successful in achieving these aims (Pentz, 1986; Robert Wood Johnson Foundation, 1993; U.S. Congress, 1991). Three out of four recent quasi-experimental studies have shown that school programs conducted in combination with mass media, parent, and community organization programs yield significant reductions in regular (weekly or daily) adolescent tobacco use that are maintained through the end of high school, 4 to 5 years after cessation of intervention, as well as reductions in occasional use as found from school programs based on social influences (Jason et al., 1991; Kelder et al., 1993; Pentz, 1994a). One of these studies also showed reductions in alcohol and marijuana use, with similar alcohol reductions and greater marijuana reductions than those found from a comprehensive school-based program (Botvin et al., 1995; Pentz, 1994a). A fourth study showed no differences between two states participating in either a multicomponent community and state intervention or no multicomponent intervention (Murray et al., 1992). A fifth study, the COMMIT collaborative trial, was a community program involving community education, cessation clinics, mass media, and community organization for reducing tobacco use, with a primary focus on adults (Bowen et al., 1995). School programs were not included. There were no significant diffusion effects on youth (Bowen et al., 1995). As noted earlier, only one school-based prevention program has shown sustained effects on adolescent substance use through the end of high school and, moreover, three successive years of continued intervention were required to achieve these effects (Botvin et al., 1995; Hansen, 1992; Tobler, 1992). The overall trend in results would suggest that multicomponent community-based prevention programs, with school programming included as a central component, may yield stronger, longer effects on decreasing adolescent substance use than school programs alone (Murray, Moscowitz, & Dent, 1996).

ARGUMENTS FOR COMMUNITY-BASED PREVENTION

Theory of Effectiveness

If we are to accept the premise that community-based prevention programs may yield the strongest possible effects on reducing youth substance use, we should examine why or how these programs yield such effects. Examination of this question constitutes a search for the appropriate theoretical premise of behavioral change on a community level, and consequently, development of hypotheses about program mediators—that is, the mechanisms by which community programs produce behavioral change. There are at least four theoretical premises or arguments for the greater effects achievable from community-based prevention programs: (a) the argument for affecting more risk factors at more levels, based on transactional theory; (b) the argument for greater message consistency, based on expectancy-value theory; (c) the argument for more dissemination channels, based on diffusion of innovation theory; and (d) the argument for addressing demand *and* supply reduction, based on skills and reinforcement principles from learning theory. Each of these will be discussed in turn.

Affecting More Risk Factors at More Levels

Transactional theory posits that an individual's personality is formed or changed as a result of the interaction of intra-, inter-, and extrapersonal factors (Magnusson, 1981). Applied to the understanding of substance use development and prevention, an adolescent's behavior toward substance use is formed or changed as a result of the interaction of personal-level factors (intrapersonal history of prior drug use, skills, support-seeking, and physiological reaction), situation-level factors (interpersonal and group influences of drug use modeling, pressures or offers to use drugs, peer and family communication and support, and peer group transitions), and environment-level factors (extrapersonal media influences, resources, community norms and policies, and demographic factors) (Hawkins, Catalano, & Miller, 1994; Murray & Perry, 1985; Pentz, 1986, 1994a, 1994b, 1995b).

The general interactional pattern of personal, situational, and environmental factors ($P \times S \times E$) is shown in Fig. 18.1 (adapted from Pentz, 1986). The most effective school-based prevention programs—those that focus on counteracting social influences to use drugs—address personal-level factors of resistance skills, and ability to appraise drug-use situations and models; and situation-level factors of perceived social norms and avoidance of drug-using groups and drug-use opportunities (Hansen, 1992; Tobler, 1992). A few also include coping and support-seeking skills (e.g., Pentz, Pentz, & Gong, 1993), or general social skills related to coping, such as problem-solving and assertiveness skills (Botvin et al., 1995). Thus, school-based programs are designed to affect psychosocial risk factors operating at the level of individual and group. Community-based programs can address individual and group-level risk factors with school and parent program components. In addition, community-based programs can address environment-level risk factors by including mass media, community organization, and policy change strategies, all of which are beyond the scope, budget, and influence of school-based programs.

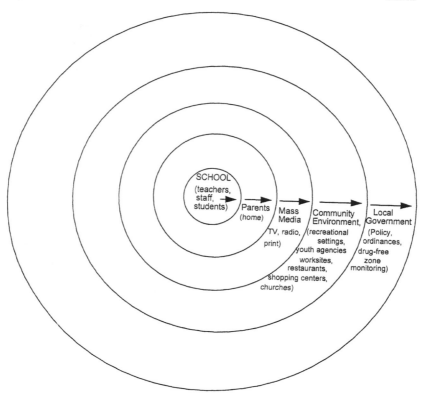

FIG. 18.1. Community influences on adolescent drug use behavior representing potential prevention program dissemination channels.

Community-based prevention programs, with their greater capacity to address personal, situation, and environment-level risk factors, are more likely than school-based programs to produce a larger, synergistic or interactive effect rather than a simple additive effect on reducing drug-use risk and, subsequently, drug-use behavior. For example, avoiding drug-use situations and peers is likely to produce a decrease in perceived social norms for drug use, and over time, an actual decrease in social norms for drug use in the community (Hansen, 1992). Lower social norms, in turn, should produce an intolerant attitude toward drug use, which results in a change in formalized drug policy. This sequential, synergistic effect is larger than the simple effect of an individual's resistance to an offer of drugs, resulting in a decrease in that individual's drug use. The synergistic effect is also larger than any additive effect derived from combining personal-, situation-, or group-level skills. For example, an individual youth's resistance plus a parent's choice to no longer model drug use (for example, cigarette smoking) in the presence of that youth may affect family members' drug use. However, youth resistance and parent behavioral choices may steer the family toward greater involvement in community prevention activities, which reinforce nonuse social norms in the community.

A few examples illustrate this synergistic effect. The youth program of the Minnesota Heart Health Project included a school program, parent education and homework activities, and changing food services in the school environment (Kelder et al., 1993). Results have shown effects on student tobacco use, parent–child communication and knowledge of healthy eating habits, and school food selection; school food selection is assumed to have had a synergistic effect with parent–child knowledge of nutrition (Kelder et al., 1993). A school–community tobacco project supported the adoption of a restrictive community tobacco policy through school and media programs (Jason et al., 1991). Results showed increased compliance as well as lower tobacco use among youth. The Midwestern Prevention Project, an adolescent community-based drug abuse prevention trial, included school, parent, community organization, mass media, and policy change components (Pentz, Dwyer, et al., 1989). Results have shown effects on decreasing adolescent drug use and parent marijuana use, increasing parent–child communications about drug use prevention, and facilitating development of prevention programs, activities, and services among community leaders (Mansergh, Rohrbach, Montgomery, Pentz, & Johnson, 1996; Pentz, Johnson, et al., 1989). These results are in contrast to results of even the most lengthy or comprehensive school-based programs, where effects have been limited to reducing youth drug use (Botvin et al., 1995; Hansen, 1992; Tobler, 1992).

Greater Message Consistency

Expectancy-value theory posits that an individual's attitudes, decisions, and intentions about future behavior are shaped by knowledge about the behavior, initial values about the behavior, and the interaction of expectancies and evaluation or subjective judgments about behavioral consequences (Azjen & Fishbein, 1980). Applied to the prevention of drug use, an adolescent's delay or reduction in using drugs will be determined by the number, frequency, and consistency of prevention messages that impart knowledge about avoiding drug use, values or advantages pertaining to this avoidance, information about consequences to expect from the use or avoidance of drugs, and decision-making guidelines by which to weigh these consequences (Flay & Petraitis, 1994; Pentz, 1994a). The greater the number, frequency, and consistency of these prevention messages, the more rapidly an adolescent will shape attitudes and normative expectations conducive to nonuse, the stronger the adolescent's intention to avoid drug use will be, and consequently, the more likely that the adolescent will delay or avoid subsequent drug use.

The general message consistency model adapted from expectancy-value theory is shown in Fig. 18.2. The model represents an abbreviated portion of more extensive models of person, situation, and environment influences (Flay & Petraitis, 1994; Pentz, 1986). The consistency of a prevention message is assumed to be positively and linearly related to the rate and strength of acquisition of knowledge, values, expectancies, and evaluations supportive of nonuse. Consistency is also assumed to be related to the speed with which the sequence of nonuse attitudes, intentions, and behavior is enacted.

School-based prevention programs depend primarily on a single channel for program delivery: through teachers in schools. Thus, the frequency, dissemination, and control of prevention messages is limited, and may or may not be consistent with messages disseminated through other channels in the community—for example, mass media messages that glamorize drug use. Alternatively, community-based prevention programs—if designed cor-

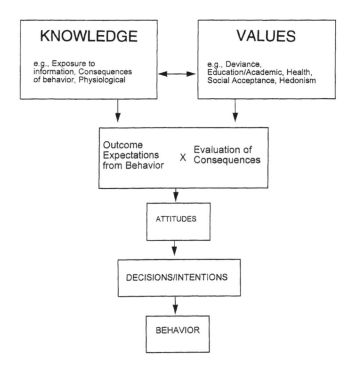

FIG. 18.2. Influences on prevention message consistency. Adapted from Flay and Petraitis (1994) and Ajzen and Fishbein (1980).

rectly—have the capacity to develop and control the content, frequency, and rate of dissemination of prevention messages through schools, parent groups, community organizations, and mass media (Pentz, 1993a). Greater message consistency is likely to translate to more rapid formulation of non-drug-use attitudes, intentions, and behavior.

At least three community-based prevention programs illustrate the use of message consistency. The Minnesota Heart Health Project coordinated mass media, educational, and screening center messages for heart health and heart disease prevention (McGovern, et al., 1996). Although the primary focus of intervention was on adults, the consistency of messages about heart disease prevention diffused to affect smoking behavior in adolescents (Kelder et al., 1993). The COMMIT trial coordinated smoking cessation messages for adults through the use of community education, smoking cessation clinics, agency services, and community coalitions (Bowen et al., 1995). There is some evidence that these messages also diffused to affect changes in community and school tobacco policies for youth (Bowen et al., 1995). The Midwestern Prevention Project serves as an example of message consistency directly aimed at youth (Pentz, Brannon, et al., 1989). Prevention messages developed for commercials, news series, and talk shows were geared toward demonstrating a youth's decision to select nonuse activities and parent–child communications showing support of nonuse activities (Pentz, 1990). The messages were consistent with the content of the school and parent programs. Frequent, varied broadcasting of these consistent messages influenced station managers to select other programs and ads that were consistent with prevention, and reduce broadcasting that appeared to glamorize drug use. The effect of planned on unplanned media coverage was also synergistic and continued for almost 5 years (Pentz, 1990). The consistency and continuation of these messages would not have been possible with a school program alone.

More Dissemination Channels

Extending the argument of greater message consistency is the argument that the use of more channels or opportunities for prevention message (program) delivery, the greater the likelihood that a new behavior will be adopted. The argument is based on diffusion of innovation theory, which posits that highly visible and credible innovators adopt a program, that a program is first implemented through a single credible channel most proximal to the population of interest, and that early program implementation be followed by sequenced implementation (dissemination) through additional channels selected on the basis of their relationship to the first channel and to the target population (Rogers, 1987). To apply this to drug-use prevention, community leaders or school administrators would adopt and promote a selected prevention program, which might be implemented first in schools, where adolescents are most easily reached. The success of school program implementation would be disseminated to parents, who would then participate in an extended prevention program at home with their adolescents following the school program. The school and parent programs—with school and home as program channels—would follow with related programs and channels. For example, mass media prevention programs could be targeted to adolescents and their parents who had participated in the school and parent programs, and simultaneously reach family members and other interested community residents who would constitute a modeling influence on adolescents.

The general model of program channels that represent successive influences on youth drug use and opportunities for program diffusion is shown in Fig. 18.3 (Pentz, 1994a). School is the first and central program channel,

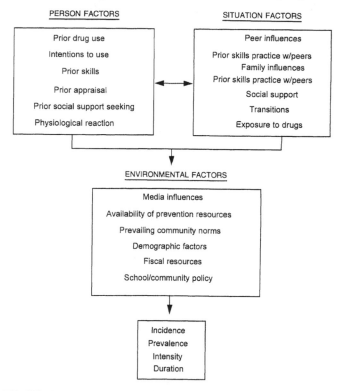

FIG. 18.3. Integrated Person × Situation × Environmental perspective to development and prevention of adolescent drug use behavior. Reprinted with permission from M. A. Pentz, Primary prevention of adolescent drug abuse. In C. B. Fisher & R. M. Lerner (Eds.), *Applied Developmental Psychology* (pp. 435–474). New York: McGraw-Hill, 1993.

because schools are where most adolescents spend the majority of their day, and where educational programming is expected (Pentz, 1993b). Also, teachers and peers serve as important models for behavior. Home is the second program channel, where parents and siblings can potentially extend prevention messages from a school program through homework activities, family discussion, and special family–school nights where parent–child skills training is provided. Parents serve as models for drug use prevention behavior as well as guides for setting risk behavior limits for youth. Mass media, particularly television, is the third program channel. Although its reach cuts across all levels shown in Fig. 18.3, the strength of mass media influence on adolescent drug use behavior may be mediated by school and home influences and programs. Community agencies, services, and settings represent a more removed influence on drug use among youth than the school or home, and where most youth spend less time. Yet the community environment may constitute the most important influence on changing perceived and actual social norms for drug use—the strongest predictors of youth drug use after previous use, and the influences most amenable to change in a prevention program (Hansen, 1992; MacKinnon et al., 1991). Finally, the social norms and normative changes effected by the community environment can, in turn, affect local tobacco, alcohol, and illicit drug use policies in the community (Pentz, 1995a). For example, there is increasing evidence to suggest that nonuse social norms in the community are related to support of restricted access policies (Forster, Hourigan, & McGovern, 1992), and that prevention- and support-oriented policies representing nonuse social norms are related to lower youth tobacco use (Pentz, Brannon, et al., 1989).

Four community-based prevention projects illustrate the use of multiple program channels to affect drug use or other health risk behavior in youth. In one opportunistic study, dissemination and support for a change that had occurred in a community tobacco policy was increased by the joint implementation of a school tobacco prevention program and positive mass media coverage of police and policy enforcement (Jason et al., 1991). In a second study, the Minnesota Heart Health Project, tobacco prevention and nutrition were simultaneously addressed in a school program, parent activities and family night at school, and cafeteria food service policy (Kelder et al., 1993). In a third study, community intervention strategies have been developed to restrict youth access to tobacco (Forster et al., 1992). To promote more rapid community adoption of restricted access policies, these strategies have been accompanied by youth activism and educational programs and messages that are delivered through the school and community. Unlike the other projects, the MPP utilized sequenced rather than simultaneous implementation of multiple program channels (Pentz, Dwyer, et al., 1989). School, home, television and print, community agency, and local government program channels for substance abuse prevention were introduced into communities at the rate of 6 months to 1 year apart over a 5-year period. The order and sequencing of program channels was based on the proximal to remote influences on youth drug use shown in Fig. 18.3, as well as on communication theories suggesting the use of variable programming to maintain high interest in the community (Farquhar et al., 1984).

Addressing Both Demand and Supply Reduction

Extending the previous three arguments is the argument that reducing youths' demand for drugs, and subsequently their use of drugs, may be easier if the supply of available drugs is also reduced. The argument for a dual focus on demand *and* supply reduction is based on several principles of experimental and social learning theory, including stimulus variability, generalization, and behavioral transfer (Bandura, 1977; Rotter, 1954). Applied to drug-use prevention, most intervention strategies have been aimed at either demand reduction (e.g., social and resistance skills training programs, parent–child communications training), or supply reduction (restricted access policies), but not to both.

A dual focus on demand and supply reduction can be achieved through one or more of the following strategies in a community-based intervention. The first strategy is the integration of prevention programs and policies. School, parent, and community educational programs that focus on promoting nonuse messages and awareness and support of existing no-use policies can be implemented. Where no-use policies do not formally exist, programs can be used to promote awareness of the need for adoption of such policies. These policies, on the other hand, would include reference and referral to prevention programs.

The second strategy is supportive enforcement of the policy. For example, a community intervention could include youth activism and community education to support local police and extend the responsibility to the community of monitoring drug-free zones. Third, a community intervention could enable or enhance the potential for strategic prevention with youth— that is, the smooth, continuous funneling of youth through primary prevention programs, to special topic or counseling programs, to broad-based, multifocus student assistance programs, to treatment and back to school (Pentz, 1993a). For example, a community organization or coalition of service providers could develop mechanisms for streamlining referrals of at-risk youth from student assistance programs to the appropriate drug abuse treatment program, and back again.

Two community-based programs illustrate the potential for effecting both demand and supply reduction through a dual focus on program and policy change. The Center for Substance Abuse Prevention (CSAP) Community

Partnership grants, actually a collection of over 200 different community-based coalitions and programs, have utilized partnerships among community leaders and agencies to promote both changes in drug policies, and implementation of various prevention programs and activities. Recent findings show an average of six drug policies implemented per community, and an insignificant trend toward lower youth drug use in communities with partnerships and programs functioning for at least 2 years compared to nonpartnership/nonprogram communities (CSAP, 1996). The Midwestern Prevention Project, in the latter 2 years of a 5-year intervention, coordinated the prevention education activities of a community organization for the prevention of drug abuse, with lobbying for local program funding and restricted access policies for youth (Pentz, Bonnie, & Shopland, 1996).

One current community program illustrates strategies for supporting enforcement of local policies (Forster et al., 1992). In this program, youth serve as community activists to promote tobacco policy change, rally support for voluntarily restricting youth access to tobacco, and monitor vendors for policy compliance.

Finally, several of the CSAP community partnerships have the potential to illustrate the effective process and outcome of strategic prevention strategies, particularly those that have targeted all youth for primary prevention as well as high-risk youth for special services or counseling (CSAP, 1996). Comparative data are not yet available for these particular partnerships.

CURRENT STATUS OF COMMUNITY-BASED PREVENTION PROGRAMS

Available data suggest that there are several advantages and disadvantages to the use of community-based substance abuse prevention programs compared to other types of prevention programs or strategies. The data are limited by the relatively few studies available on these programs for youth, the lack of experimental comparisons between community and other programs such as school programs, and the relative lack of experimental studies using community as the unit of analysis and a sufficient number of communities to detect program effects.

In terms of advantages, as noted earlier, there is some evidence that community-based programs may have longer-lasting effects on youth substance use compared to school or other single-channel programs (Murray et al., 1996; Pentz, 1994a). Community-based programs also appear to contribute to and sustain prevention coalition-building in the community, whereas there is no published evidence to suggest that school or other single-channel prevention programs achieve this end (Mansergh et al., 1996). Similarly, there is evidence to indicate that community-based programs develop methods, resources, and funding to institutionalize prevention programming after an initial research phase and funding has ended, whereas there is little evidence to suggest that institutionalization occurs with single-channel prevention programs (CSAP, 1996; Mansergh et al., 1996; Mittelmark, 1990; McGovern et al., 1996; Wandersman & Giamartino, 1980). Finally, there is increasing evidence that community-based prevention programs increase the empowerment of community leaders to design and implement new prevention initiatives as an offshoot or extension of the original community program (CSAP, 1996; Mansergh et al., 1996; Wandersman & Giamartino, 1980). While there are few findings on empowerment from single-channel programs such as school programs, the lack of data suggests that empowerment from these programs is low and is not expected.

There are several disadvantages to community-based prevention programming that render it difficult to implement compared to school-based and other single-channel programs. First is the expense. Although estimates differ, rough comparisons suggest that community programs may cost about four times as much as a school program—approximately $24 versus $6 per student per year (Pentz, 1995b, in press). Second, both programmatically and experimentally, a community as a unit of implementation is much more diverse and difficult to control than a school in terms of confounds, standards of implementation, and rates of program adoption (Pentz, 1994a). The diversity of strategies and timelines for coalition-building, and progress from coalition-building to program implementation experienced in the CSAP community partnerships, illustrate this disadvantage (Mansergh et al., 1996). Third, related to diversity, is communities' tendency to adopt and implement grass-roots prevention strategies that are unique or individually tailored to the needs of a particular community, rather than programs that are standardized across several communities (Pentz, 1995a). This tendency was illustrated by the Robert Wood Johnson Fighting Back communities, which opted to design their own individual programs and strategies rather than those developed from research (Robert Wood Johnson Foundation, 1993). Fourth, substance abuse, and any program aimed at its prevention, competes with other problems and programs that surface in communities. Although schools face a similar competition of interests, the problem is particularly acute for communities, which represent multiple rather than single bureaucratic and political pressures. The intensity of competition increases in direct relationship to the length of time a drug abuse prevention program has already been in effect and the extent to which a competing program is perceived as more novel (Farquhar et al., 1984). Both the Midwestern Prevention Project and the Minnesota Heart Health Project have experienced this competition with other health interests after the first 7 years (Mittlemark, 1990; Pentz, 1994a).

FUTURE DIRECTIONS

Future directions for community-based drug abuse prevention can be classified as recommendations for practice and recommendations for research. In reality, they are interrelated.

In terms of practice, community-based prevention programs could benefit significantly from developing local expertise in evaluating outcomes. The recent experiences of the CSAP and Robert Wood Johnson communities, where local outcome evaluations were delayed or poor in quality, bear this point out. Following the logic of strategic prevention, existing community coalitions and organizations could develop better information sharing and referral procedures for linking primary prevention, secondary or selective prevention, and treatment services than they have been able to show thus far. Finally, in recognition of competing interests and the community's need for novelty, community-based prevention programs could plan, after the first three or more years, a sequential phase-in of programming for other health and social problems known to be related to substance abuse; for example, violence or accident prevention. Given that etiologic and epidemiologic research has already shown evidence for a common set of risk factors underlying substance abuse, unsafe sex, violence, and school failure, it would appear logical for communities to plan for prevention programs that address these behaviors and their common risk factors (Jessor, 1982; Perry & Jessor, 1985).

In terms of research, experimental methods could be developed to provide better controls over a community's maintenance of its assigned experimental condition (e.g., commitment of a community to retain its control status and not adopt other similar programs during a study), or to restrict a community sampling pool to communities that provide strong evidence of readiness for programming (Boruch & Shadish, 1983). More attention should be paid to the routine analysis of unplanned national or community events that would be expected to affect a community's intervention or control status, or behavioral outcomes. For example, recent national mass media coverage suggests that tobacco companies have increased the level of nicotine in cigarettes. The effect of this phenomenon on prevention program effects on adolescent daily smoking rates could be analyzed in time series analyses, or in repeated measures analyses of variance that code time periods for before or after tobacco company patents for increased nicotine in cigarettes. Finally, community-based prevention research should routinely analyze the main and interactive effects of existing local tobacco, alcohol, and other drug policies with program effects, on adolescent drug use, and the potential effects of programming on local policy change at the community and school levels. This research direction will first require several advance steps before causal hypotheses about the relationship between program, policy, and drug use can be developed. These steps include the development and validation of a typology of demand- and supply-oriented policies, and epidemiological studies of the relationship of high community drug use levels to the adoption of restrictive or punitive policies versus supportive policies.

ACKNOWLEDGMENTS

This research was supported by grants from the National Institute on Drug Abuse (DA03976).

REFERENCES

Ajzen, I., & Fishbein, M. (1980). *Understanding attitudes and predicting social behavior*. Englewood Cliffs, NJ: Prentice-Hall.

Bandura, A. (1977). *Social learning theory*. Englewood Cliffs, NJ: Prentice-Hall.

Boruch, R. F., & Shadish, W. R. (1983). Design issues in community intervention research. In E. Seidman (Ed.), *Handbook of social intervention* (pp. 73–98). Beverly Hills, CA: Sage.

Botvin, G. J., Baker, E., Dusenbury, L., Botvin, E. M., & Diaz, T. (1995). Long-term follow-up results of a randomized drug abuse prevention trial in a white middle-class population. *Journal of the American Medical Association, 273*, 1106–1112.

Bowen, D. J., Kinns, S., & Orlandi, M. (1995). School policy in COMMIT: A promising strategy to reduce smoking by youth. *Journal of School Health, 65*, 140–144.

Bukoski, W. J. (1990). The federal approach to primary drug abuse prevention and education. In J. A. Inciardi (Ed.), *Handbook of drug control*. Westport, CT: Greenwood.

Center for Substance Abuse Prevention. (1996, August 1–2). *National evaluation of the community partnership demonstration program*. Technical assistance meeting. Washington, DC.

Farquhar, J. W., Fórtmann, S. P., Maccoby, N., et al. (1984). The Stanford Five-City Project: An overview. In J. D. Matarazzo, et al. (Eds.), *Behavioral health: A handbook of health enhancement and disease prevention*. New York: Wiley.

Flay, B. R., & Petraitis, J. (1994). The theory of triadic influence: A new theory of health behavior with implications for preventive interventions. *Advances in Medical Sociology 4*, 19–44.

Forster, J. L., Hourigan, M. E., & McGovern, P. (1992). Availability of cigarettes to underage youth in three communities. *Preventive Medicine, 21*, 320–328.

Hansen, W. B. (1992). School-based substance abuse prevention: A review of the state of the art in curriculum, 1980–1990. *Health Education Research, 7*, 403–430.

Hawkins, J. D., Catalano, R. F., & Miller, J. Y. (1992). Risk and protective factors for alcohol and other drug problems in adolescence and early adulthood: Implications for substance abuse prevention. *Psychological Bulletin, 11*, 64–105.

Jason, L. A., Ji, P. Y., Anes, M. D., & Birkhead, S. H. (1991). Active enforcement of cigarette control laws in the prevention of cigarette sales to minors. *Journal of the American Medical Association, 266*, 3159–3161.

Jessor, R. (1982). Problem behavior and developmental transition in adolescence. *Journal of School Health, 52*, 295–300.

Johnson, E. M., Amatetti, S., Funkhoser, J. E., & Johnson, S. (1988). Theories and models supporting prevention approaches to alcohol problems among youth. *Public Health Reports, 103,* 578–586.

Johnston, L. D. (1995, July). *Changing trends, patterns and nature of marijuana use.* Paper presented at the NIDA, National Conference on Marijuana Use: Prevention, Treatment, and Research, Arlington, VA.

Kelder, S. H., Perry, C. L., & Klepp, K. I. (1993). Community-wide youth exercise promotion: Long-term outcomes of the Minnesota Heart Health Program and the Class of 1989 study. *Journal of School Health, 63,* 218–223.

MacKinnon, D. P., Johnson, C. A., Pentz, M. A., Dwyer, J. H., Hansen, W. B., Flay, B. R., & Wang, E. Y. I. (1991). Mediating mechanism in a school-based drug prevention program: First-year effects of the Midwestern Prevention Project. *Health Psychology, 10,* 164–172.

Magnusson, D. (Ed.). (1981). *Toward a psychology of situations: An international perspective.* Hillsdale, NJ: Lawrence Erlbaum Associates.

Mansergh, G., Rohrbach, L., Montgomery, S. B., Pentz, M. A., Johnson, C. A. (1996). Process evaluation of community coalitions for alcohol and other drug prevention: Comparison of two models. *Journal of Community Psychology, 24,* 118–135.

McGovern, P. G., Pankow, J. S., Shahar, L., Doliszny, K. M., Folsom, A. R., Blackburn, H., & Luepker, R. V. (1996). For the Minnesota Heart Survey Investigators. Recent trends in acute coronary heart disease mortality, morbidity, medical care, and risk factors. *New England Journal of Medicine, 334,* 884–890.

Mittlemark, M. (1990). Balancing the requirements of research and the need, of communities. In N. Bracht (Ed.), *Health promotion at the community level.* Newbury Park, CA: Sage.

Murray, D. M., Moskowitz, J. M., & Dent, C. W. (1996). Design and analysis issues in community-based drug abuse prevention. *American Behavioral Scientist, 39,* 853–867.

Murray, D. M., & Perry, C. L. (1985). The prevention of adolescent drug abuse: Implications of etiological, developmental, behavioral, and environmental models. In C. L. Jones & R. J. Battjes (Eds.), *Etiology of drug abuse: Implications for prevention* (NIDA Research Monograph No. 56).

Murray, D. M., Perry, C. L., Griffin, G., Harty, K. C., Jacobs, D. R., Schmid, L., Daly, K., & Pallonen, U. (1992). Results from a state-wide approach to adolescent tobacco use prevention. *Preventive Medicine, 21,* 449–472.

Pentz, M. A. (1986). Community organization and school liaisons: How to get programs started. *Journal of School Health, 56,* 382–388.

Pentz, M. A. (1990). Mass media campaigns for drug abuse prevention. In T. E. Backer, E. M. Rogers, & P. Sopory (Eds.), *Comparative synthesis of mass media campaigns for health behavior change* (pp. 88–93). Rockville, MD: Office for Substance Abuse Prevention.

Pentz, M. A. (1993a). Comparative effects of community-based drug abuse prevention. In J. S. Baer, G. A. Marlatt, & R. J. McMahon (Eds.), *Addictive behaviors across the lifespan: Prevention, treatment, and policy issues* (pp. 69–87). Newbury Park, CA: Sage.

Pentz, M. A. (1993b). Primary prevention of adolescent drug abuse. In C. B. Fisher & R. M. Lerner (Eds.), *Applied developmental psychology* (pp. 435–474). New York: McGraw-Hill.

Pentz, M. A. (1994a). Adaptive evaluation strategies for estimating effects of community-based drug abuse prevention programs. *Journal of Community Psychology, (Special issue),* 26–51.

Pentz, M. A. (1994b). Target populations and interventions in prevention research: What is high risk? In A. Cazares & L. A. Beatty (Eds.), *Scientific methods for prevention intervention research,* (NIDA Res Mono No. 139, NIH Publication No. 94-3631, pp. 75–94).

Pentz, M. A. (1995a). Alternative models of community prevention research. In P. Langton & M. A. Orlandi (Eds.), *Challenge of Participatory Research: Preventing Alcohol Related Problems in Ethnic Communities. CSAP Cultural Competence Series 3,* Rockville, MD: Center for Substance Abuse Prevention.

Pentz, M. A. (1995b). The school-community interface in comprehensive school health education. In S. Stansfield (Ed.), *1995 Institute of Medicine annual report*, Committee on Comprehensive School Health Programs, Institute of Medicine, Bethesda, MD. Washington, DC: National Academy Press.

Pentz, M. A. (in press). Cost benefit and cost effectiveness research in drug abuse prevention: Implications for programming and policy. In W. Bukoski & R. I. Evans (Eds.). NIDA Res Mono.

Pentz, M. A., Bonnie, R. J., & Shopland, D. S. (1996). Integrating supply and demand reduction strategies for drug abuse prevention. *American Behavioral Scientist, 39*(7): 897–910.

Pentz, M. A., Brannon, B. R., Charlin, V. I., Barrett, E. J., MacKinnon, D. P., & Flay, B. R. (1989). The power of policy: The relationship of smoking policy to adolescent smoking. *American Journal of Public Health, 79,* 857–862.

Pentz, M. A., Dwyer, J. H., MacKinnon, D. P., Flay, B. R., Hansen, W. B., Wang, E. Y. I., & Johnson, C. A. (1989). A multi-community trial for primary prevention of adolescent drug abuse: Effects on drug use prevalence. *Journal of the American Medical Association, 261,* 3259–3266.

Pentz, M. A., Johnson, C. A., Dwyer, J. H., MacKinnon, D. P., Hansen, W. B., & Flay, B. R. (1989). A comprehensive community approach to adolescent drug abuse prevention: Effects on cardiovascular disease risk behaviors. *Annals of Medicine, 21,* 219–222.

Pentz, M. A., Pentz, C. A., & Gong, A. (1993, March). *Different strokes for different folks? Effects of two adolescent smoking prevention programs on different racial/ethnic groups.* Annual Meeting of the Society of Behavior Medicine (Special Citation), San Francisco, CA.

Perry, C. L., & Jessor, R. (1985). The concept of health promotion and the prevention of adolescent drug abuse. *Health Education Quarterly, 12,* 170–184.

Rice, D. P., Kelman, S., Miller, L. S., & Dunmeyer, S. (1990). *The economic costs of alcohol and drug abuse and mental illness: 1985.* San Francisco, University of California.

Rice, D. P., Max, N., Novotony, T., Schultz, J., & Hodgson, T. (1992, November). *The cost of smoking revisited.* Paper presented at the Annual American Public Health Association Meeting, Washington, DC.

Robert Wood Johnson Foundation. (1993). *Evaluation meeting of fighting back.* Princeton, NJ.

Rogers, E. M. (1987). The diffusion of innovations perspective. In N. D. Weinstein (Ed.), *Taking care: Understanding and encouraging self-protective behavior* (pp. 79–94). New York: Cambridge University Press.

Rotter, J. B. (1954). *Social learning and clinical psychology.* New York: Prentice-Hall.

Tobler, N. S. (1992). Drug prevention programs can work: Research findings. *Journal of Addictive Diseases, 11,* 1–28.

U.S. Congress, Office of Technology Assessment. (1991). *Adolescent health, Volume I: Summary and policy options.* (OTA-H-468). Washington, DC: U.S. Government Printing Office.

Wandersman, A., & Giamartino, G. A. (1980). Community and individual difference characteristics as influences on initial participation. *American Journal of Community Psychology, 8,* 217–228.

19

Prevention in the Military

Robert M. Bray
Research Triangle Institute

Mary Ellen Marsden
Brandeis University

John F. Mazzuchi
Roger W. Hartman
Department of Defense

Substance abuse—heavy alcohol use, illicit drug use, and cigarette smoking—has substantial negative effects on the health, productivity, and welfare of military personnel. It not only detracts from the well-being of both military personnel and civilians, but it may also decrease the readiness of military personnel to perform their mission. Further, because of the special conditions of military life, such as living away from family and friends or working in high-risk environments, substance use rates may be higher among military personnel than among civilians and the negative effects associated with use may be correspondingly higher. Accordingly, the Department of Defense (DoD) set forth a series of policy directives to decrease the impact of substance abuse on military personnel. Recent DoD policies largely are based on preventing problems from occurring rather than treating problems after they occur. The DoD recognizes that prevention is the most effective policy, and preventive efforts are initiated at recruitment and continue throughout military service.

This chapter examines both military policy and the prevention programs designed to combat substance abuse. Findings from the 1980 to 1995 World-

---

The views, opinions, and findings contained in this chapter are those of the authors and should not be construed as an official Department of Defense position, policy, or decision, unless so designated by other official documentation.

wide Survey series that examine substance use and health behaviors among military personnel (six surveys in all) are presented on trends in substance use and (based on information from the latest survey in the series) on the impact of specific programs.

IMPACT OF SUBSTANCE ABUSE

Substance abuse is a major contributor to mortality and morbidity for all Americans. Of the 2 million deaths in the United States each year, more than one in four is attributable to the use of alcohol, illicit drugs, or tobacco (Institute for Health Policy, 1993). Tobacco use accounts for 400,000 deaths, alcohol use for 100,000 deaths, and illicit drug use for about 20,000 deaths each year (McGinnis & Foege, 1993). These deaths arise from chronic diseases associated with use and from unintentional injuries occurring while under the influence of alcohol or other drugs.

Substance abusers are also less healthy than nonusers (Marsden, Bray, & Herbold, 1988). They not only suffer from serious chronic diseases, such as liver cirrhosis resulting from long-term use of alcohol, but also their overall level of health may be lower than that of individuals who do not abuse drugs or alcohol. Excessive alcohol consumption affects almost every part of the body; it results in liver damage, pancreatitis, cardiovascular injury, and depression of the immune system among other health effects (National Institute on Alcohol Abuse and Alcoholism, 1993). Untreated alcoholics may incur health care costs 100% higher than nonalcoholics (Holder, 1987). Drug abusers are vulnerable to acquiring a host of infectious diseases, including the acquired immune deficiency syndrome (AIDS), hepatitis, sexually transmitted diseases, and tuberculosis (Haverkos, 1991; Haverkos & Lange, 1990). The negative health effects of smoking and passive smoking are well known (U.S. Department of Health and Human Services, 1986, 1989).

Substance abuse also affects family and social relationships and performance in the workforce. Substance abuse is implicated in many cases of divorce, domestic violence, and child abuse and neglect (Institute for Health Policy, 1993). Alcohol and drug abuse are strongly related to absenteeism, fatal and nonfatal accidents of transportation workers, and job turnover (Normand, Lempert, & O'Brien, 1994). Drug abusers are absent about 1.5 times as often, consume almost twice the medical benefits, and make over twice the number of worker's compensation claims as nonusers (National Institute on Drug Abuse [NIDA], 1990). About 10% of young adults who used marijuana in the past year had restricted activity due to illness or injury; about 16% of those who used marijuana and cocaine had restricted activity (Keer et al., 1994).

The estimated annual cost of these negative effects of substance abuse to our nation is enormous. Alcohol abuse is estimated to cost $98.6 billion per year, smoking $72.0 billion, and drug abuse $66.9 billion from lost productivity, medical expenditures, and costs related to crime and victimization. The major burden of alcohol abuse is productivity loss associated with illness and death; the major component for drug abuse is crime-related costs; and the major component for smoking is losses associated with premature death (Institute for Health Policy, 1993; Rouse, 1995).

These costs of substance abuse are largely preventable. Indeed, substance abuse has been called our nation's number one preventable health problem, and the value of preventive efforts in decreasing the harm associated with substance abuse has been increasingly recognized. Decreases in substance abuse and associated negative effects are goals of both military and civilian policy and are to be attained largely through preventive efforts.

EVOLUTION OF MILITARY POLICY TOWARD SUBSTANCE ABUSE

The DoD's comprehensive series of policy directives to monitor, regulate, and eliminate substance abuse among military personnel began during the Vietnam War era. A concerted policy toward decreasing and possibly preventing drug and alcohol abuse originated in the early 1970s (DoD, 1970, 1972), while policies directed toward smoking prevention have been more recent (DoD, 1986a, 1986b, 1987, 1994). Current substance abuse policy emphasizes prevention, with a policy of zero tolerance toward drug and alcohol abuse and those who use or possess illegal drugs (DoD, 1980a, 1980b, 1983, 1985a, 1985b, 1986a). Earlier policies more strongly focused on treatment than prevention, but the current policy of detection and deterrence is based on a strong stance toward preventive efforts during recruitment and active service.

1960s and 1970s: Emphasis on Rehabilitation

Military policy toward drug abuse was largely developed in response to concerns about illicit drug use among American servicemen returning from Vietnam. Heroin and opium were widely used among American servicemen in Vietnam, and although few continued using when they returned home (Robins, 1975), there were concerns about addiction. To investigate the problem of drug abuse in the military, the DoD convened a task force in 1967. Congress, however, charged that alcohol abuse should be accorded the same level of attention as drug abuse and imposed this stipulation on the task force. Based on the findings and recommendations of the task force, a policy directive was set forth in 1970 that guided military efforts to confront drug and alcohol abuse for the next decade (DoD, 1970).

The policy emphasized the prevention of drug and alcohol abuse through education and law enforcement procedures focusing on detection and early intervention. However, treatment was provided for problem users, and the emphasis was on returning problem users to service. The individual service branches were to implement programs consistent with overall military policy, but that met the distinctive needs of their personnel. Overall policy was implemented with several new directives in the early 1970s that clarified how treatment and prevention were to be set in motion (Bray, Marsden, Herbold, & Peterson, 1993).

In response to continuing public concern about reports of serious drug addiction among U.S. forces in Southeast Asia, President Nixon in 1971 directed the DoD to take additional measures to address the drug problem. The result was the establishment of a urinalysis testing program that grew almost immediately to include service members returning from Vietnam who were addicted to heroin. The program tested for opiates, barbiturates, and amphetamines and was a massive undertaking. It not only consisted of mandatory testing for service members leaving all of Southeast Asia, but also grew to include random mandatory urinalysis for all U.S. forces worldwide. To carry out this program, the military departments established a Tri-Service drug screening laboratory system. Each laboratory was required to provide drug testing services for all military personnel within a geographic region, and by 1980, the military was routinely testing for six drugs by thin-layer chromatography (opiates, barbiturates, amphetamines, methaqualone, phencyclidine [PCP], and cocaine). The Armed Forces Institute of Pathology (AFIP) was designated to serve as the reference laboratory to determine each individual laboratory's capability to detect drugs and to determine a false positive rate.

The mid-1970s proved a difficult time for the fledgling urinalysis program. In June 1974, the military drug-testing program was challenged in the courts (*U.S. v. Ruiz*, 1974). The core of the argument was whether the Fifth Amendment protection against self-incrimination was being violated. The court ruled that because general discharge was considered to have a potentially adverse effect on an individual's status, service members could refuse to submit a urine sample for testing. In 1975, the DoD issued new guidelines for its drug-testing program. Although drug testing was mandatory, the results could be used only to support entry into a drug rehabilitation program, and those personnel identified by urinalysis testing could be given only an honorable discharge. In 1976, Congress discouraged the use of large-scale random drug testing as not cost-effective. Consequently, from 1976 until 1981, the military's drug-testing program was dormant. By 1977, however, there were widespread reports, particularly in the Federal Republic of Germany, of increased drug use among military personnel. The House Select Committee on Narcotics Abuse and Control conducted a series of observational surveys that gave supporting evidence to growing abuse. The overwhelming drug of choice appeared to be marijuana. At that time, however, the DoD had no reliable confirmatory test for marijuana and thus had no effective way of addressing the problem.

Early 1980s: Shift to Prevention and Zero Tolerance

Comprehensive policies on alcohol and drug abuse were set forth in a 1980 directive, superseding the 1970 and 1972 directives (DoD, 1980a). The new directive stressed prevention and was a significant shift away from the earlier policies that promoted rehabilitation. The goal stated in the new directive was for the DoD to "be free of the effects of alcohol and drug abuse; of the possession and trafficking in illicit drugs by military and civilian members of the Department of Defense; and of the possession, use, sale, or promotion of drug abuse paraphernalia." The DoD clearly stated that drug and alcohol abuse were incompatible with the maintenance of high standards of performance, military discipline, and readiness. Alcohol- and drug-dependent persons were not to be inducted into the military, and continuing education and training were to be provided to military personnel. Treatment was provided but did not receive the central focus it had previously. The policy, which defined drug and alcohol abuse in terms of its negative consequences to the individual and society, was consistent with federal guidelines established by the Office of Drug Abuse Policy in 1979.

The greater emphasis on prevention, according to Allen and Mazzuchi (1985), was largely the result of the recognition that deterrence was not fully effective and that not all drug abusers were addicts in need of treatment. The findings from the 1980 Worldwide Survey showed little evidence of drug dependence. It further showed that those most likely to use drugs were 18- to 25-year-olds who had not developed a more mature lifestyle that would preclude drug use (Burt, Biegel, Carnes, & Farley, 1980). The drug problem was then reinterpreted to be a lack of discipline rather than addiction. Accordingly, greater emphasis was placed on prevention programs directed at all military personnel and more on punitive policies for drug and alcohol abusers. Also, as a result of findings from the 1980 Worldwide Survey, the military began to focus on alcohol and marijuana, the two drugs most often abused by military personnel. Moreover, the emphasis came to be placed more on encouraging healthy lifestyles.

The crash of a jet on the flight deck of the aircraft carrier *Nimitz* in 1981 riveted public attention on the military's drug problem. Autopsies of 14 Navy personnel killed in the crash showed evidence of marijuana use among 6 of the 13 sailors and nonprescription antihistamine use by the pilot. The Congress demanded action by the Secretary of Defense. In response, the DoD announced a 10-point program to control drug abuse that called for increased drug testing, discharge of repeat offenders, improved rehabilitation programs, and a massive education effort. In the summer of 1981, a major scientific breakthrough provided an important impetus for the DoD's antidrug efforts. Scientists at AFIP developed procedures to confirm the presence of tetrahydrocannabinol (THC), the active ingredient in marijuana, using gas chromatography. The Assistant Secretary of Defense for Health Affairs issued instructions to the services to begin a 6-month evaluation of this drug-testing procedure and required a 1-year evaluation of new portable drug-testing equipment. In December 1981, the Deputy Secretary of Defense issued a major policy change to evidentiary use of drug testing. Test results could be used as evidence if properly obtained and if a strict chain of custody was maintained for all. These modifications were based on a late 1980 Court of Military Appeals ruling (*U.S. v. Armstrong*, 1980) that reversed some aspects of the *Ruiz* case.

In December 1981, the Department of the Navy launched its War on Drugs. This aggressive program involved extensive use of urinalysis that included 100% testing of all samples for marijuana, widespread use of portable drug-testing equipment, unit-wide sweep testing, and testing of all recruits during accession. The Navy also included intense drug education as part of its program with the unequivocal message that drug use would not be tolerated. The Navy's program marked the beginning of DoD's emphasis on zero tolerance. The other services also soon responded with related programs. Although help was offered to those on drugs who sought it, the message was clearly stated that those who did not follow the zero tolerance policy would be discharged.

Expanded drug testing introduced unexpected problems, and 1982 proved to be a difficult year. The entire military laboratory system became strained. There was a backlog of more than 100,000 samples, and the AFIP found it difficult to maintain an adequate quality control system. In May 1982, the Deputy Assistant Secretary of Defense for Drug Abuse and Alcohol Prevention convened a meeting of nationally recognized experts in toxicology under the auspices of the White House Policy Advisor, Dr. Carlton Turner, and with NIDA's support. The conference produced a series of recommendations that were accepted by the DoD. These included requiring two separate chemical methodologies of identification to protect against false positives and the expansion of the AFIP quality control program. The conference also agreed that the gas chromatography confirmation test was adequate legally, provided that tight external quality control was maintained. The services were given greater latitude to tailor drug testing to their own needs.

In November 1982, a second White House drug-testing conference was convened that refined the program by standardizing minimal levels for both screening and confirmatory testing. During 1982 and 1983, there were numerous court challenges to DoD's program, although most sustained the department's position. In December 1983, a third White House drug-testing conference was convened that resulted in additional refinements of AFIP's demanding quality control standards and further strengthened the credibility of the DoD's drug-testing program. The DoD policy became not only zero tolerance for drug abuse, but also zero tolerance of any false positive test result.

In 1984, the Senate Armed Services Committee directed the DoD to review its drug-testing program. As part of this review, the urinalysis testing program underwent close scrutiny from the Congress and the American public. The report submitted to the Congress in October 1984 concluded that the drug-testing program was sound and that the services had taken all necessary steps to address and prevent procedural problems. Although drug testing was a major factor in the department's efforts to reduce drug abuse among military personnel, it was placed within a framework that sent a clear message that drug use was incompatible with military life and that assistance was available to those who had abused drugs.

Mid-1980s and the 1990s: Substance Abuse Within a Health Promotion Framework

Beginning in 1986 and continuing into the 1990s, policies on drug and alcohol abuse have been placed in the broader perspective of a coordinated, comprehensive policy on health promotion that recognizes the value of good health and healthy lifestyles for military performance and readiness. A 1986 directive defined health promotion as those activities designed to support and influence individuals in managing their health through lifestyle decisions and self-care (DoD, 1986a). Smoking prevention and cessation, as well as alcohol and drug abuse prevention, physical fitness, nutrition, stress management, and prevention of hypertension, were included in the directive. Smoking prevention and cessation programs were to include information on the health consequences of smoking provided at initial entry and permanent change of station. The health promotion strategy was developed to encourage changes in lifestyle to make healthy behavior practices the norm and thereby foster the belief that unhealthy behaviors, such as smoking and drug and alcohol abuse, were incompatible with military service.

During this period, the DoD also examined the impacts of the sale of tobacco in the military, including the impact of increasing prices of tobacco products. The resulting report clearly recognized the negative health impacts of smoking and the importance of individual choice (DoD, 1986b). In 1986, the Secretary of Defense issued a memorandum calling for an intensive antismoking campaign, with an emphasis on the negative health impact of smoking. Smoking rates and effects on health continued to be monitored, and positive steps were taken to reduce the impact of passive smoking, including restrictions on smoking in certain common areas and prohibition of smoking by medical personnel in the presence of patients (Ballweg & Bray, 1989; DoD, 1987). All of the services now prohibit smoking on base except in designated smoking areas and offer smoking cessation programs to encourage smokers to quit (DoD, 1994; Kroutil, Bray, & Marsden, 1994).

In 1987, a DoD conference was called by the Assistant Secretary of Defense for Health Affairs to review progress in reducing drug and alcohol abuse. The conference confirmed the substantial reduction in use of illicit drugs but highlighted the less impressive accomplishments in reducing alcohol abuse and related medical and disciplinary problems. Progress in reducing alcohol abuse was not as great in the higher enlisted ranks as in other military ranks. The findings raised awareness of the alcohol problem and have resulted in a number of new initiatives toward alcohol abuse. For example, the Secretary of the Navy in 1996 created a high-level Standing Committee on Alcohol Abuse Prevention and Alcohol Use Deglamorization in the Department of the Navy. This committee, chaired by an Assistant Secretary of the Navy, is to evaluate Navy and Marine Corps policies and education programs to ensure that all members maintain a maximum state of personal readiness by avoiding the abuse of alcohol and deglamorizing its use. The Navy campaign, called "Right Spirit," and the Marine Corps campaign, called "Semper Fit," are to carry out the initiatives of this committee.

Beginning with *Healthy People: The Surgeon General's Report on Health Promotion and Disease Prevention* (Public Health Service [PHS], 1979) and continuing in 1980 with *Promoting Health/Preventing Disease: Objectives for the Nation* (PHS, 1980), the federal government adopted a national health agenda. Broadly speaking, the agenda is aimed at taking steps to prevent unnecessary disease and disability and to achieve a better quality of life for all Americans. These initial efforts were followed by *Healthy People 2000: National Health Promotion and Disease Prevention Objectives* (PHS, 1991).

Health objectives for the nation were set forth in 22 priority areas in four major categories: health promotion (including alcohol and other drugs, and tobacco), health protection (including unintentional injuries and occupational safety and health), preventive services (including maternal and infant health and human immunodeficiency virus [HIV] infection), and surveillance and data systems. In 1992, the DoD identified a subset of these objectives that were of highest importance for near-term measurement. Some of these objectives were considered amenable to measurement by surveys and began to be monitored with the DoD Worldwide Survey series described in the following paragraphs, beginning in 1992 and 1995.

NATURE AND EXTENT OF SUBSTANCE USE PROBLEM

To understand whether prevention efforts are having a positive effect in reducing substance use, it is necessary to provide systematic evaluations of prevention efforts, programs, and their associated interventions. This can be a rather formidable task for an organization as large and complex as the DoD because programs are developed, operated, and managed by the individual services. Even though prevention programs may all have the same broad objectives to prevent, reduce, and control substance abuse as established by the DoD, there can be considerable variation in terms of the specifics of the interventions and the rigor and effectiveness with which they are implemented. Consequently, it has not been practical for the DoD to conduct large-scale program evaluations to assess the effectiveness of prevention efforts. Specific studies of program effectiveness have been left to the services.

Rather than conduct large-scale evaluations of programs, the DoD has elected to obtain a broad perspective about the nature and extent of substance use and its related negative effects in the military and then to use these data to inform program and policy decisions. This has been done through a continuing series of worldwide surveys of military personnel that, to date, have been conducted from 1980 to 1995 to assess the prevalence, correlates, and negative effects of substance use among active-duty military personnel. Although these surveys are not formal evaluation studies, they provide the most systematic information available about military trends in the use of tobacco, illicit drugs, and alcohol. The trends across the surveys serve as a barometer to the DoD about the effectiveness of broad policies and, in combination with other data provided by the services, are used to assess program directions and needed changes.

DoD Worldwide Survey Series*[1]

In 1980, under the direction of the Office of the Assistant Secretary of Defense for Health Affairs, the DoD initiated a series of recurrent surveys to (a) improve understanding of the nature, causes, and consequences of substance use and health in the military; (b) determine the appropriateness of the emphasis placed on program elements; and (c) examine the impact of current and future program policies. Six such surveys have been conducted between 1980 and 1995. Burt Associates, Incorporated, of Bethesda, Maryland, conducted the 1980 survey (Burt et al., 1980), and Research Triangle Institute (RTI) of Research Triangle Park, North Carolina, conducted the 1982, 1985, 1988, 1992, and 1995 surveys (Bray et al., 1983, 1986, 1988, 1992; Bray, Kroutil, Wheeless, et al., 1995; see also Bray, Kroutil, & Marsden, 1995).

Editors Note: A seventh woldwide survey is currently underway in 1998.

The sampling designs and data collection methods have been similar throughout the survey series and are described in detail in Bray, Kroutil, Wheeless, et al. (1995). For each survey, the eligible survey population consisted of all U.S. active-duty military personnel except recruits, service academy students, persons absent without official leave, and persons who had a permanent change of station at the time of data collection. Participants were selected to represent men and women in all pay grades of the active force throughout the world, using a probability design that first sampled installations and then selected personnel within installations. Respondents anonymously completed self-administered questionnaires that took about 50 minutes on average to answer. Survey sample sizes were 15,268 in 1980; 21,936 in 1982; 17,328 in 1985; 18,673 in 1988; 16,395 in 1992; and 16,193 in 1995. Response rates ranged from 70% to 84%. Data for each survey were weighted to represent all active-duty personnel, and adjustments were made for the potential effects of nonresponse.

Several measures of substance use and negative effects were included in the Worldwide Survey questionnaires. *Illicit drug use* in the past 30 days was measured in terms of the prevalence of nonmedical use of marijuana or hashish, PCP, lysergic acid diethylamide (LSD) or other hallucinogens, cocaine, amphetamines or other stimulants, tranquilizers or other depressants, barbiturates or other sedatives, heroin or other opiates, analgesics or other narcotics, inhalants, and "designer drugs." A summary index for estimating the prevalence of use of any illicit drug referred to nonmedical use of 1 or more of the 11 categories of drugs. *Heavy alcohol use* was defined as consuming five or more drinks per typical drinking occasion at least once a week and was based on a drinking-level classification scheme adapted from Mulford and Miller (1960). *Cigarette smokers* were defined as military personnel who reported that they smoked at least 100 cigarettes in their lifetime and who smoked at least once in the 30 days prior to the survey.

Negative effects were measured in terms of serious consequences, productivity loss, and dependence symptoms (alcohol only). The measure of *serious consequences* referred to the occurrence of one or more of the following problems in the past 12 months: Uniform Code of Military Justice punishment, loss of a week or more from duty because of a substance-related illness, substance-related injury, spouse left, arrests for driving while impaired or other incidents, incarceration, fights, not getting promoted, and needing detoxification. *Productivity loss* referred to one or more occurrences in the past 12 months of being late for work or leaving early, not coming to work at all, being drunk or high at work, or performing below a normal level of productivity because of alcohol or drug use. The *dependence symptoms* indicator was based on the number of occurrences in the past 12 months of withdrawal symptoms (e.g., the "shakes"), inability to recall things that happened while drinking, inability to stop drinking before becoming drunk, and morning drinking. The number of occurrences were summed across items, and persons with scores of 48 or more were classified as dependent (Polich & Orvis, 1979).

Trends in Substance Use: 1980–1995

Figure 19.1 presents trends from 1980 to 1995 in heavy alcohol use, any illicit drug use, and any cigarette use during the past 30 days for active-duty military personnel. As shown, use of all three substances declined significantly over time, although the rate of decline varied for each substance and between each of the six surveys.

Heavy alcohol use during the month prior to the survey declined significantly from 20.8% for all military personnel in 1980 to 17.1% in 1995. Heavy drinking increased from 1980 to 1982, was relatively stable from 1982 to 1985, decreased significantly between 1985 and 1988, then remained at about the same level from 1988 to 1995. Although these data show a small but significant decline over the 15-year period, standardized comparisons over the period indicated that much of observed decline can be attributed to changes in the sociodemographic composition of the military since 1980 (Bray, Kroutil, Wheeless, et al., 1995).

Illicit drug use during the past 30 days declined sharply from 1980 to 1995. Military personnel showed a fairly steep decline from 1980 (27.6%) to 1988 (4.8%), but a more gradual drop and tapering off to 1995 (3.0%). This repre-

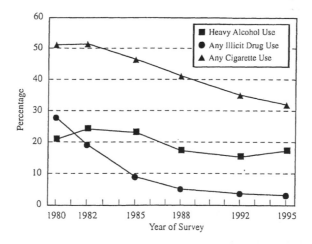

FIG. 19.1. Trends in Substance Use, Past 30 Days, Total DoD, 1980–1995. Source: Worldwide Surveys of Substance Use and Health Behaviors Among Military Personnel, 1980 to 1995.

sents a striking decrease in illicit drug use of 89.1% over the 15-year period. It is likely that these findings reflect, in part, societal trends toward reduced drug use (Substance Abuse and Mental Health Services Administration, 1995) and the strong emphasis on zero tolerance for drug use in the military.

The percentage of military personnel who smoked cigarettes in the past 30 days also decreased during the 15-year period, from 51.0% in 1980 to 31.9% in 1995. Smoking rates showed no significant change between 1980 and 1982, but decreased significantly between each of the later surveys, including between 1992 and 1995. Nonetheless, despite clear progress in reducing the prevalence of smoking, the 1995 rate is considerably higher than the *Healthy People 2000* objective of 20% adopted for the military (PHS, 1991). In contrast to the findings for heavy alcohol use, standardized comparisons of rates of illicit drug use and smoking suggest that little of the decline was related to changes in the demographic composition of the military (Bray, Kroutil, Wheeless, et al., 1995).

Overall, findings indicate that the military made steady and notable progress during the 15 years from 1980 to 1995 in combating substance abuse. The most dramatic results occurred with reductions in illicit drug use and cigarette smoking. The DoD made less progress in reducing heavy drinking. Despite progress, there is still room for considerable improvement in some areas. Cigarette smoking remained common, affecting about one in every three military personnel, and the rate of heavy drinking affected slightly more than one in six active-duty personnel. Further, findings suggest that observed declines in heavy drinking from 1980 to 1995 were largely a function of changes in the demographic composition of the military, although declines in drug use and smoking were likely associated with other factors. Societal trends in illicit drug use or the impact of military programs are alternative explanations.

Trends in Alcohol- and Drug-Related Negative Effects

The substantial negative consequences of alcohol use on the work performance, health, and social relationships of military personnel have been a continuing concern of the military and were assessed in the DoD surveys. Figure 19.2 presents trends in alcohol- and drug-related negative effects for active military personnel during the survey series. Alcohol-related negative effects are shown for 1980 to 1995, and drug-related negative effects are shown for 1980 to 1992. (Data for drug-related negative effects were not obtained in the 1995 survey because of the low rates observed in 1992.)

Consistent with the decline in heavy drinking between 1980 and 1995 observed in Fig. 19.1, all three measures of negative effects due to drinking displayed in Fig. 19.2a also showed a decline. Serious consequences associated with alcohol use declined from 17.3% in 1980 to 7.6% in 1995. Productivity loss resulting from alcohol use decreased from 26.7% in 1980 to 16.3%

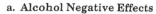

a. Alcohol Negative Effects

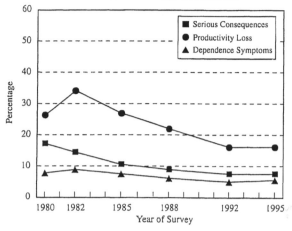

b. Drug Negative Effects

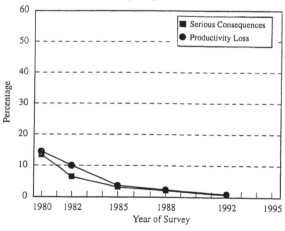

FIG. 19.2. Trends in Alcohol and Drug Use Negative Effects, Past 12 Months, Total DoD, 1980–1995. Source: Worldwide Surveys of Substance Use and Health Behaviors Among Military Personnel, 1980 to 1995.

in 1995. Although less pronounced, symptoms of alcohol dependence also declined significantly from 8.0% in 1980 to 5.7% in 1995.

As shown in Fig. 19.2b, drug-related negative effects also declined consistent with declines in illicit drug use (Fig. 19.1) from 1980 to 1992. In 1980, 13.3% of military personnel reported experiencing a drug-related serious consequence during the year; by 1992, only 0.4% reported this. The percentage who reported experiencing productivity loss associated with illicit drug use also decreased significantly between 1980 and 1992, from 14.4% of all military personnel to 0.7%. By 1992, the percentage of military personnel reporting any serious consequences or productivity loss associated with drug use was minimal.

Healthy People 2000 and Substance Abuse

The 1992 Worldwide Survey provided some information about a limited number of *Healthy People 2000* objectives among military personnel, and the 1995 Worldwide Survey expanded this emphasis. The objectives related to substance abuse include

- reduce cigarette smoking to a prevalence of no more than 20% among military personnel,
- reduce smokeless tobacco use by males aged 24 and younger to a prevalence of no more than 4%, and
- increase abstinence from tobacco use by pregnant women to at least 90% and increase abstinence from alcohol by at least 20%.

As shown in Table 19.1, findings from the 1995 Worldwide Survey indicate (a) a prevalence of cigarette smoking of 31.9%, notably higher than the

TABLE 19.1
Healthy People 2000 Objectives for Substance Abuse

Behavior	Goal	Result
Cigarette smoking, past 30 days—All personnel	20% or less	31.9%
Smokeless tobacco use, past 30 days—Males, ages 18–24	4% or less	21.9%
Substance use during last pregnancy[a]		
No alcohol use	Increase by at least 20%	85.2%[b]
No cigarette use	90% or more	83.9%

Note: Total $N = 16,193$.

[a]Estimate made for women who were pregnant in the past 5 years.

[b]Estimate provides baseline rate against which to compare subsequent rates of abstinence from alcohol during pregnancy.

Source: Worldwide Survey of Substance Use and Health Behaviors Among Military Personnel, 1995.

objective; (b) a smokeless tobacco prevalence among males 24 and younger of 21.9%, about five times the objective; and (c) a cigarette abstinence rate of 83.9% among pregnant women. The 1995 survey also established the baseline for measurement of progress toward the alcohol abstinence rate. About 15% of all military women who were pregnant during the past 5 years consumed some alcohol during their last pregnancy (Bray, Kroutil, Wheeless, et al., 1995). These findings suggest the need for improvement in these substance abuse behaviors.

These data on trends in substance use, negative effects associated with that use, and *Healthy People 2000* objectives provide key information for the military in considering the emphasis and directions of its prevention programs.

CURRENT MILITARY SUBSTANCE ABUSE PREVENTION PROGRAMS

To effectively carry out its policies regarding substance abuse prevention, the DoD provides overall guidance and direction to the individual services and charges them to develop programs to meet policy objectives. As noted earlier, DoD directives set forth general policy guidelines, whereas service instructions make these policies operational within the military and in some cases expand upon or add policies.

Although efforts aimed at preventing illicit drug use, tobacco use, and alcohol abuse are discussed separately, they often overlap. For example, one of the military's broad substance abuse prevention tools is the national campaign called "Put Prevention Into Practice" developed by the PHS. The campaign is designed to achieve the goals of *Healthy People 2000* by improving the delivery of clinical preventive services. Its kit of materials is tailored for various subpopulations, such as health care providers, office staff, and health care consumers (i.e., military members). As part of this effort, clinicians are encouraged to use patient contacts as an opportunity to discuss the patient's use of alcohol, drugs, and tobacco products. Military members are encouraged to constantly monitor their use of these substances and to seek assistance when necessary.

Illicit Drug Use Prevention

The prevention of drug abuse can take many forms. All services include drug abuse prevention information as part of general military training, ranging from the earliest days of recruit training to various other points along one's military path. Education includes information on the hazards of drug use, administrative and punitive consequences, responsible decision making, and healthy alternatives to drug use. Many commands use drug-detection dogs to periodically search barracks and vehicles at installation gates. Selected high-risk target groups, such as units preparing to deploy to areas where drug use is prevalent, often receive tailored drug abuse prevention information and education.

One of the military's most potent weapons against drug abuse is its drug-testing program, commonly referred to as urinalysis. The purpose of drug testing is to deter service members from using drugs and to permit commanders to detect drug abuse and assess the security, readiness, and discipline of their commands. Drug testing is conducted under a number of different premises; the most common, and probably the most effective as a deterrent to drug abuse, is random testing, with the minimum rate being one sample per active-duty member each year. Drug testing also may be called for during inspections, probable-cause searches, when members are enrolled in substance abuse rehabilitation programs, following any incident that may be considered a safety mishap, when the commander has reason to suspect the member's competence for duty (e.g., when the member exhibits aberrant, bizarre, or uncharacteristic behavior, or after a period of unauthorized absence), or during any valid medical examination, including emergency room treatment. Depending on the premise of the test, drug-testing results may be used as evidence in disciplinary actions under the Uniform Code of Military Justice and in adverse administrative actions.

Although there has been no formal evaluation of the effectiveness of the urinalysis testing program, data from the 1995 Worldwide Survey suggest that the program is having its intended effect of preventing some personnel from using illicit drugs. As shown in Table 19.2, most personnel (76.9%) were

TABLE 19.2
Beliefs About Urinalysis Testing

Item	User[a] (n = 759)	Nonuser (n = 15,430)	Total (n = 16,189)
I would not use drugs even if there were no urinalysis testing.	30.8	80.1	76.9
I would be more inclined to use drugs if the military did not have urinalysis testing.	52.6	11.4	14.1
People in my unit would be more inclined to use drugs if the military did not have urinalysis testing.	73.4	46.1	47.8
I can usually predict when I'm going to be selected for urinalysis testing.	17.6	5.4	6.2
Some people get away with using drugs because they know when they're not likely to be tested.	55.2	25.9	27.8

Note: Entries are percentages who "agreed" or "strongly agreed" with the item.

[a]"User" refers to reports of any drug use in the past 12 months.

Source: Worldwide Survey of Substance Use and Health Behaviors Among Military Personnel, 1995.

not inclined to use drugs and would not do so even if there were no testing program. Some 14% of military personnel believed that they would be more inclined to use drugs without testing, and 48% thought people in their unit would be more inclined to use drugs if the military did not have urinalysis testing. Comparisons of responses from past-year drug users and nonusers showed that users were over 4.5 times more likely than nonusers to report that testing reduced their likelihood of using drugs (52.6% vs. 11.4%). Similarly, users were over 1.5 times more likely than nonusers to indicate that people in their unit were likely to use drugs (73.4% vs. 46.1%). This suggests that testing is reaching its intended audience, the potential users. Only 6% thought they personally could predict when they would be selected for testing, although over a fourth (28%) thought that some people get away with using drugs because they know when they are likely to be tested. Although not definitive, these data support the belief that urinalysis testing has a desired deterrent effect on illicit drug use by military personnel.

Prevention of Tobacco Use

The DoD recognizes the harmful effects that result both from the use of tobacco products, including smokeless tobacco, and exposure to environmental tobacco smoke. It is DoD policy to provide personnel with effective tobacco-cessation programs and to protect all personnel from the health hazards caused by exposure to tobacco smoke. Accordingly, the DoD policy is to ban smoking of tobacco products in all DoD workplaces. Commands can designate outdoor smoking areas that are reasonably accessible to personnel and provide a measure of protection from the elements. Because environmental tobacco smoke is classified as a potential occupational carcinogen, outdoor smoking areas are designated so as to reduce exposure to environmental tobacco smoke to the lowest feasible concentration (i.e., not near air intakes or entrances). The DoD prohibits indoor designated smoking areas, such as hallways, stairways, restrooms, and private offices.

The DoD requests all commands to provide their personnel with effective tobacco cessation programs. These programs are designed to encourage DoD personnel not to start using tobacco, as well as to motivate current users to quit. Anti-tobacco education messages are routinely made available to all personnel. High-risk personnel, such as those with chronic respiratory and cardiac conditions, and those who are part of special occupational groups, such as asbestos workers, receive special medical counseling about the risks of smoking. Lectures, films, pamphlets, and other forms of health promotion incorporate the latest available medical research information on tobacco, smoking, health, and treatment.

Tobacco-cessation programs take many different forms, and local installation commanders are authorized to implement whatever activities are appropriate to their sites and populations. Most bases offer some form of tobacco-cessation classes, generally presented by personnel from the installation hospital or clinic, substance abuse counseling facility, or family service center. Physicians and other health care providers are expected to evaluate all their patients for use of tobacco products and, where indicated, to recommend appropriate cessation activities. When clinically determined as safe and appropriate, nicotine replacement therapy is prescribed. This includes the use of nicotine gum or the nicotine patch. Nicotine replacement therapy is most effective when used in combination with other cessation activities, including the counseling, social support, and skills training that enable one to achieve and maintain abstinence. "Committed Quitters," for example, is a commercial smoking-cessation program that incorporates all three elements.

Some likely effects from these prevention and cessation efforts are noted in Table 19.3, which presents findings from the 1995 Worldwide Survey on attempts to stop smoking cigarettes during the past year. As shown in the top half of the table, over half (54.6%) of military personnel never smoked. In the total DoD, some 13.8% of personnel successfully stopped smoking, 10.6% over a year ago and 3.2% within the past year. An additional 15.4% made a serious, but unsuccessful attempt to quit smoking within the past year, whereas 16.2% did not try to quit. The lower half of Table 19.3 shows smokers' attempts to quit during the past year. For the total DoD, 9.3% of smokers quit within the past year, 44.3% tried to quit but continued smoking, and 46.4% did not try to quit. Overall, then, over half (53.6%) of past-year smokers made an attempt to quit, but of those who tried to quit, only about one out of four was successful. These data suggest considerable interest in cessation of smoking and a relatively large potential audience for programs

TABLE 19.3
Serious Attempt to Stop Smoking Cigarettes During the Past Year

Group/Status	Total DoD
Among all personnel	
Never smoked[a]	54.6
Former smoker, quit over a year ago	10.6
Former smoker, quit within past year	3.2
Current smoker, tried to quit	15.4
Current smoker, didn't try to quit	16.2
Among smokers, past year	
Former smoker, quit within past year	9.3
Current smoker, tried to quit	44.3
Current smoker, didn't try to quit	46.4

Note: Entries are column percentages. Total $N = 16,180$.
[a]Smoked fewer than 100 cigarettes in the lifetime.
Source: Worldwide Survey of Substance Use and Health Behaviors Among Military Personnel, 1995.

designed to help military personnel stop smoking. However, the 46.4% of smokers in the military who did not try to quit during the past year may represent a more formidable target for policies and programs designed to reduce or eliminate smoking.

Alcohol Abuse Prevention

Prevention of alcohol abuse has been a key component of military substance abuse programs for the past 25 years. Clearly, the most effective way to deal with problems associated with the abuse of alcohol is to prevent them from occurring in the first place. Alcohol abuse prevention can best be viewed from three different levels: the services, commands and installations, and the individual service member.

All services now test for the presence of alcohol in those seeking entrance into the military, in much the same way that drugs are tested for. A member's on-base driving privileges are revoked if the member is convicted of driving while intoxicated (DWI). Each service stresses the importance of alcohol abuse prevention through various training and education classes. The Navy, for example, offers a 4-hour command-level course called "Alcohol Aware" that is designed to provide all members with basic information on alcohol and alcohol abuse. "Alcohol Impact" is a 20-hour intervention course for first-time offenders who do not require formal counseling or rehabilitation but whose alcohol use has caused a problem (e.g., DWI, assault, family violence). All services emphasize early detection and early intervention as critical in the prevention of alcohol abuse.

Local bases and installations have a great amount of flexibility to develop alcohol abuse prevention initiatives. Many commands, for example, offer safety stand-downs and red ribbon campaigns prior to holidays and the vacation season, reminding members of the dangers of drinking and driving. National Drunk and Drugged Driving Awareness week is another opportunity that commands use to make members aware that drinking and driving don't mix. Commands encourage their personnel to use designated drivers for situations where alcohol will be available, and most bases provide server training for employees of clubs and on-base restaurants that serve alcohol. Some base commanders require their junior personnel to complete an alcohol awareness course before they are allowed to receive an on-base driving permit. It is common for bases to set up driving mazes at gates and other checkpoints to detect intoxicated drivers, especially on weekends. Alcohol deglamorization campaigns stress the importance of food and non-alcoholic beverages at command-sponsored social events. Happy hours, where they still exist, do not allow for alcoholic beverages to be sold at a reduced price, unless nonalcoholic beverages have a similar discount.

At the individual service member level, personal responsibility and taking care of your buddy are stressed. Individuals are encouraged to volunteer for alcohol education and awareness classes that are not mandatory. Designated drivers often receive free nonalcoholic beverages from clubs and on-base restaurants. Supervisory personnel are expected to lead by example and be role models for junior personnel, both on and off duty. Alcohol abuse and drinking to intoxication are incompatible with the core values of the services, and individual service members understand that these behaviors can be avoided by making sound decisions that reflect a healthy lifestyle.

Although the military has a strong emphasis on alcohol prevention, there have been few attempts at formal evaluation of the military's alcohol prevention programs. One recent study of Navy programs using interviews and focus groups examined perceptions of the effectiveness of alcohol prevention efforts (Bishop, Alaimo, Baker, Goodwin, & Leyrer, 1993). Results were somewhat mixed about the program's effectiveness. Some 29% rated it as below average, 32% as average, and 39% as above average. Despite this, respondents also indicated that the military prevention program surpassed comparable efforts in the civilian world (Bishop et al., 1993). These results suggest that even though the programs have many positive elements, additional improvements are needed to provide a more uniform positive perception of prevention policies and practices.

SUMMARY

Heavy alcohol use, illicit drug use, and cigarette smoking constitute a significant detriment to the health, productivity, and welfare of not only military personnel, but also all other Americans. Substance abuse is a major contributor to mortality and morbidity and also adversely affects work performance. These effects are largely preventable, and substance abuse has been called our nation's number one preventable health problem.

The DoD has since 1970 set forth a series of policies designed to decrease the impact of substance abuse on military personnel. Current policies emphasize prevention as the most effective approach to reducing substance abuse, although treatment is provided to those for whom prevention efforts are not successful. The military's drug abuse policy originated in response to concerns about drug use among service members returning from Vietnam. An early emphasis in the 1970s on rehabilitation gave way during the 1980s to the present focus on prevention and zero tolerance of those who continue to use. Education coupled with broad-based aggressive use of urinalysis are provided at recruitment and throughout service. As with illicit drug use, early policies on alcohol abuse also focused on rehabilitation; current policies still offer treatment, but place greater emphasis on prevention of problems.

Restrictions on smoking and adoption of smoking-cessation programs began in the mid-1980s. In 1986, alcohol and drug abuse and smoking policies were included in a broader health promotion framework that encourages healthy lifestyles to promote high-level military performance and readiness.

The services have developed substance abuse prevention programs consistent with overall DoD policy. Findings from the Worldwide Survey series show important progress in reducing substance abuse among military personnel; they are generally consistent with the conclusion that these programs are having their intended effects, although more rigorous evaluation studies are needed. Heavy alcohol use, illicit drug use, and cigarette smoking all decreased significantly between 1980 and 1995 as did alcohol- and drug-related negative effects. In addition, findings suggest that the urinalysis program is an effective deterrent and indicate that many military personnel have made attempts to quit smoking. Data on alcohol prevention efforts are somewhat mixed and indicate that programs need to be made more coherent and consistent to be fully effective.

Despite substantial progress, there is still room for improvement. More concerted efforts are now needed to decrease heavy drinking (which affects about one in six military personnel) and smoking (which affects about one in three). Continued vigilance will be needed to maintain low rates of drug use. Without question, prevention programs will continue to play a key role in reducing alcohol and other drug problems in the military.

REFERENCES

Allen, J., & Mazzuchi, J. (1985). Alcohol and drug abuse among American military personnel: Prevalence and policy implications. *Military Medicine, 150,* 250–255.

Ballweg, J. A., & Bray, R. M. (1989). Smoking and tobacco use by U.S. military personnel. *Military Medicine, 154,* 165–178.

Bishop, S., Alaimo, L., Baker, S., Goodwin, M., & Leyrer, C. (1993). *Baseline needs assessment for the Navy alcohol abuse and treatment programs: Final report* (Pers-63, Bureau of Personnel Navy Alcohol and Drug Program). Fairfax, VA: Caliber Associates.

Bray, R. M., Guess, L. L., Mason, R. E., Hubbard, R. L., Smith, D. G., Marsden, M. E., & Rachal, J. V. (1983). *1982 Worldwide Survey of Alcohol and Non-medical Drug Use Among Military Personnel* (RTI/2317/01-01F). Research Triangle Park, NC: Research Triangle Institute.

Bray, R. M., Kroutil, L. A., Luckey, J. W., Wheeless, S. C., Iannacchione, V. G., Anderson, D. W., Marsden, M. E., & Dunteman, G. H. (1992). *1992 Worldwide Survey of Substance Abuse and Health Behaviors Among Military Personnel.* Research Triangle Park, NC: Research Triangle Institute.

Bray, R. M., Kroutil, L. A., & Marsden, M. E. (1995). Trends in alcohol, illicit drug, and cigarette use among U.S. military personnel: 1980–1992. *Armed Forces & Society, 21,* 271–293.

Bray, R. M., Kroutil, L. A., Wheeless, S. C., Marsden, M. E., Bailey, S. L., Fairbank, J. A., & Harford, T. C. (1995). *1995 Department of Defense Survey of Health Related Behaviors Among Military Personnel* (DoD Contract No. DASWO1-94-C-0140). Research Triangle Park, NC: Research Triangle Institute.

Bray, R. M., Marsden, M. E., Guess, L. L., Wheeless, S. C., Pate, D. K., Dunteman, G. H., & Iannacchione, V. G. (1986). *1985 Worldwide Survey of Alcohol and Nonmedical Drug Use Among Military Personnel.* Research Triangle Park, NC: Research Triangle Institute.

Bray, R. M., Marsden, M. E., Guess, L. L., Wheeless, S. C., Iannacchione, V. G., & Keesling, S. R. (1988). *1988 Worldwide Survey of Substance Abuse and Health Behaviors Among Military Personnel.* Research Triangle Park, NC: Research Triangle Institute.

Bray, R. M., Marsden, M. E., Herbold, J. R., & Peterson, M. R. (1993). Progress toward eliminating drug and alcohol abuse among U.S. military personnel. In J. Stanley & J. D. Blair (Eds.), *Challenges in military health care: Perspectives on health status and the provision of care* (pp. 33–53). New Brunswick, NJ: Transaction.

Burt, M. A., Biegel, M. M., Carnes, Y., & Farley, E. C. (1980). *Worldwide Survey of Non-medical Drug Use and Alcohol Use Among Military Personnel: 1980.* Bethesda, MD: Burt Associates.

Department of Defense. (1970, October 23). Directive No. 1300.11. *Illegal or improper use of drugs by members of the Department of Defense.* Washington, DC: Author.

Department of Defense. (1972, March). Directive No. 1010.2. *Alcohol abuse by personnel of the Department of Defense.* Washington, DC: Author.

Department of Defense. (1980a, August 25). Directive No. 1010.4. *Alcohol and drug abuse by DoD personnel.* Washington, DC: Deputy Secretary of Defense.

Department of Defense. (1980b, December 5). Instruction No. 1010.5. *Education and training in alcohol and drug abuse prevention.* Washington, DC: Author.

Department of Defense. (1983, August 10). Directive No. 1010.7. *Drunk and drugged driving by DoD personnel* (rev. 7 June 1985). Washington, DC: Author.

Department of Defense. (1985a, March 13). Instruction No. 1010.6. *Rehabilitation and referral services for alcohol and drug abusers.* Washington, DC: Author.

Department of Defense. (1985b, September 23). Directive No. 1010.3. *Drug and alcohol abuse reports.* Washington, DC: Author.

Department of Defense. (1986a, March 11). Directive No. 1010.10. *Health promotion.* Washington, DC: Author.

Department of Defense. (1986b). *Smoking and health in the military.* Washington, DC: Author.

Department of Defense. (1987). *Department of Defense updated report on smoking and health in the military (prepared by the Office of the Assistant Secretary of Defense [Health Affairs]).* Washington, DC: Author.

Department of Defense. (1994, March 7). Instruction No. 1010.15. *Smoke-free workplace.* Washington, DC: Author.

Haverkos, H. W. (1991). Infectious diseases and drug abuse: Prevention and treatment in the drug abuse treatment system. *Journal of Substance Abuse Treatment, 8,* 269–275.

Haverkos, H. W., & Lange, R. (1990). Serious infections other than human immunodeficiency virus among intravenous drug abusers. *Journal of Infectious Diseases, 161,* 894–902.

Holder, H. D. (1987). Alcoholism treatment and potential health care cost saving. *Medical Care, 25,* 52–71.

Institute for Health Policy. (1993). *Substance abuse: The nation's number one health problem: Key indicators for policy.* Princeton, NJ: Robert Wood Johnson Foundation.

Keer, D. W., Colliver, J. D., Kopstein, A. N., Hughes, A. L., Gfroerer, J. C., Rice, S. C., Jr., & Schoenborn, C. A. (1994). *Restricted activity days and other problems associated with the use of marijuana or cocaine among persons 18 to 44 years of age: United States 1991* (NCHS Advance Data No. 246, April 8). Hyattsville, MD: National Center for Health Statistics.

Kroutil, L. A., Bray, R. M., & Marsden, M. E. (1994). Cigarette smoking in the U.S. military: Findings from the 1992 worldwide survey. *Preventive Medicine, 23,* 521–528.

Marsden, M. E., Bray, R. M., & Herbold, J. R. (1988). Substance use and health among U.S. military personnel: Findings from the 1985 Worldwide Survey. *Preventive Medicine, 17,* 366–376.

McGinnis, J. M., & Foege, W. H. (1993). Actual causes of death in the United States. *Journal of the American Medical Association, 270,* 2207–2212.

Mulford, H. A., & Miller, D. A. (1960). Drinking in Iowa: 2. The extent of drinking and selected sociocultural categories. *Quarterly Journal of Studies on Alcohol, 21,* 26–39.

National Institute on Alcohol Abuse and Alcoholism. (1993). *Eighth special report to the United States Congress on alcohol and health.* Rockville, MD: Author.

National Institute on Drug Abuse. (1990). *Research on drugs and the workplace (NIDA Capsules).* Rockville, MD: Author.

Normand, J., Lempert, R. O., & O'Brien, C. P. (Eds.). (1994). *Under the influence? Drugs and the American workforce.* Washington, DC: National Academy Press.

Polich, J. M., & Orvis, B. R. (1979). *Alcohol problems: Patterns and prevalence in the U.S. Air Force.* Santa Monica, CA: Rand Corporation.

Public Health Service. (1979). *Healthy people: The Surgeon General's report on health promotion and disease prevention* (DHEW Publication No. PHS 79-55071). Washington, DC: U.S. Department of Health, Education, and Welfare.

Public Health Service. (1980). *Promoting health/preventing disease: Objectives for the nation.* Washington, DC: U.S. Department of Health and Human Services.

Public Health Service. (1991). *Healthy people 2000: National health promotion and disease prevention objectives—full report, with commentary* (DHHS Publication No. PHS 91-50212). Washington, DC: U.S. Department of Health and Human Services.

Robins, L. N. (1975). Narcotic use in Southeast Asia and afterwards. *Archives of General Psychiatry, 32,* 955–961.

Rouse, B. A. (Ed.). (1995). *Substance abuse and mental health statistics sourcebook* (DHHS Publication No. SMA 95-3064). Washington, DC: Superintendent of Documents, U.S. Government Printing Office.

Substance Abuse and Mental Health Services Administration. (1995, September). *Preliminary estimates from the 1994 National Household Survey on Drug Abuse* (Advance Report No. 10). Rockville, MD: Author.

U.S. v. Armstrong, 9 M.J. 374 (C.M.A. 1980).

U.S. v. Ruiz, 23 U.S.C.M.A. 181, 48 C.M.R. 797 (1974).

U.S. Department of Health and Human Services, Public Health Service, Centers for Disease Control. (1986). *The health consequences of involuntary smoking: A report of the Surgeon General.* Atlanta, GA: Author.

U.S. Department of Health and Human Services, Public Health Service, Centers for Disease Control, Center for Chronic Disease Prevention and Health Promotion, Office of Smoking and Health. (1989). *Reducing the health consequences of smoking: 25 years of progress: A report of the Surgeon General* (DHHS Publication No. CDC 89-8411). Atlanta, GA: Author.

20

Prevention in Prisons

Holly P. Wald
Michael T. Flaherty
Janice L. Pringle
St. Francis Medical Center

America's drug problem and its relationship to increased criminal activity has been well documented in the literature. The linkage between drugs and violence is manifested in a variety of different ways. Some drug users engage in criminal activities, either violent or nonviolent, for economic gain, while others commit their offenses to acquire money for drugs. Other violent acts occur while the person is under the influence: drugs can affect cognitive ability, mood, and physiological functioning, which may contribute to the type of violent action committed. Additional violent acts may arise out of conflict with or disagreement between drug traffickers.

Surveys conducted for the Bureau of Justice Statistics (1992) indicate that 49% of state prisoners reported that they were under the influence of alcohol or other drugs at the time they committed their offense. Fifty percent of violent offenders reported that they were under the influence when their crimes were committed. In addition, a large proportion of incarcerated offenders have a history of substance use: 60% of federal prisoners, 79% of state prisoners, and 78% of jail inmates.

CASA/Columbia (1998a) found that 77% of jail inmates, 80% of federal, and 81% of state prisoners possess all or some of the following characteristics: regular use of illegal drugs (at least weekly for 1 month); being under the influence of alcohol or other drugs at the time of the offense; incarcerated for alcohol abuse violations, including driving under the influence (DUI), drug selling, or possession; commitment of the crime to obtain money for drugs; and a history of alcohol abuse.

Between 1980 and 1996 the number of individuals incarcerated has tripled and is primarily attributed to the criminal activity related to substance abuse. During this time period, there was a 229% increase in the number of males and a 439% increase in the number of females who were incarcerated (CASA, 1998). Incarceration without treatment results in increased rates of criminal recidivism and subsequent reincarceration. This results in increased costs to society on a variety of levels including law enforcement, adjudication, corrections, medical care, social welfare, and to the families of the offenders.

When added together, the total annual cost of substance abuse to the American way of life is estimated to be $188 billion. It is widely recognized that substance abuse is America's number one health and budgetary problem (e.g., CASA/Columbia, 1992). However, substance abuse treatment is rarely provided in the criminal justice system. This greatly increases the likelihood of a return to addiction and crime, an expensive cycle that is depleting limited resources.

However, inroads have been made to demonstrate the effectiveness of treatment in reducing (1) further use of alcohol and other drugs, (2) commitment of additional criminal acts, and (3) the subsequent costs to society. The provision of sufficient and appropriate treatment models serve as effective vehicles of preventing additional criminal acts, as well as the recurrence of addiction.

EFFECTIVE PRISON-BASED TREATMENT MODELS

The notion that prison-based treatment is ineffective has permeated through the field of corrections and substance abuse. The underlying sentiment is that the environment in prisons is not conducive to treatment. Many individuals have access to drugs while in prison, making it difficult for them to abstain from using during their period of incarceration or even to motivate an interest in participation in treatment (Mahon, 1997). Career criminals have difficulty letting down their defenses, as it makes them prime game for the other inmates. Inmates find it difficult to attend treatment or counseling sessions, where they are expected to address difficult personal issues, and then be returned to a jail cell with the general population.

A number of investigations present the components necessary of these programs to enhance the likelihood of efficacious outcomes (De Leon & Ziegenfuss, 1986; Field, 1985, 1992a; Wexler, 1992; Wexler, Falkin, & Lipton, 1990). Others examine the recidivism rates for individuals who received treatment while in prison and present impressive reductions in the rates of recidivism. Overall, the results indicate that treatment of the offender is effective in reducing rates of relapse, rearrests, convictions, and reincarcerations.

The residential therapeutic community (TC) model has been operational in a variety of prison settings. According to Wexler (1995), this approach to treatment evolved from the self-help tradition. Incarcerated substance abusers typically come from environments characterized by poverty, gangs, and involvement in physical, emotional, and sexual abuse. They have not learned how to take responsibility for their problems and take charge of their lives. Most professionally trained counselors come from more functional backgrounds and oftentimes find it difficult to relate to or feel comfortable with individuals from such a different background. However, with appropriate training, counselors (including recovering persons) generally have the background and insight to work with this population. Recovering persons have a special penchant for being part of the treatment field as it also gives them the opportunity to give something back to the system that helped them.

Another benefit of the TC is that the residents are housed in a special community, segregated from the general prison population. Such a protective environment supports the intellectual, physical, and emotional growth of the resident, which is contrary to the alienation, secrecy, paranoia, and fear that is fostered in the prison environment. It also helps to sustain a sense of camaraderie amongst the residents, as they have the opportunity to share common experiences and change together. Moreover, the TC modality encourages residents to participate in the treatment of other residents, an especially effective approach for the substance-abusing offender.

A renowned program in the Oregon prison system is Cornerstone, an intensive residential modified TC model. The program, which serves about 80 individuals each year, seeks to provide treatment to individuals who have extensive chronic addiction and criminal histories. Prison counselors identify and refer potential clients to the program. The eligibility criteria include the following: an extensive history of substance abuse; 6 to 18 months remaining on the prison sentence; willingness to participate in community-based aftercare programming upon release from treatment and prison; and authorized minimum security status by the prison superintendent (Field, 1992a).

Cornerstone's programming consists of four phases of treatment. The first two phases, inpatient orientation and intensive, span a 5- to 9-month time period. The approaches included in the program are an examination of the relationship between substance abuse and crime, cognitive and behavioral therapy, appropriate use of recreational time, 12-step meetings, and others. Residents earn privileges and learn to develop a recovery support system. The next two phases, transition and aftercare, prepare the client for re-entry into the community. During the transition stage, the client performs community volunteer work and obtains community employment. At the aftercare level, the program staff facilitates meetings with a community treatment provider, family members, and parole officers, in order to develop an aftercare plan.

Cornerstone's outcome studies (Field, 1985, 1992b) yield impressively low recidivism rates as defined by arrests, convictions, and prison incarcerations. There was also a documented direct relationship between the length of time in treatment and outcome (i.e., the longer an individual remained in treatment the longer the person remained out of the criminal justice system). It was found that after a 3-year period, only 26% of program graduates who remained in treatment for 11 months returned to prison. However, 85% of the nongraduates (those who remained in the program for less than 60 days) were reincarcerated.

The Stay 'N Out model is located in two prisons in the New York system, the Arthur Kill Correctional Facility for Men in Staten Island and the Bayview Correctional Facility for Women in Manhattan. The 143-bed modified TC at Arthur Kill consists of four phases of treatment: orientation, main treatment, re-entry, and training. The Bayview program consists of three phases: orientation, main treatment, and re-entry. Upon release from prison, all clients are referred to community-based aftercare services (Wexler, Williams, Early, & Trotman, 1996).

Admission criteria consist of the following: over 18 years of age, no history of sex crimes or mental illness, a history of drug abuse, and a positive record of institutional participation. The average length of stay is 6 to 9 months. Many of the counselors are ex-offenders who graduated from the program and who serve as role models for efficacious rehabilitation. All programming focuses on teaching residents how to take responsibility for their behavior and attitudes, including the development of an understanding of their thinking and motivations. Residents also learn relapse prevention/recovery techniques to be used upon return to the community.

Studies of the Stay 'N Out program indicate a direct relationship between the time spent in treatment and recidivism (Wexler, Falkin, & Lipton, 1990). Wexler et al. divided substance-abusing offenders into three groups: inmates who volunteered for treatment but did not participate, inmates participating in a therapeutic community setting, and those involved in a counseling treatment modality. Results indicated that the therapeutic community setting led to better outcomes (i.e., decreased recidivism and increased positive parole discharges), and that the positive effects increased in conjunction with greater amounts of time in the program (9–12 months). It was found that the success rate declined for those individuals who remained in treatment for greater than 1 year. The authors interpreted this finding as being part of a nonlinear dose response effect, whereby after a certain period, yield from treatment is no longer significant.

Another example of an effective prison-based TC is the Amity Prison program, located at the R. J. Donovan medium security facility in California. Its characteristics are similar to Stay 'N Out and Cornerstone: participants are housed in a separate unit, the eligibility criteria are the same, and the programming is stratified into phases. The course of treatment, spanning 12 months, utilizes a developmental process approach, whereby the resident's responsibilities within the program increase over time. The uniqueness of the Amity program is the provision of aftercare services in its community based residential TC. The curriculum of this program is individualized for each resident and builds upon what occurred in the prison program. Outcome studies of this program indicate that the lowest recidivism rates were in residents who participated in both the prison and community based programs. Twelve months following parole, 26.2% of this group was reincarcerated. In contrast, 63% of nonparticipants were reincarcerated at the 12-month interval.

Delaware's Key Crest (K-C) program is structured as a three-stage treatment model utilizing a continuum of care approach to treatment. The first or primary stage of treatment is Key, an intensive 12-month prison-based residential TC for men. (A similar program, W.C.I. Village, is located at the Women's Correctional Institution in Delaware.) Crest, the second stage, is a transitional TC/work release program for men and women. Community-based aftercare is provided to parolees who have been released from Key and Crest. Individuals eligible for the Crest program must be approaching the end of their sentence and are provided the opportunity to continue to reside in and participate in the treatment program, while being employed in the community. The third stage, aftercare, is provided to recently released inmates who have completed the Key and Crest programs. During this phase, parolees participate in community-based outpatient individual and group counseling, and spend 1 day a month at the Crest program.

To address the individual needs of the client, three types of therapy are utilized in the Key program: behavioral, cognitive, and emotional. Behavioral therapy is employed to help residents behave in a prosocial instead of an antisocial manner. Cognitive therapy helps to increase the residents' awareness of their thinking errors and to develop alternative thinking patterns. Emotional therapy focuses on the feelings and behaviors that have arisen due to unresolved conflicts with other individuals.

Participants in the Crest Outreach Center adhere to a five-phase program that focuses on helping the individual adjust to the treatment community, participate in treatment, participate in programs that will help the individual obtain gainful employment and subsequently reenter the community. During the last phase, residents obtain jobs and work in the community while residing in the facility. As most individuals are placed on probation or parole on release, they have the opportunity to participate in an aftercare program. They are also encouraged to participate in community-based 12-step programs.

Outcome studies comparing participants in only the Key, only the Crest, both Key and Crest, and no treatment/work release groups yield impressive results. At the 6-month interval, individuals who participated in any of the treatment programs had outcomes that are more favorable over the no treatment/work release group. The Key-Crest graduates were reported to be 100% drug-free and 100% crime-free. In contrast, 48% of the no treatment/work release group was drug-free and 72% of the same group was crime-free (Inciardi, 1996). At the 18-month postrelease interval, offenders who participated in 12–15 months of residential and 6 months of work release were more than twice as likely to be drug-free compared to those who only participated in the Key program (75% vs. 34%). The results suggest that length of stay and participation in a continuum of services increases the probability that a client will remain drug-free and crime-free (Inciardi, 1996a; Lipton, 1995).

The Parole Transition Release Project examined offenders who began treatment while incarcerated and then continued their participation in treatment after being released into the community on parole. The study compared the arrest and conviction rates for treated clients 1 and 2 years after release from prison, with the rates 6 months prior to the incarceration leading to treatment. Results indicated a significant reduction in arrests and convictions after involvement with this treatment project (i.e., over 70% of the clients were not rearrested 2 years after their release from prison; Field & Karecki, 1992).

In Pittsburgh, Pennsylvania, inmates are given several treatment alternatives that surround incarceration. Attendant to a Drug Court model, nonviolent substance-abusing offenders may be referred to "pre-sentenced" intensive outpatient or residential treatment tailored to the offender. Failure at this stage leads to sentencing and likely incarceration. Even when incarcerated, inmates may again be afforded the opportunity for a community residential referral during the final 6 months of incarceration. This model of "wraparound" treatment alternatives has earned high marks for offering the court both cost- and clinically effective alternatives, pre- and post-incarceration, while still insuring that substance abuse issues are addressed. This approach also keeps open the court's latitude in making decisions regarding how to best provide support for the overburdened probation officers and enhance the motivation of offenders in need of treatment along the correction continuum. The clinical and cost-effectiveness of this model has been well documented locally and nationally. Outcome studies indicate that, 6 months post-discharge, over 95% of the respondents were crime-free, 73% were drug-free, and between 65% and 70% were employed (Flaherty, Wald, Pringle, & Singerman, 1996; Gerstein et al., 1994).

The Federal Bureau of Prisons (FBP) has developed and implemented a three-tier drug abuse treatment strategy consisting of alcohol and other drug education, outpatient treatment, and unit-based residential programs. The underlying premise is that substance use contributes to the criminal lifestyle of the individual and the individual must be willing to take responsibility for and be willing to make the changes in behavior (Arcidiacono & Saum, 1995; Hayes & Schimmel, 1993).

The drug education program is compulsory for all inmates who have a history of substance abuse, whose substance use contributed to the commission of the crime, whose parole was revoked due to substance usage, or if it is court-recommended. Individuals who do not fit these categories may also participate in the programs. Inmates must complete the course during the first 6 months of incarceration, and successful completion is based upon attendance and passage of a written exam. The primary aim of this component is to foster an understanding of the reasons individuals abuse substances, the potential effects of continued substance use, the effectiveness of treatment, and the availability of treatment both within the prison and in the community. Participation in these programs is seen as a first step toward motivating an individual to enroll in an alcohol and other drug treatment program.

Outpatient alcohol and drug counseling services are available to inmates at all institutions. There are no eligibility requirements and inmates may receive the services at any time during their incarceration. The program consists of a variety of different services including AA/NA, individual and group therapy, personal development and stress management, and vocational and prerelease planning.

Thirty-three comprehensive residential-unit-based treatment programs are in existence in the federal prison system. Each unit houses 100 to 125 inmates who participate in treatment over a 9-month period (Murray, 1996). The program content is divided into eight core modules: orientation, assessment, and treatment planning, which are used to identify needs and develop a treatment plan; cognitive skills, targeting and correcting the antisocial thinking patterns; interpersonal and communication skills, addressing social deficits; criminal lifestyle confrontation, exploring criminal causation; relapse prevention; wellness; group and individual counseling; and transitional issues. Included in the last module is preparation for transition in the community, including placement in Community Corrections Centers, where participants have an opportunity to continue with treatment in community-based settings (Hayes & Schimmel, 1993).

CHARACTERISTICS OF SUCCESSFUL PROGRAMS

Some studies have examined those program characteristics that are associated with efficacious outcomes. The appropriate selection of clients to match the program services has been demonstrated to be an important consideration in developing a treatment program for addicted offenders. Clients who are more motivated, externally or internally, are thought to show greater improvement in treatment. The internal motivator, as described by Yochelson and Samenow (1979), is "choosing" to change. Addiction and the resulting commitment of unlawful acts result from individual choice. Consequently, a prerequisite for succeeding in treatment is by making a commitment to change.

External motivation, in the form of incentives and sanctions, may also help the offender achieve successful treatment outcomes. For example, a person may prefer to participate in a residential TC as it provides them with an opportunity to address issues while residing in a section of the prison that is separate from the general population. The offender chooses to remain drug-free or to stay in treatment when he/she knows the sanction for failing a drug screen is return to the general population. In addition, the individual who has been released into the community on parole or probation may choose to remain drug-free when the sanction is reincarceration. In general, it is believed that an external motivator may be very effective with offenders until they can achieve adequate internal motivation to make longer-term changes.

Other matching criteria for this population include assessment of mental health problems, previous treatment history, and whether the individual is violent. Clients with concomitant mental health disorders have poorer outcomes and require specialized programming (Chiles, Von Cleve, Jemelka, & Trupin, 1990). Clients who have a history of failing previous alcohol and other drug treatment usually require increasingly restrictive levels of care at subsequent treatment experiences. Clients who have a history of violent behavior require specialized programming that imposes structure to the client's behavior.

Research has examined the relationship between specific program characteristics and outcomes. Wexler (1992) investigated the different rates of recidivism by the type of treatment program. Program types included milieu therapy, counseling, and therapeutic community. Results indicated that the lowest rate of recidivism was found in the therapeutic community. This level of care provides long-term residential programming that seeks to change the client's life skills, values, and coping mechanisms to better support recovery.

Programming that is offered to offenders varies, regardless of level of care. Programs may employ the psychoeducational approach to addiction treatment. Such programs operate under the premise that multiple biological, psychological, and social factors contribute to the development of substance abuse problems (Peters, 1992). It is believed that by addressing these factors in a psychoeducational manner, individuals will learn to achieve long-term abstinence. With this programming, offenders have been helped to develop self-management skills to solve problems independently.

Cognitive behavioral techniques, whereby the offender is taught to recognize and respond appropriately in situations involving drug use, is a successful approach to use with the offender population. This form of treatment focuses on helping the client develop more effective problem-solving and thinking skills (Husband & Platt, 1993; Inciardi, 1996b; Leukefeld & Tims, 1990; Peters, Kearns, Murrin, Dolente, & May, 1993). Typically one or more of the following strategies are used: skills training, rational emotive therapy, problem solving, negotiation skills training, interpersonal skills training, role playing and modeling, and behavior modification (Husband & Platt, 1993). Both the Stay 'N Out, Cornerstone, and Key Crest programs have been recognized for including this approach as part of the TC program.

Other programs employ a multimodal approach to treatment (Peters, 1992). Program components include individual and group counseling, family involvement, AIDS prevention, educational and vocational counseling and job skill development, medical and mental health assessment (often including a psychiatric consultation), relapse prevention, and case management. The multimodal approach is regarded as the most efficacious method for treating this population (Leukefeld & Tims, 1990; Peters, 1992).

An example of multimodal programming is the Criminal Justice Substance Abuse Treatment Program in Jacksonville, Florida. Included in the programming are 12-step meetings, family programs, and parenting skills training. In addition, the program participants are required to participate in aftercare meetings with case managers, and are placed in outpatient services. The goal of this program is to help the individual develop new skills that can help him/her become a more productive member of society, thereby reducing the need to use and abuse drugs and to commit crime.

Several authors have maintained that aftercare services are vital to the effective treatment of offenders (e.g., Rouse, 1991). Inherent in the provision of aftercare service is the inclusion of an aftercare plan, the development of relapse awareness skills, and referral to community-based aftercare services. The purpose is to provide the supports needed to help the offender upon release from treatment, and to enhance adjustment to the community.

Successful programs include the provision of services along a continuum of care, ranging from the most intensive (i.e., intensive residential) to the least intensive (i.e., community-based aftercare). The strength of this approach is the ability to provide services according to the offender's needs and to be able to reward individuals as they step down through the various levels of care. It also provides clients with the continued support needed when re-entering the community.

FUTURE DIRECTIONS

The provision of treatment programs is a necessary element towards stemming the tide with regard to increasing rates of crime related to substance abuse. By providing education and prevention services in prisons, inmates, who are a captive audience, will have the opportunity to learn how to understand themselves, their actions and behaviors, and make the necessary changes. As described above, the primary model found in prisons is the therapeutic community, which emphasizes personal responsibility and confrontation. However, they also include alcohol and other drug education, HIV education, psychosocial rehabilitation, counseling, and vocational and life skills training. Such programs are most successful as self-contained isolated units within the prison. In addition, former addicts and offenders work in the communities and serve as effective role models.

Treatment is most efficacious if provided immediately prior to release from incarceration. In addition, it is important to have prerelease and aftercare planning, as well as linkages to support placement in the community, including step down into Community Corrections Centers and halfway houses. This should include continuing care, self-help and peer support groups in the community, assistance with education, medical care, and other ancillary support services. Providing a continuum of care, as evidenced by the Key Crest program, has yielded impressive outcomes in the form of low relapse and recidivism rates.

In addition to supporting prison-based programs, increased effort should be placed on developing programs that are alternatives to incarceration. It is more costly to incarcerate individuals than it is to place them in an alternative setting in conjunction with treatment. Examples include incorporating work release and treatment in a secure setting, such as a community corrections center, or placing an offender on intensive supervision and including treatment as a condition of sentence. Violation of probation would result in incarceration; successful completion of treatment could result in early release. Drug courts are being developed in communities as another vehicle for providing alternatives to incarceration. Offenders are evaluated for alcohol and other drug needs, referred to the treatment program offering the most appropriate level of care, and are required to meet with the judge every two weeks to monitor progress. If individuals continue to use drugs or to commit crimes, they are incarcerated.

Finally, increased funding opportunities should be made available to support programs that target the substance involved offender as they result in significant savings in human lives and in dollars. CASA/Columbia (1998b) estimates that the additional cost of providing residential treatment in conjunction with vocational and educational training, psychological services and aftercare, is $6,500 per year. It is also estimated that the economic benefit for each person who returns to the community, remains sober and employed and crime-free, is $68,800. The savings is in the form of potential earnings, health care savings, and reduced offense, arrest, prosecution, and incarceration costs. This is one of the most effective mechanisms for breaking the insidious cycle of crime and addiction.

REFERENCES

Arcidiancono, A., & Saum, C. A. (1995). Substance abuse treatment options: A federal initiative. *The Journal of Psychoactive Drugs, 27*, 105–107.

Aukerman, R. B., & McGarry, P. (1994). *Combining substance abuse treatment with intermediate sanctions for adults in the criminal justice system* (Treatment Improvement Protocol [TIP] Services, 12). Washington, DC: Substance Abuse and Mental Health Services Administration, Center for Substance Abuse Treatment.

Brown, B. S. (1992). Program models. In C. Leukefeld & F. Tims (Eds.), *Drug abuse treatment in prisons and jails*. Washington, DC: The National Institute on Drug Abuse Research Monograph Series, Monograph 118, pp. 31–37.

Bureau of Justice Statistics. (1992, December). *Drugs, crime, and the justice system*. Washington, DC: U.S. Government Printing Office.

CASA/Columbia. (1998a). Costs of substance abuse. *Behind bars: Substance abuse and America's prison population, introduction and executive summary* [on-line]. Available: http://www. casacolumbia. org/pub/jan98/summary.htm#most

CASA/Columbia. (1998b). *Costs of substance abuse* [on-line]. Available: http://www.casacolumbia. org/costs/menu1.htm

Chaiken. (1995). *Drugs and crime facts, 1994* (Office of National Drug Control Policy Drugs and Crime Clearinghouse) [on-line]. Available: http://www.ojp.usdoj.gov/bjs/pub/ascii/dcfacts. txt

Chiles, J. A., Von Cleve, E., Jemelka, R. P., & Trupin, E. W. (1990). Substance abuse and psychiatric disorders in prison inmates. *Hospital and Community Psychiatry, 41*, 1132–1134.

DeLeon, G. J., & Ziegenfuss, J. (1986). *Therapeutic communities for addiction: Readings in theory, research and practices*. Springfield, IL: Thomas.

Falkin, G. P., Prendergast, M., & Anglin, M. D. (1994). Drug treatment in the criminal justice system. *Federal Probation, 58*, 31–36.

Field, G. (1985). The Cornerstone Program: A client outcome study. *Federal Probation, 48*, 50–55.

Field, G. (1992a). Oregon prison drug treatment programs. In C. Leukefeld & F. Tims (Eds.), *Drug abuse treatment in prisons and jails* (The National Institute on Drug Abuse Research Monograph Series, Monograph 118, pp. 142–155).

Field, G. (1992b). *Preliminary outcome study of the Powder River Alcohol and Drug Program*. Unpublished manuscript. Oregon Department of Corrections.

Field, G., & Karecki, M. (1992). *Outcome study of the Parole Transition Release Project*. Unpublished manuscript. Oregon Department of Corrections.

Flaherty, M. T., Wald, H. P., Pringle, J. L., & Singerman, B. (1996). Punishing the sick? *The St. Francis Journal of Medicine, 2*, 11–14.

Gerstein, D. R., Johnson, R. A., Harwood, H. J., Fountain, D., Suter, N., & Malloy, K. (1994). *Evaluating recovery services: The California Drug and Alcohol Treatment Assessment (CALDATA)*. Sacramento, CA: State of California Department of Alcohol and Drug Programs.

Gorski, T. T. (1994). *Relapse prevention therapy with chemically dependent criminal offenders*. Independence, MO: Herald House/Independence Press.

Hayes, T. J., & Schimmel, D. J. (1993). Residential drug abuse treatment in the Federal Bureau of Prisons. *The Journal of Drug Issues, 23*, 61–73.

Husband, S. D., & Platt, J. J. (1993). The cognitive skills component in substance abuse treatment in correctional settings: A brief review. *The Journal of Drug Issues, 23*, 31–42.

Inciardi, J. A. (1996a). Corrections-based continuum of effective drug abuse treatment. *National Institute of Justice Research Preview* [on-line]. Available: http://www.ncjrs.org/txtfiles/contfrug. txt

Inciardi, J. A. (1996b). The therapeutic community: An effective model for corrections-based drug abuse treatment. In K. E. Early (Ed.), *Drug treatment behind bars: Prison-based strategies for change* (pp. 65–74). Westport, CT: Praeger.

Institute for Health Policy. (1993). *Substance abuse: The nation's number one health problem: Key indicators for policy.* Waltham, MA: Brandeis University.

Leukefeld, F., & Tims, F. (1990). Compulsory treatment for drug abuse. *The International Journal of the Addictions, 25,* 621–640.

Lipton, D. S. (1995). *The effectiveness of treatment for drug abusers under criminal justice supervision. A National Institute of Justice research report.* Presented at the 1995 Conference on Criminal Justice Research and Evaluation, Washington, DC.

Lipton, D. S., Falkin, G. P., & Wexler, H. K. (1992). Correctional drug abuse treatment in the United States: An overview. In C. Leukefeld & F. Tims (Eds.), *Drug abuse treatment in prisons and jails.* Washington, DC: The National Institute on Drug Abuse Research Monograph Series, Monograph 118, pp. 8–30.

Mahon, N. (1997). Treatment in prisons and jails. In J. H. Lowinson, P. Ruiz, R. B. Millman, & J. G. Langrad (Eds.), *Substance abuse: A comprehensive textbook, 3rd ed.* (pp. 455–458). Baltimore: Williams and Wilkins.

Mullen, R. (1996). Therapeutic communities in prisons: Dealing with toxic waste. In K. E. Early (Ed.), *Drug treatment behind bars: Prison-based strategies for change* (pp. 45–64). Westport, CT: Praeger.

Murray, D. W. (1992). Drug abuse treatment programs in the Federal Bureau of Prisons: Initiatives for the 1990s. In C. Leukefeld & F. Tims (Eds.), *Drug abuse treatment in prisons and jails.* Washington, DC: The National Institute on Drug Abuse Research Monograph Series, Monograph 118, pp. 62–83.

Murray, D. W. (1996). Drug abuse treatment in the Federal Bureau of Prisons: A historical review and assessment of contemporary initiatives. In K. E. Early (Ed.), *Drug treatment behind bars: Prison-based strategies for change* (pp. 89–100). Westport, CT: Praeger.

Pelissier, B., & McCarthy, D. (1992). Evaluation of the Federal Bureau of Prisons' drug treatment programs. In C. Leukefeld & F. Tims (Eds.), *Drug abuse treatment in prisons and jails.* Washington, DC: The National Institute on Drug Abuse Research Monograph Series, Monograph 118, pp. 261–278.

Peters, R. H. (1992). Referral and screening for substance abuse treatment in jails. *The Journal of Mental Health Administration, 19,* 53–75.

Peters, R. H., & Kearns, W. D. (1992). Drug abuse history and treatment needs of jail inmates. *American Journal of Drug and Alcohol Abuse, 18,* 355–366.

Peters, R. H., Kearns, W. D., Murrin, M. R., Dolente, A. S., & May, R. L. (1993). Examining the effectiveness of in-jail substance abuse treatment. *Journal of Offender Rehabilitation, 19,* 1–39.

Peters, R. H., & May, R. (1992). Drug treatment services in jails. In C. Leukefeld & F. Tims (Eds.), *Drug abuse treatment in prisons and jails.* (The National Institute on Drug Abuse Research Monograph Series, Monograph 118, pp. 38–50.)

Rouse, J. J. (1991). Evaluation research on prison-based drug treatment programs and some policy implications. *The International Journal of the Addictions, 26,* 29–44.

Singer, S. F. (1996). Essential elements of the effective therapeutic community in the correctional institution: A director's perspective. In K. E. Early (Ed.), *Drug treatment behind bars: Prison-based strategies for change* (pp. 75–88). Westport, CT: Praeger.

Vigdal, G. L. (1995). *Planning for alcohol and other drug abuse treatment for adults in the criminal justice system* (Treatment Improvement Protocol [TIP] Services, 17). Washington, DC: Substance Abuse and Mental Health Services Administration, Center for Substance Abuse Treatment.

Vigdal, G. L., & Stadler, D. W. (1996). Assessment, client treatment matching, and managing the substance abusing offender. In K. E. Early (Ed.), *Drug treatment behind bars: Prison-based strategies for change* (pp. 17–43). Westport, CT: Praeger.

Wexler, H. K. (1992). Overview of correctional drug treatment evaluation research. *The Psychotherapy Bulletin, 27,* 25–27.

Wexler, H. K. (1994). Progress in prison substance abuse treatment: A five year report. *The Journal of Drug Issues, 24*, 349–360.

Wexler, H. K. (1995). The success of therapeutic communities for substance abusers in American prisons. *The Journal of Psychoactive Drugs, 27*, 57–66.

Wexler, H. K., Falkin, G. P., & Lipton, D. S. (1990). Outcome evaluation of a prison therapeutic community for substance abuse treatment. *Criminal Justice and Behavior, 17*, 71–92.

Wexler, H. K., Williams, R. A., Early, K. E., & Trotman, C. D. (1996). In K. E. Early (Ed.), *Prison treatment for substance* (pp. 101–108). Westport, CT: Praeger.

Winett, D. L., Mullen, R., Lowe, L. L., & Missakian, E. A. (1992). Amity Righturn: A demonstration drug abuse treatment program for inmates and parolees. In C. Leukefeld & F. Tims (Eds.), *Drug abuse treatment in prisons and jails*. Washington, DC: The National Institute on Drug Abuse Research Monograph Series, Monograph 118, pp. 84–98.

Yochelson, S., & Samenow, S. (1979). *The criminal personality, Volume 3*. New York: Aronson.

Prevention in Medical Services Systems

Mark G. Fuller
Highmark Blue Cross Blue Shield

The abuse of alcohol and other drugs represents one of society's greatest challenges to health care. Many serious medical and psychiatric disorders are caused or exacerbated by substance abuse. For example, the incidence of accidents, myocardial infarctions, strokes, seizures, birth defects, hypertension, liver failure, and cancers are all heavily impacted by chemical use. Managed care organizations (MCOs) and other organized systems of care are in a unique position to make an impact on the prevention of substance use disorders.

SCOPE OF THE PROBLEM

In the general population, the lifetime prevalence of alcohol and other drug abuse and dependence is between 10% and 15% (Robins et al., 1984). Nicotine dependence represents an even greater problem, with approximately 25% of the population being regular smokers (Bartecchi, MacKenzie, & Schrier, 1994). Patients with psychoactive substance use disorders average a much greater than expected rate of medical care (Zook & Moore, 1980). Regular use of alcohol and other drugs results in significant health problems (Adams, Yuan, Barboriak, & Rimm, 1993; Gill, Zezulka, Shipley, Gill, & Beevers, 1986; Moushmoush & Abi-Monsour, 1991). The incidence of trauma and liver disease is also greatly exacerbated by the use of alcohol and other drugs (Guohua, Smith, & Baker, 1994; Lieber, 1995). Similarly, tobacco is linked to a number of serious health consequences including hypertension, myocardial infarction, stroke, and cancer (Bartecchi et al., 1994; MacKenzie, Bartecchi, & Schrier, 1994). As these associations have become increasingly clear, so has the opportunity for prevention activities. Unfortunately, because of the current lack of emphasis on prevention, little has been accomplished in providing high-quality, widely available substance abuse prevention efforts.

Under a fee-for-service system there is little incentive to provide preventative services. In fact, there is a financial disincentive to prevent disease. The traditional reimbursement system, which only pays for health care services after a person becomes ill, overlooks prevention services. The fee-for-service system is more accurately described as a "disease care system" rather than a true health care system, because this system is organized around illness, not wellness. Historically, third-party payers have insisted that a person demonstrate signs and symptoms of disease prior to reimbursement for those services. Thus, the current financial structure creates a system that has no mechanism of encouraging or financing prevention activities. The few prevention programs that do exist are usually funded by research grants or charitable foundations rather than health care dollars.

In fairness, health insurance companies that were organized around indemnity strategies have been skeptical about the benefits of prevention activities. And, clearly, not all prevention programs have been shown to be effective (Tobler, 1992). However, recent research into effective prevention activities has yielded some successes (Botvin, Baker, Dusenberry, Botvin, & Diaz, 1995).

CURRENT STATE OF AFFAIRS

MCOs have a tremendous opportunity to profoundly influence the health and quality of life of a substance abuser. Most MCOs are organized around primary care physicians and their relationships with patients. From this basis of trust and respect there exists a powerful opportunity for altering the course of a patient's substance use. Twenty percent of the patients who visit a physician's office have an alcohol use disorder (NIAAA, 1990). Similarly, approximately 30% of all patients hospitalized for any reason have an alcohol problem (NIAAA, 1990). This situation creates a natural opportunity to intervene with substance-abusing patients.

Even though patients who have psychoactive substance abuse disorders come in regular contact with their primary care physician, the physician often does not diagnose or treat the disorder (Deitz, Rohde, Bertolucci, & Dufour, 1994; Moore et al., 1989). In a recent study of patients referred to a drug and alcohol treatment program (Walsh et al., 1992) this fact was highlighted. In this study, less than one fourth of the patients admitted to a drug and alcohol rehabilitation center could recall receiving a warning about their drinking from their family physician despite the fact that three quarters of the patients had seen their doctor in the year prior to admission. This finding has been replicated by other studies of the same phenomenon. Also, the same studies that demonstrated a lack of physician warnings regarding excessive drinking (Walsh et al., 1992), also demonstrated that those patients who had been counseled by their doctors regarding their substance abuse disorders were found to have better medical outcomes.

Similar findings hold true for cigarette smoking and physician intervention. While Cummings, Rubin, and Oster (1989) demonstrated the effectiveness of physician counseling for smoking cessation, Frank, Winkleby, Altman, Rockhill, and Fortmann (1991) found that less than half of smokers stated that their primary care physicians had advised them to quit, and only 3.6% reported their physicians had helped them quit. At first glance, these findings may seem difficult to reconcile. On the one hand, there is demonstrated opportunity and efficacy of physician intervention with substance abusers. However, this fact is coupled with the consistent finding that when presented with the opportunity, most physicians choose not intervene.

Although the explanation for this phenomenon is multifactorial, the root cause lies in training programs that do not adequately prepare health care professionals for dealing with substance abuse. Many clinicians complete their education with little exposure to high quality learning experiences regarding the detection, intervention, and successful treatment of patients with substance abuse. Thus, the beginning clinician's misconceptions about substance abuse often go unchallenged throughout their training period. To further compound this problem, the attitude of the health care system in general is quite negative about substance abuse. Some health care professionals do not even consider psychoactive substance abuse and dependence to be a disease. Rather, some clinicians still view psychoactive substance abuse disorders as moral failings, not occasions for treatment. These judgmental and moralistic attitudes, when not offset by appropriate education and training, can come to be adopted by young trainees. The lack of acceptance of the disease model of addiction, accompanied by the belief that chemically dependent patients do not belong in the health care system and are not deserving of high-quality care, are just two instances of attitudes that need to be changed in medical school education.

The lack of accurate information about chemical dependency, coupled with unchanged prior attitudes and exposure to negative role models, prevents many health care professionals from being able to reach out and effectively intervene with the substance-abusing patient. The clinician's uncertainty and discomfort with this area of medicine may result in a conspiracy of silence. That is, when a substance-abusing patient who wants help but does not know how to ask for it encounters a well-intentioned but inadequately prepared health care professional, the clinician might look the other way to avoid facing the obvious but awkward diagnosis of alcoholism or drug abuse.

This conspiracy of silence results in the deaths of hundreds of thousands of people every year. Each time a physician sees unexplained elevated liver functions and other signs of alcoholism but neglects to question the patient about their alcohol intake, an important opportunity is missed. Similarly, every time a clinician looks at nicotine-stained fingers and sees a pack of cigarettes in a shirt pocket but remains silent about the dangers of smoking, he or she loses another chance to make a difference. The fee-for-service model of health care has done a poor job of preventing, identifying, intervening with and treating substance abuse. The question arises as to whether a managed care model could do better.

OPPORTUNITIES FOR GROWTH

If money were no object, what kind of substance abuse services would our health care system create? The obvious starting point is with our society's needs. Given the high rate of substance abuse, there is a significant need for high-quality, efficacious, readily accessible prevention programs. Tarter (1992) outlines a number of key characteristics that must be taken into consideration when designing prevention programs. These key ingredients include targeting the intended group, individualizing the intervention to the person's needs and susceptibilities, and covering the life span with the prevention efforts. These factors are critical to the success of any comprehensive prevention system.

Since children and adolescents initiate their first substance use between ages 12 and 20 with a peak age of 15 (Office of Substance Abuse Prevention, 1989a), it is important to intervene early. The importance of reaching children early is highlighted by the finding that the younger a person is when they first begin their chemical use, the more likely they are to develop a substance abuse disorder (Office of Substance Abuse Prevention). Primary prevention services are critical at this stage. Ideally, in order for prevention programs to provide maximum exposure, they would be provided at a variety of different locations such as schools, churches, health care facilities, and workplaces (Office of Substance Abuse Prevention, 1989a, 1989b). In addition, prevention programs should be targeted to persons of all age groups and social classes. While it is important to address substance abuse in children and adolescents, it is also important to address substance abuse in the elderly. Researchers (Adams et al., 1993) demonstrated that hospitalization of elderly patients with alcohol problems cost over $230 million dollars in one year! The need for a broad-based approach cannot be underestimated.

A key piece of this primary prevention has to be provided by the health care system. As MCOs take on the financial risk of people's health along with the responsibility to provide high-quality medically necessary services, primary prevention activities should expand considerably. The high turnover of patients in many health plans works against the idea of investing in primary preventative services. But the concept of portability of health care insurance may insure the likelihood that patients and insurers will stay together long enough for primary prevention to become economically viable. Also, as consolidation within the managed care industry continues, it is possible that a small number of insurers and providers will be responsible for much of the nation's health care costs and thus will have a significant stake in effective prevention programs.

In addition, the issue of secondary and tertiary prevention has already been demonstrated to have medical as well as economic advantages that are observable within one year (Goodman, Holder, & Nishiura, 1991; Holder & Blose, 1986). Identifying substance abuse patients and motivating them to enter treatment in health care settings has been demonstrated to be effective (Fuller & Jordan, 1994; Goldberg, Mullen, Ries, Psaty, & Ruch, 1991). The lack of enthusiasm for these approaches in the vast majority of health care settings reflects both educational and attitudinal problems as well as financial issues. Currently, the average health care professional is not responsible for the future care costs of their patients. They receive little if any reimbursement for time spent on prevention and education activities. On the other hand, the MCO is directly responsible for future illnesses and their subsequent health care costs. Thus, the MCO has a significant stake in altering the trajectory of a chemically dependent patient's disease process.

In order for this paradigm shift to occur, it is incumbent upon MCOs to properly educate and provide incentives to clinicians in their network to recognize the early signs and symptoms of substance abuse and to intervene as early as possible. Substance abuse, like many other chronic diseases, is far more amenable to treatment if detected and treated at an early stage. End-stage addicts who have lost key social supports (family, friends, employment) and who may be experiencing significant neurocognitive problems have a much worse prognosis for recovery (Fein, Bachman, Fisher, & Davenport, 1990).

The most recent evolutionary phase of managed care has not focused on prevention activities. The high rates of overutilization in behavioral health care has been the initial focus of MCOs. This problem has been addressed by MCOs through selective contracting with efficient and effective providers, alternative payment strategies (capitation, case rates, etc.), and rigorous utilization review. Initially, these approaches produce a significant reduction in costs. However, over time, as MCOs saturate a market and the provider community becomes more mature in terms of using outpatient services flexibly and creatively, there will be fewer gains to be made with respect to utilization management. At this point in the evolutionary process, prevention activities may have their best chance of success. It is in the best interest of the patient as well as the health care system to maximize every patient's opportunity for a healthy life.

THE FUTURE OF PREVENTION

The future of prevention activities in health care systems has enormous potential. For the first time, a single organization (or system of organizations) has both the opportunity as well as the incentive (if not the moral obligation) to begin addressing some of society's fundamental health care problems. It may be tempting for some organizations to remain conservative in their strategy and continue to define their role as "disease care responders." These organizations will remain on the sidelines of their members' lives until such time as the member is both ill and willing to consult a clinician. Depending on how far the disease process has advanced (and what resources remain), the patient has a better or worse chance for recovery. These more conservative MCOs will hope their members do not become too ill, or consume too many resources.

Each MCO will probably approach their mission differently. As health care markets mature and behavioral health utilization approaches optimum numbers, behavioral health MCOs will be seeking out new and different opportunities to be effective. Some of them will explore prevention activities in a significant way. The companies that fully exploit the prevention potential will want to become an integral part of their members' lives. Rather than waiting for the member to become ill, the MCO will become proactively involved in health promotion not just disease prevention. The MCO will seek out opportunities to inform their members about healthy choices as well as risk avoidance. In the near future a significant amount of an MCO's limited resources will be focused on their members' individual needs and risk factors in order to be cost effective.

A model behavioral health MCO that chooses to approach substance abuse from a prevention as well as a treatment approach may look something like the following.

Primary Prevention

The MCO's initial prevention activities begin prior to the member's conception. With a clear understanding of the risks of prenatal exposure to alcohol and other drugs, all of the health plan's primary care physicians and obstetrician/gynecologists (ob-gyns) have attended continuing medical education seminars (at the plan's expense) on the hazards of substance use during pregnancy. Most of the physicians' waiting rooms and all of the obstetricians' rooms contain literature on substance abuse and pregnancy. In addition, as part of the routine gynecological exam, all physicians and ob-gyn's will inquire about substance abuse in women of childbearing age. Any woman who is planning to become pregnant or who is having unprotected sex receives additional education, literature, and screening regarding substance abuse and other risks that are especially relevant to pregnancy. This intervention may result in a follow-up evaluation or referral to a substance abuse specialist for further screening or treatment if necessary. Moreover, the MCO will be targeting women of childbearing age with specific newsletters on a variety of topics of interest, including the risks of maternal substance abuse not only during pregnancy but during conception.

After becoming pregnant, further screening and education by both the ob-gyn as well as the home health nurse increases the likelihood of early identification and intervention in substance abuse problems. This MCO understands the tremendous damage that can be done to a fetus that is exposed to chemicals via maternal use, while also realizing that it is in everyone's best interests to avoid a preterm delivery of an infant with multiple birth defects. A lot of education and screening activities can take place for the price of a couple of days in a neonatal intensive care unit (Chasnoff, 1991).

The next stage of prevention arrives in a variety of different forms. The MCO is a leading one in the community and thus has a major stake in the health of many of its citizens. Hence, the health plan sponsors a number of community-wide substance abuse prevention programs. In addition, through its primary care physicians, the MCO cosponsors substance abuse prevention activities in the local school system. Also, as children come in for routine vaccinations and check-ups, the physician and other health care professionals in the practice screen the child and educate the patient (as well as the family) about the risks of substance abuse. The combination of a variety of prevention programs coupled with educated parents and a concerned physician will not prevent all cases of psychoactive substance use disorders, but it will prevent some. And, it will also significantly increase the potential for early detection of these disorders.

The use of well-researched substance abuse prevention programs continues throughout the life cycle. Because of the patient's ability to maintain their health insurance regardless of employer, assuming the true portability of health insurance, the MCO knows that it is very likely to be at risk for this individual's health care costs throughout his or her life. Thus, the company is very aggressive about pursuing prevention activities targeted to all stages of the member's life. The MCO does this through partnerships with local employers as well as through community groups. For senior citizens, the MCO has a number of intervention and detection programs that are age-appropriate and run year-round.

At the heart of each of these programs is the doctor–patient relationship. One of the most powerful tools for detecting and intervening with substance abuse is the primary care physician. This MCO is fully aware of this opportunity and empowers its network of physicians through continuing education opportunities as well as appropriate feedback of information on the physician's patients. This partnership between the MCO and the primary care physician is one of the primary reasons this MCO is so effective at promoting health and decreasing health care costs.

Secondary Prevention

Due to the underlying structure of the MCO, which places the primary care physician at the center of coordinating all aspects of a patient's care, the physician is continually aware of which patients are accessing health care services and for what reasons. This continual monitoring allows the physician to spot signs of substance abuse much earlier, because patients are receiving coordinated, continuous care rather than the old-style, fee-for-service, disconnected and uncoordinated treatment. In addition, the physician has received extensive training in recognizing and intervening with the substance-abusing patient and has access to other behavioral health care professionals located within or nearby to the practice who can provide essential and rapid support for difficult cases.

With the patient's permission, the physician is updated on the patient's status while in rehabilitation. The patient remains under the physician's care while progressing in rehabilitation. This continuation of service reinforces the connection between physician and patient.

Effective and convenient drug and alcohol rehabilitation is readily available to all members of the health plan who have been identified with substance abuse problems. As the MCO wants to encourage attendance and completion of the program, there are no copayments. Twelve-step programs are strongly encouraged and are available at the MCO's community health centers after hours. Each patient has an individualized plan tailored to the patient's needs, which is developed and implemented by the plan's substance abuse program. Ongoing follow-up is coordinated through the primary care physician as well as the rehabilitation program as long as needed, as the health plan has eliminated benefit limits on substance abuse treatment in an attempt to fully address this serious medical problem.

Tertiary Prevention

Despite their outstanding prevention and treatment programs, some of the health plan members develop end stage signs and symptoms of chronic substance use. These patients have significant medical and psychiatric sequelae and are beyond rehabilitation, or they have repeatedly failed traditional treatment programs and appear unresponsive to conventional interventions. In order to meet the needs of these members, the MCO offers a variety of tertiary prevention services targeted at preventing further consequences of substance use. One of these programs is a nearby methadone maintenance program, which the health plan contracts with on behalf of its opioid-dependent patients who have failed conventional treatment on multiple occasions. There are also a series of halfway houses and chemical-free personal care homes aimed at providing an environment in which the patient may consolidate their gains in rehabilitation as well as protecting the patient from further exposure to chemicals.

CONCLUSIONS

Model programs such as this depend on the likelihood of the MCO becoming responsible for a person's health care costs for a long enough period to make intensive, effective prevention programs worthwhile. If health insurance becomes truly portable, this will significantly increase the possibility of programs, such as the one described above, to become reality. The other trend that is likely to impact upon prevention activities is the rapid consolidation that is taking place in the health insurance industry. With the development of several large insurance companies, the likelihood of long-term coverage by any one company increases significantly. This change will greatly increase an MCO's willingness to expend resources on the kind of prevention programs that take years to fully realize their benefit. In addition, as the quality revolution in U.S. industry sweeps through health care, it is possible that MCOs will take on serious prevention activities in order to significantly enhance the quality of their services. At this juncture, it is too early to predict all of the influences that will subsequently decide how actively MCOs will pursue prevention activities. However, the stage is set for a dramatic turnaround in the way prevention is approached and financed in all areas of health care, especially in the area of substance abuse. While some of the suggested activities listed above may seem unrealistic, it is worth noting that some health care plans are already implementing innovative substance abuse prevention activities (Del Toro, Larsen, & Carter, 1994; Hollis, Lichtenstein, Vogt, Stevens, & Biglan, 1993).

REFERENCES

Adams, W. L., Yuan, Z., Barboriak, J. J., & Rimm, A. A. (1993). Alcohol-related hospitalizations of elderly people: Prevalence and geographic variation in the United States. *Journal of the American Medical Association, 270,* 1222–1225.

Bartecchi, C. E., MacKenzie, T. D., & Schrier, R. W. (1994). The human costs of tobacco use. *New England Journal of Medicine, 330,* 907–912.

Botvin, G. J., Baker, E., Dusenberry, L., Botvin, E. M., & Diaz, T. (1995). Long-term follow-up results of a randomized drug abuse prevention trial in a white middle-class population. *Journal of the American Medical Association, 273,* 1106–1112.

Chasnoff, I. J. (1991). Drugs, alcohol, pregnancy and the neonate: Pay now or pay later. *Journal of the American Medical Association, 266,* 1567–1568.

Cummings, S. R., Rubin, S. M., & Oster, G. (1989). The cost-effectiveness of counseling smokers to quit. *Journal of the American Medical Association, 261,* 75–79.

Deitz, D., Rohde, F., Bertolucci, D., & Dufour, M. (1994). Screening for alcohol use by physicians during routine physical examinations. *Alcohol Health and Research World, 18,* 162–168.

Del Toro, I. M., Larsen, D. A., & Carter, A. P. (1994). A new approach to alcoholism detection in primary care. *Journal of Mental Health Administration, 21,* 124–135.

Fein, G., Bachman, L., Fisher, S., & Davenport, L. (1990). Cognitive impairments in abstinent alcoholics. *Western Journal of Medicine, 152,* 531–537.

Frank, E., Winkleby, M. A., Altman, D. G., Rockhill, B., & Fortmann, S. P. (1991). Predictors of physician's smoking cessation advice. *Journal of the American Medical Association, 266,* 3139–3144.

Fuller, M. G., & Jordan, M. L. (1994). The role of a substance abuse consultation team in a trauma center. *Journal of Studies on Alcohol, 56,* 267–271.

Gill, J. S., Zezulka, A. V., Shipley, M. J., Gill, S. K., & Beevers, D. G. (1986). Stroke and alcohol consumption. *New England Journal of Medicine, 315,* 1041–1046.

Goldberg, H. I., Mullen, M., Ries, R. K., Psaty, B. M., & Ruch, B. P. (1991). Alcohol counseling in a general medical clinic. A randomized controlled trial of strategies to improve referral and show rates. *Medical Care, 29,* 49–56.

Goodman, A. C., Holder, H. D., & Nishiura, E. (1991). Alcoholism treatment offset effects: A cost model. *Inquiry, 28,* 168–178.

Guohua, L., Smith, G. S., & Baker, S. P. (1994). Drinking behavior in relation to cause of death among U.S. adults. *American Journal of Public Health, 84,* 1402–1406.

Holder, H. D., & Blose, J. O. (1986). Alcoholism treatment and total health care utilization and costs: A four-year longitudinal analysis of federal employees. *Journal of the American Medical Association, 256,* 1456–1460.

Hollis, J. F., Lichtenstein, E., Vogt, T. M., Stevens, V. J., & Biglan A. (1993). Nurse-assisted counseling for smokers in primary care. *Annals of Internal Medicine, 118,* 521–525.

Lieber, C. S. (1995). Medical disorders of alcoholism. *New England Journal of Medicine, 333,* 1058–1065.

MacKenzie, T. D., Bartecchi, C. E., & Schrier, R. W. (1994). The human costs of tobacco use. *New England Journal of Medicine, 330,* 975–980.

Moore, R. D., Bone, L. R., Geller, G., Mamon, J. A., Stokes, E. J., & Levine, D. M. (1989). Prevalence, detection and treatment of alcoholism in hospitalized patients. *Journal of the American Medical Association, 261,* 403–407.

Moushmoush, B., & Abi-Monsour, P. (1991). Alcohol and the heart: The long-term effects of alcohol on the cardiovascular system. *Archives of Internal Medicine, 151,* 36–42.

National Institute on Alcohol Abuse and Alcoholism. (1990, April). Screening for alcoholism. *Alcohol Alert,* 1–4.

Office of Substance Abuse Prevention. (1989a). *Stopping alcohol and other drug use before it starts: The future of prevention* (DHHS Publication Number ADM 89-1645). Rockville, MD: U.S. Department of Health and Human Services.

Office of Substance Abuse Prevention. (1989b). *You can help your community get rid of drugs* (DHHS Publication Number ADM 89-1562). Rockville, MD: U.S. Department of Health and Human Services.

Robins, L. N., Helzer, J. E., Weissman, M. M., Orvaschel, H., Gruenberg, E., Burke, J. D., & Regier, D. A. (1984). Lifetime prevalence of specific psychiatric disorders in three sites. *Archives of General Psychiatry, 41*, 949–958.

Tarter, R. E. (1992). Prevention of drug abuse: Theory and application. *American Journal of Addictions, 1*, 2–20.

Tobler, N. S. (1992). Drug prevention programs can work: Research findings. *Journal on Addictive Diseases, 11*, 1–28.

Walsh, D. C., Hingson, R. W., Merrigan, D. M., Levenson, S. M., Coffman, G. A., Heeren, T., & Cupples, L. A. (1992). The impact of a physician's warning on recovery after alcoholism treatment. *Journal of the American Medical Association, 267*, 663–667.

Zook, C. J., & Moore, F. D. (1980). High-cost users of medical care. *New England Journal of Medicine, 302*, 996–1002.

Author Index

H

403

Stephens, R. C., 143
Stevens, V. J., 391
Stewart, K., 188, 191
Stewart, R., 126, 135
Stitzer, M. L., 101
Stoduto, G., 120
Stokes, E. J., 384
Stoltzfus, J. A., 310
Stonier, R. J., 263
Stover, S. L., 156
Straus, M. A., 190
Strecher, V. J., 103
Streff, F. M., 271
Strumpf, F., 153
Substance Abuse and Mental Health
      Services Administration
      (SAMHSA), 128, 132, 133, 134,
      356
Sugarman, D., 6
Sullivan, K. A., 166, 167, 169, 170, 175
Sun, P., 290, 294, 295
Sunderland, T., 102
Sung, H., 255
Susser, M., 97
Sussman, S., 290, 294, 295
Suter, N., 179, 374
Suurvali, H., 310
Swann, J. P., 224
Swartz, J., 186
Sweeney, T. T., 155
Swisher, J. D., 288, 289
Sykora, K., 269
Szasz, T., 230

T

Tabon, F., 76
Tahtela, R., 82
Tanaka, K., 85
Tapasak, R. C., 290
Tariot, P. N., 102
Tarter, R. E., 5, 8, 10, 12, 14, 17, 21, 386
Task Force on Education of Young Ad-
      olescents, 282, 287
Tauchen, G., 268
Taylor, A. H., 226
Taylor, I. K., 98
Tebes, J. K., 290

Teer, P., 251
Telch, M. J., 290, 295
Telles, P., 128, 129, 130, 139
Temin, P., 223, 224
Tenhu, M., 110
Tenner, S., 70
Teplin, L. A., 186
Terblanche, J., 69
Terhune, K. W., 119
Tharp, M., 249
Thomas, D. L., 141
Thomas, G. A. O., 102
Thomas, J. C., 141
Thompson, A., 288
Thompson, W. L., 84
Thomson, M., 173
Thomson, R. A., 136
Thomson, S. J., 295
Thum, D., 284
Thun, M., 93
Thuyns, H., 128
Tillerman, R. C., 75
Tims, F., 377
Tirch, D., 152, 158
Titus, S., 143
Tobler, N. S., 298, 328, 330, 331, 333,
      384
Todak, G. G., 99
Tolan, P., 187
Toledano, E., 213
Toneatto, T., 245
Tortu, S., 135, 294
Toskes, P. P., 75
Toth, V., 294
Toye, P. A., 82
Trapido, E. J., 143
Travis, K. M., 173, 177
Treat, J. R., 114, 119
Trebach, A. S., 229
Trice, H. M., 317, 320
Trotman, C. D., 372
Trotter, R. T., 135
Trudeau, J., 310
Trupin, E. W., 376
Tsukazaki, N., 85
Tucker, L., 245
Tunninen, R., 82
Tunving, K., 126
Turner, G. S., 186, 187, 190, 191

Subject Index